Chinese Herbal Medicines
Comparisons and
Characteristics

Commissioning Editor: Mary Law/Karen Morley
Development Editor: Ewan Halley
Project Manager: Joannah Duncan
Designer/Design Direction: Kirsteen Wright
Illustrator: Chartwell

Chinese Herbal Medicines

中药比较与中药特性

Comparisons and Characteristics

SECOND EDITION

Yifan Yang MD MSc
Practitioner and Lecturer in Traditional Chinese Medicine,
The Netherlands

Foreword by

Mazin Al-Khafaji
Doctor of Chinese Medicine (Shanghai, China);
FRCHM,
Avicenna Centre for Chinese Medicine, UK

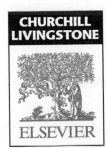

Edinburgh London New York Oxford Philadelphia St Louis Sydney Toronto 2010

CHURCHILL LIVINGSTONE
ELSEVIER

© 2010, Elsevier Limited. All rights reserved.
© 2002, Harcourt Publishers Ltd. All rights reserved.

First edition 2002
Second edition 2010

ISBN: 978 07020 3133 5

British Library Cataloguing in Publication Data
A catalogue record for this book is available from the British Library

Library of Congress Cataloging in Publication Data
A catalog record for this book is available from the Library of Congress

Notice
Neither the Publisher nor the Author assumes responsibility for any loss or injury and/or damage to persons or property arising out of or related to any use of the material contained in this book. It is the responsibility of the treating practitioner, relying on independent expertise and knowledge of the patient, to determine the best treatment and method of application for the patient.

The Publisher

Printed and bound in the United Kingdom
Transferred to Digital Print 2011

Contents

(See Notes on the second edition for an explanation of asterisks that appear alongside herb names)

Fig. 2.1 Comparison of the temperature of the warm herbs.
Fig. 2.2 Comparison of the herbs that induce sweating.
Fig. 2.3 Comparison of the light and dispersing features of the warm herbs.
Fig. 2.4 Comparison of the herbs that expel exogenous Cold.
Fig. 2.5 Comparison of the herbs that expel exogenous Dampness.
Fig. 2.6 Comparison of the temperature of the cold herbs.
Fig. 2.7 Comparison of the light and dispersing features of the cold herbs.

Chapter 4 Herbs that drain downwards 63

Chapter 6 Herbs that transform Dampness 81

Fig. 17.1 Comparison of the substances that anchor the Liver-Yang.

Fig. 17.2 Comparison of the herbs that extinguish Liver-Wind and subdue the Liver-Yang.

Fig. 17.3 Comparison of the herbs that cool the Liver or disperse Liver-Heat and extinguish Wind.

Fig. 17.4 Comparison of the substances that open the collaterals and extinguish Wind.

Chinese herbal medicine is a medical system that has evolved empirically over many thousands of years, with countless millions contributing to its development and systemisation. Its' roots reach back to the very dawn of history, when all manner of methods, including trial and error played a roll in the gradual amassment of the myriad facts that have passed down to us today.

When first embarking on its study, all but the hardiest of students will pale at the sheer quantity of information that has to be committed to memory. Their excitement at first encountering the wonders of this vast body of knowledge, that ultimately form the backbone of treatment, is soon swamped by the dawning realisation of the efforts required to master it. Knowledge of each and every one of the ingredients' many attributes, such as the temperature, flavour, channel association, nature, action, movement, toxicity, interaction with other ingredients (both antagonistic and enhancing) and dosage needs to be grasped and assimilated.

As study continues, the student soon discovers that even once all this information has been secured, the surface has barely been scratched, for now the hundreds of commonly used formulas have also to be memorised and understood. As this proceeds, it emerges with even greater clarity that it is indeed the combinations of these medicinal substances in precise quantities, which form one of the defining factors to an ultimately successful outcome to treatment. Just as in a well-crafted gourmet dish, it is the skillful combining of ingredients, that in turn accentuate and enhance some flavours, whilst subduing and downplaying others, that ultimately lead to the pleasing taste we experience when we consume it. So too with a medicinal formula, it is the precise interaction of ingredients in the correct quantity that makes the difference between an efficacious formula and one that will ultimately prove ineffective.

The biggest challenge facing any serious practitioner, having undergone this lengthy and arduous process, is the understanding of how to modify classical prescriptions into useful and effective formulas, suitable to the presenting clinical picture—how to judge the synergies of the different herbs when combined in different groups or dosages, how to choose a particular herb over another in any given situation. The answers, after dedicated study of the theoretical essentials, can usually only be gleaned after many years of clinical practice and the observation of thousands of patients. At Chinese hospitals where junior doctors are under the clinical supervision of old and experienced physicians, this type of knowledge is more readily available to those who seek to develop their own style of practice. In the West however, such opportunities can still be extremely hard to come by. Most useful source material is accessible only to those with a solid grasp of the Chinese language, and openings for extensive clinical practice under supervision are limited.

It is for this reason that I welcome the republication of this delightful work by Dr Yifan Yang. This book offers an extremely useful grid by which to systemize the practitioner's understanding of the 'real life' qualities of the medicinal substances, by categorizing them into groups according to their energetic properties, presenting their characteristics and clinical uses and then comparing them through finer analysis of their individual strengths. This is information compiled from many sources, with the unmistakable stamp 'clinical practice' written all over it. It will act as a reference work for serious students and experienced practitioners alike, to deepen their understanding of Chinese medicine in a most productive way, and to apply this understanding as it links to the principles and fundamental concepts of Chinese medical theory.

Mazin Al-Khafaji, 2010

When I was a medical student, endeavoring to study traditional Chinese herbal medicine, it was quite challenging to memorize, within the space of one semester, the properties and functions of at least 300 commonly used herbs. As a junior doctor I still hesitated to select herbs to make my own formulae. I was amazed to hear my teacher's precise and vivid explanations: 'Oh, this is a wonderful herb, it is pungent and warm, yet not drying in nature, it moves in a quick, yet gentle way, it can tonify the body without cloying; the perfect choice for chronic diseases.' 'This herb is very hot, so it can quickly spread the warmth to the entire body, dispelling the Damp-Cold just like the sun with the fog' and 'This is the strongest herb among herbs that regulate the Qi.'

The above way of teaching, to compare the strength and characteristics of herbs, is applied, but unfortunately it is not used regularly. The primary teaching method in books and lectures in the last few decades still simply states the basic functions and provides elementary examples of applications. However, this method lacks precision in quality and quantity, and is not vivid and emphatic in nature, and as a result students have to spend much more time on study and practice to really master the characteristics of herbs and to grasp strategies to make their own formulae skillfully.

First as a student, then as a teacher and doctor of traditional Chinese herbal medicine, I have searched for a new way of studying and teaching. In this book, I have aimed to discuss the features of herbs instead of enumerating the common functions. Comparison is used as the main tool in explaining the fine differences between herbs that have the same or similar functions. Moreover, 117 figures are provided to show the differences in temperature and strength of single herbs that have the same function. The theories and concepts of Chinese herbal medicine are used as principles throughout the analysis and explanation. The *clinical applications* of single herbs are presented according to the differentiation of syndromes in the traditional Chinese medical way and the diagnosis in Western medicine. The whole book is written in a *questions and answers* style and it follows the chapter content of most commonly used textbooks in Chinese herbal medicine. Each *question and answer* form a small unit, so the book can be read all the way through, or each question can be studied individually.

This book is written for serious practitioners and students who have already learned the basic functions of the Chinese herbs and want to master Chinese herbal therapy step by step. The information in the discussion of clinical applications can be used to enrich the understanding of the characteristics of the herbs rather than to discuss the treatment of certain diseases both in the sense of Traditional Chinese Medicine and Western medicine.

For students and junior practitioners, this book offers a method of learning and memorizing the functions of herbs through the approach of comparing the characteristics and the strength of herbs with related functions or natures. Each question may be used to stimulate discussion and in reviewing lectures. The answers might just clarify confusions and help the student delve deeper.

For experienced practitioners, this book offers a comprehensive knowledge of Chinese herbal medicine and a deeper understanding of the theories and concepts of Traditional Chinese Medicine. The fine analysis of the characteristics of herbs helps the practitioner to make a formula with better quality and results. The discussion of clinical applications can be used in clinical practice to enlarge the treatment range.

The knowledge gained of each herb is not solely developed from my own experience. During my work in the Department of Chinese Herbal Formulas at Beijing University of Traditional Chinese Medicine, the study of herbs was largely done through discussion and debate with colleagues and from a large number of ancient medical texts. From practicing what I have learned, first on patients in China and now in the West, I have developed a deeper understanding of the herbs and gained experience and confidence in Chinese herbal therapy. I have tried to bring together my understanding of herbs and a new way of studying in this book, and I hope it can be of benefit both to those who have studied and those who wish to study Chinese

herbal medicine: the ancient, yet effective therapy, and an art that is full of wisdom, philosophy and strategies.

Yifan Yang
The Netherlands 2002

Notes on the second edition

In the second edition of this book, as well as keeping to the concise writing style of the first edition, I have improved and added more on the safe use of Chinese herbal medicine in Chapter 1 (The theory and concepts of Chinese herbal medicine). I have also added precautions for the use of herbs in several chapters. Moreover, three specific lists are given as appendices to assist practitioners in their daily clinical work: (1) Daily dosages for individual crude herbs above 6–9 grams; (2) Commonly used herbal combinations and their applications; (3) Commonly used Chinese words in herbal names.

In the second edition, the pharmaceutical names of herbs are given in parentheses after the Chinese Pinyin names and follow the current commonly used style.

Throughout the book, banned toxic herbs are marked with an asterisk (*) following the name of the herb. Banned and protected substances are marked with two asterisks (**). Please note that Traditional Chinese Medicine takes the standpoint that all harsh herbs that have strong effects on pathogenic factors in the body can easily cause side-effects and that these herbs all belong to the toxic herbs group. Practitioners should always keep firmly in mind, not only the banned toxic herbs that are potential causes of damage to the liver, kidney and heart in Western medicine, but also the herbs (which are not always flagged with an asterisk in this book) with strong properties and functions that may bring the same risks if they are not used in the correct situation, at the correct dosage and for the correct duration of time.

Yifan Yang
The Netherlands 2009

- At the end of each chapter, a group of figures are presented. There are more herbs listed and compared in the figures than are in the text since it is easier and clearer to compare the temperature and the strength of many herbs in this way. These figures can be used as a supplement to the text, but they can also be used separately from the text.
- The dark red, medium red and pink bars represent the temperatures, *very hot*, *warm* and *slightly warm* respectively of the herbs.
- The black, gray and light gray bars represent the temperatures, *very cold*, *cold* and *slightly cold* respectively of the herbs.
- The white bar represents a neutral temperature.

- The herbs which will be compared are presented on the abscissa.
- The strength of a particular action of the herbs is indicated on the ordinate.
- If the herbs are very similar in strength of a particular action, the strength is summed up from the temperature, meridians they enter, tendency of action and other functions.

Note on Chinese herb names
In the text, herb names are given in Pinyin. In each question, the pharmaceutical name of the herb follows the first mention of the herb. In the figures, the pharmaceutical names are given in the caption only. A full list of Pinyin and pharmaceutical names appears as Appendix IV.

Acknowledgements

I would like to express my gratitude to my teachers at Beijing University of Traditional Chinese Medicine, where I studied and worked for 13 years. I am especially grateful to Professor Wang Mianzhi. He was my first teacher of Chinese herbal formulas when I was a medical student, my tutor for my Master's degree in medical science, and the director of the department where I worked. I was amazed by his lectures, particularly the detailed analysis on the characteristics of herbs, the combinations of herbs and the structure of formulas, which came from his deep understanding, knowledge and experience of Traditional Chinese Medicine. I learned a lot from his lectures and during the time when I was his assistant. Furthermore, his devoted spirit on the work of Chinese medicine, his principles of life, and his tireless and kind manner to patients always encouraged me in the endless study and practice.

I would also like to thank Dr X. Yang BA, MB, BChir from the University of Cambridge, UK, Dr D. Zajac PhD from the University of Reading, UK, Mr M. Tjioe MD, Mr A. Van Dinteren MD, Mrs K. N. Tan MD and Mrs B. E. Sciarone MD from The Netherlands, for checking the manuscript and for their indispensable advice, and Dr J. Weng PhD from the University of Reading, UK for the beautiful figures and for his valuable suggestions. I would like to thank my friend Dr Gao Yuan from China for helping me to check some text in the original ancient books, and Mr Charles Wauters from The Netherlands for helping me to check the pharmaceutical names of the herbs with his knowledge as a pharmacist. I am also grateful to the team at Elsevier Ltd for their expertise and efficiency in the procedure of publishing this book.

Finally, I am still grateful to my daughter Chuan for her understanding, love and support.

PART 1

Theory and concepts

中药理论和基本概念

Chapter One

The theory and concepts of Chinese herbal medicine

中药理论和基本概念

1 What are the four flavors of Chinese herbs? What are their applications in clinical practice?

The four flavors are called 'Si Qi' in Chinese. 'Si' means 'four', and 'Qi' means 'the special quality of the herb'. In this context it indicates the temperature of the herbs, namely hot, warm, cold and cool. Hot and cold herbs are opposite in nature, and correspond to the Yang and Yin. Cool and warm herbs have the same nature as cold and hot, but to a lesser degree. Each herb possesses one of these four temperatures. However, there are also herbs that are neither hot nor cold, and are not included in the four flavors. They are classified as 'Ping', meaning 'neutral'.

In clinical practice, hot or warm herbs are used to warm the body and to treat Cold syndromes. For example, Gan Jiang (*Zingiberis rhizoma*) is able to warm the Middle Jiao and treat abdominal cramp and diarrhea; Dang Gui (*Angelicae sinensis radix*) can warm the Blood and alleviate pain due to Cold in the Blood. A cold or cool herb is used to clear Heat and to treat Heat syndromes. For instance, Shi Gao (*Gypsum*) can clear Heat in the Lung and Stomach and therefore it can reduce fever, wheezing and thirst; Sheng Di Huang (*Rehmanniae radix*) can reduce Heart-Fire in order to treat restlessness and insomnia. A neutral herb can be used when the syndrome is not characterized by Heat or Cold. For instance, Fu Ling (*Poria*) can promote urination and reduce edema. A neutral herb can also be used in

either a Cold or Heat syndrome in combination with other hot or cold herbs. For instance, Fu Ling (*Poria*) can be used with Fu Zi (*Aconiti radix lateralis preparata*)* to warm the Kidney-Yang and reduce edema; it can also be used with Xiao Ji (*Cirsii herba*) to treat painful urinary dysfunction due to Heat in the Bladder. These are the basic applications of the four flavors.

The four flavors are amongst the primary properties of herbs but, in fact, the number is not confined to four. Like many other theories in Traditional Chinese Medicine (TCM), the four flavors primarily indicate the temperature quality of the herbs. The theory also suggests that these temperatures can be subdivided into different degrees, but does not indicate the details of these degrees. The terms 'very hot', 'hot', 'warm' and 'slightly warm' are sometimes used. In practice, differences in temperature between herbs are usually found out from the explanations of the function, from applications given in books and from personal experience.

Moreover, hot herbs can be divided into thin-hot and thick-hot. A thin-hot herb possesses a lighter hot nature, which leads to a quicker action; it is often used to expel exterior pathogenic Cold—examples are Ma Huang (*Ephedrae herba*)*, Gui Zhi (*Cinnamomi cassiae ramulus*) and Xin Yi (*Magnoliae flos*). A thick-hot herb possesses a strong hot nature that leads to a strong and steady action; it is used to warm the Interior and treat interior Cold syndrome—examples include Fu Zi (*Aconiti radix lateralis preparata*)*, Rou Gui (*Cinnamomi cassiae cortex*) and Gan Jiang (*Zingiberis rhizoma*). Cold herbs can likewise be divided into thin-cold and thick-cold. A thin-cold herb can gently but quickly disperse and clear Heat in the Upper Jiao or in the superficial level of the body—examples are Bo He (*Menthae herba*), Chai Hu (*Bupleuri radix*), Sang Ye (*Mori folium*) and Ju Hua (*Chrysanthemi flos*). A thick-cold herb can strongly clear Heat and reduce Fire—examples include Huang Lian (*Coptidis rhizoma*), Huang Qin (*Scutellariae radix*), Huang Bai (*Phellodendri cortex*) and Long Dan Cao (*Gentianae radix*).

2 What are the five tastes of herbs? What are their clinical applications?

The five tastes of herbs are pungent, sour, bitter, salty and sweet. Each herb has at least one taste and most have two or three. Some herbs have no specific taste, and so are considered bland herbs. There are also herbs which have a special aromatic smell; these are called aromatic herbs. Another exception is that there are also some herbs or substances which give an astringent sensation in the mouth, so these are called astringent substances.

Originally, the tastes of herbs were defined directly from the perception in the mouth and stomach. People found that Gan Jiang (*Zingiberis rhizoma*) is pungent, Gan Cao (*Glycyrrhizae radix* is sweet, Huang Lian (*Coptidis rhizoma*) is bitter, Wu Mei (*Mume fructus*) is sour, Zhi Mu (*Anemarrhenae rhizoma*) is salty, Fu Ling (*Poria*) is bland and Long Gu (*Mastodi fossilium ossis*) is astringent. In early medical practice, it was also found that a specific taste caused a specific reaction in the body; as medical experience increased, the study of the tastes of herbs changed. As a result, some tastes are ascribed to herbs not according to their perception in the mouth, but to their action in the body. Therefore, the five tastes of herbs no longer simply describe the taste properties of herbs but have also become a part of the theory of herbal medicine and are used to analyze and study herbs.

According to experience from medical practice, each taste possesses specific properties, which can bring about specific actions in the body. The basic actions from the tastes are as follows.

Pungency

A pungent herb has moving and dispersing characteristics, which are able to disperse Wind, Cold, Heat and Dampness and therefore treat corresponding disorders. For instance, Ma Huang (*Ephedrae herba*)* can disperse the Lung-Qi, Shi Gao (*Gypsum*) is able to disperse Heat from the Lung and the Stomach, Fu Zi (*Aconiti radix lateralis preparata*)* can expel Cold from the Kidney, Fang Feng (*Saposhnikoviae radix*) is able to expel Wind from the superficial region of the body and Chai Hu (*Bupleuri radix*) can lift the Qi from the Liver and Gall Bladder.

Since pungent herbs can move quickly and expel pathogenic factors, they can also promote Qi movement, Blood circulation and water metabolism, open the meridians and reduce stagnation. For instance, Mu Xiang (*Aucklandiae radix*)**, Chen Pi (*Citri reticulatae pericarpium*), Sha Ren (*Amomi xanthioidis fructus*) and Hou Po (*Magnoliae cortex*) can promote Qi movement; Chuan Xiong (*Chuanxiong rhizoma*), Dang Gui (*Angelicae sinensis radix*), Chi Shao Yao (*Paeoniae radix rubra*) and Yan Hu Suo (*Corydalidis rhizoma*) are able to invigorate the Blood; Di Fu Zi (*Kochiae fructus*) and Qin Jiao (*Gentianae macrophyllae radix*) can eliminate Dampness; Jiang Can (*Bombyx batrycatus*) and Quan Xie (*Scorpio*)* can open the meridians.

The moving and dispersing ability of the pungent taste can also break up and eliminate pathological products. Many herbs that are able to break up congealed Blood, reduce food stagnation and dissolve Phlegm are also pungent, such as Mo Yao (*Myrrhae*), E Zhu (*Curcumae rhizoma*), Lai Fu Zi (*Raphani semen*), Bing Lang (*Arecae semen*), Ban Xia (*Pinelliae rhizoma*) and Xing Ren (*Armeniacae semen*).

Sweetness

A sweet herb possesses tonifying qualities. It can tonify and nourish the body, and especially its substantial aspect. Most of the herbs that tonify the Qi, Blood, Yin and Yang are sweet. For example, Ren Shen (*Ginseng radix*) and Huang Qi (*Astragali radix*) can tonify the Qi; Shu Di Huang (*Rehmanniae radix praeparata*) and Da Zao (*Jujubae fructus*) can tonify the Blood; Mai Men Dong (*Ophiopogonis radix*) can nourish the Yin; Ba Ji Tian (*Morindae radix*) and Rou Gui (*Cinnamomi cassiae cortex*) can tonify the Yang.

A sweet herb also possesses moderate quality. It can relieve acute stomach ache, abdominal pain or cramping pain of muscles, because sweetness can nourish the Yin of tendons and therefore relaxes the muscles; Zhi Gan Cao (*Glycyrrhizae radix preparata*) is a good example in such situations.

The moderate quality gives the sweet taste an ability to reduce stress, harmonize emotions and bring a relief from deep anger, fear or sorrow. Zhi Gan Cao (*Glycyrrhizae radix preparata*), Xiang Fu (*Cyperi rhizoma*), Bai He (*Lilii bulbus*) and Sheng Di Huang (*Rehmanniae radix*) are often used for this purpose.

Moreover, sweetness can also reduce the speed of a progressive pathological change, stabilize the condition and give time to restore the body resistance and to recover the function of the internal organs; therefore it can be used in critical situations. For instance, Ren Shen (*Ginseng radix*) and Huang Qi (*Astragali radix*) can restore the Qi; Zhi Gan Cao (*Glycyrrhizae radix preparata*) and Fu Zi (*Aconiti radix lateralis preparata*)* used together can rescue the Yang; Zhi Gan Cao (*Glycyrrhizae radix preparata*) and Bai Shao Yao (*Paeoniae radix lactiflora*) are used together to nourish the Yin.

The moderating nature of the sweet taste can also reduce the side-effects of harsh herbs and moderate the speed of other herbs, turning a harsh and quick action into a steady and constant action. For example, Zhi Gan Cao (*Glycyrrhizae radix preparata*) can moderate the cathartic action of Da Huang (*Rhei rhizoma*) and Mang Xiao (*Natrii sulfas*) to treat constipation; it can moderate the quick action of Fu Zi (*Aconiti radix lateralis preparata*)* and Gan Jiang (*Zingiberis rhizoma*) to strengthen the Yang.

In addition, a sweet herb is often used to harmonize the herbs whose functions are on different directions and levels in one formula; for example, Zhi Gan Cao (*Glycyrrhizae radix preparata*) is used in more than ninety percent of formulas as a harmonizing herb.

Sourness

A sour herb is astringent. It can stabilize the Qi, Blood, Essence and Body Fluids and prevent their leakage in pathological situations. Because it can stabilize the essential substances of the body, it is also considered to have a nourishing function in the body. For example, Wu Wei Zi (*Schisandrae fructus*), Shan Zhu Yu (*Corni fructus*) and Bai Shao Yao (*Paeoniae radix lactiflora*) can stabilize the Body Fluids and treat spontaneous sweating and night sweating; Wu Wei Zi (*Schisandrae fructus*)

and Wu Bei Zi (*Chinensis galla*) are able to stabilize the Lung-Qi to treat severe cough and shortness of breath; Suan Zao Ren (*Ziziphi spinosae semen*) can stabilize the Heart-Qi, nourish the Blood and treat palpitations, restlessness and insomnia; Bai Shao Yao (*Paeoniae radix lactiflora*) is able to nourish and stabilize the Liver-Yin to treat irritability; Shan Zhu Yu (*Corni fructus*) can stabilize the essence of the Kidney and treat poor memory, inability to concentrate and spermatorrhea; Wu Mei (*Mume fructus*) can nourish the Stomach-Yin and improve the appetite; Jin Ying Zi (*Rosae laevigatae fructus*) and Wu Bei Zi (*Chinensis galla*) are able to bind up the intestines and stop diarrhea as well as treat rectal prolapse.

Sour herbs are also considered to have a function of relieving toxicity and reducing swelling. For instance, Wu Mei (*Mume fructus*) and vinegar are used to inhibit some parasites, fungi, bacteria and viruses.

Bitterness

A bitter herb possesses drying, reducing and downward-moving capabilities. It can dry Dampness and dissolve Phlegm. For instance, Bai Zhu (*Atractylodis macrocephalae rhizoma*) can dry Dampness in the Middle Jiao and strengthen the function of the Spleen; Cang Zhu (*Atractylodis rhizoma*) can dry Dampness and relieve heavy sensations in the head and the limbs; Ban Xia (*Pinelliae rhizoma*) and Xing Ren (*Armeniacae semen*) can direct the Lung-Qi to descend, dissolve Phlegm and relieve cough.

Bitterness is very often used to reduce Heat from the internal organs. For instance, Huang Lian (*Coptidis rhizoma*) can clear Stomach-Fire and treat Excessive hunger, heartburn and toothache; Zhu Ye (*Bambusae folium*) can clear Heat from the Heart and lead it out of the body through the urine; Long Dan Cao (*Gentianae radix*) can clear Heat, reduce Fire and dry Dampness from the Liver organ and meridian, and is effective in treating tinnitus, acute eczema and infections of the eyes and ears; Huang Bai (*Phellodendri cortex*) can clear Heat from the Kidney and Bladder and therefore treats spermatorrhea and painful urinary dysfunction due to Damp-Heat in the Lower Jiao.

A bitter herb has a downward-moving tendency in its action, and therefore it can be used to direct the Qi and Blood downward in a specific region or in the whole body. For example, Xing Ren

(*Armeniacae semen*) can direct the Lung-Qi downward; Ban Xia (*Pinelliae rhizoma*) can direct the Stomach-Qi downward; Bing Lang (*Arecae semen*), Hou Po (*Magnoliae cortex*) and Da Huang (*Rhei rhizoma*) can direct the Qi in the intestines downward; Chuan Niu Xi (*Cyathulae radix*) can direct the Blood downward; San Leng (*Sparganii rhizoma*) and E Zhu (*Curcumae rhizoma*) can direct congealed Blood downward.

Saltiness

A salty substance possesses softening and reducing qualities. As it can soften hardness, it is often used to treat chronic inflammations as well as masses, such as goiter, scrofula, hepatocirrhosis and tumors. For instance, Xuan Shen (*Scrophulariae radix*) is often used for chronic pharyngitis; Mang Xiao (*Natrii sulfas*) is used to soften the feces and promote bowel movement; Zhe Bei Mu (*Fritillariae thunbergii bulbus*) and Hai Fu Shi (*Pumex*) are able to dissolve sticky sputum; Mu Li (*Ostrea concha*), Hai Zao (*Sargassum*) and Kun Bu (*Eckloniae thallus*) are used in treating goiter and scrofula. All of these can be used in formulas to treat tumors.

A salty substance also has a downward-moving tendency in action and it can direct the Qi, Blood and Body Fluids downwards. For instance, Xue Jie (*Daemonoropsis resina*) and Su Mu (*Sappan lignum*) can disperse and reduce congealed Blood; Xuan Shen (*Scrophulariae radix*) can reduce Fire from the Heart and Kidney.

Blandness

A bland substance has the function of promoting urination and leaching out Dampness. For instance, Fu Ling (*Poria*), Yi Yi Ren (*Coicis semen*), Tong Cao (*Tetrapanacis medulla*) and Hua Shi (*Talcum*) can treat urinary retention and painful urinary dysfunction; they can also treat edema.

Aromatic herbs

An aromatic herb has similar functions to those of a pungent herb. It possesses moving and dispersing properties. Furthermore, an aromatic herb has a lighter but more remarkable smell, which brings about the function of penetrating the turbidity of Dampness, reviving the Spleen and transforming Dampness. It is especially used in conditions where Dampness accumulates in the Middle Jiao and the Spleen fails to transform and transport Dampness, the Spleen-Qi is not able to ascend and the Stomach-Qi is not able to descend. This pathological change leads to symptoms such as poor appetite, nausea, vomiting, diarrhea and a sticky sensation in the mouth. Huo Xiang (*Agastachis herba*), Pei Lan (*Eupatorii herba*), Cang Zhu (*Atractylodis rhizoma*) and Sha Ren (*Amomi xanthioidis fructus*) are the most commonly used aromatic herbs and are used to treat these disorders.

There are other aromatic herbs which can transform the turbidity of Dampness and harmonize the Qi and Blood in certain organs and areas besides the Spleen. For example, Yu Jin (*Curcumae radix*), Qing Hao (*Artemisiae annuae herba*) and Yin Chen Hao (*Artemisiae scopariae herba*) can transform the Dampness from the Liver and Gall Bladder and treat distension in the hypochondriac region, nausea and irritability; Shi Chang Pu (*Acori graminei rhizoma*), Su He Xiang (*Styrax*) and Bing Pian (*Borneol*) can transform Dampness, revive the Heart and open the orifices to treat Closed syndrome; Bo He (*Menthae herba*) and Ju Hua (*Chrysanthemi flos*) can clear Wind-Heat from the head to treat headache and a heavy and distending sensation of the head and eyes.

Moreover, since aromatic herbs are light and have a moving ability, they are often used to unblock Qi and Blood obstructions and relieve pain. For instance, Su He Xiang (*Styrax*), Tan Xiang (*Santali albi lignum*) and Sha Ren (*Amomi xanthioidis fructus*) can treat severe pain in the chest and are used for angina pectoris; Mu Xiang (*Aucklandiae radix*)** and Sha Ren (*Amomi xanthioidis fructus*) can treat abdominal pain; Yu Jin (*Curcumae radix*), Chuan Xiong (*Chuanxiong rhizoma*) and Wu Yao (*Linderae radix*) can treat lower abdominal pain due to disorders in the Liver meridian; Qiang Huo (*Notopterygii rhizoma*), Chuan Xiong (*Chuanxiong rhizoma*) and Bai Zhi (*Angelicae dahuricae radix*) can relieve headache; Ru Xiang (*Olibanum*) and Mo Yao (*Myrrhae*) can treat pain due to Blood stagnation.

Since aromatic herbs can penetrate into the deeper regions of the body to regulate the Qi and Blood, they are also often used topically in herbal plasters, lotions or creams to treat muscular pain. The commonly used aromatic herbs are Chuan Xiong (*Chuanxiong rhizoma*), Ru Xiang (*Olibanum*), Rou Gui (*Cinnamomi cassiae cortex*), Qiang Huo (*Notopterygii rhizoma*) and Bo He (*Menthae herba*). In addition, aromatic herbs are also often used topically to promote the healing process of wounds, especially the Yin-type ulcers, because the herbs can reach the deep regions of the wound, transform turbidity of Dampness and regulate the Qi and Blood. The commonly used herbs are Ding Xiang (*Caryophylli flos*), Ru Xiang (*Olibanum*), Chen Xiang (*Aquilariae lignum*), Bai Zhi (*Angelicae dahuricae radix*) and Bing Pian (*Borneol*).

Astringency

An astringent herb or substance has the same characteristics as a sour substance, but no sour taste. It can stabilize the essential substances of the body and prevent the leakage of them in pathological conditions. For instance, Long Gu (*Mastodi fossilium ossis*) can stabilize the Heart-Qi and calm the Liver-Yang to treat palpitations, restlessness and insomnia; Mu Li (*Ostrea concha*) can stabilize the Body Fluids and treat night sweating; Shi Liu Pi (*Granati pericarpium*) and Zao Xin Tu (*Terra flava usta*) can bind up the intestines and treat diarrhea; Sang Piao Xiao (*Mantidis oötheca*) and Shan Yao (*Dioscoreae rhizoma*) can stabilize the Essence, treat spermatorrhea and enuresis.

3 Which characteristics exist in the combinations of the temperature and taste of herbs?

It often happens that there is more than one taste in one herb; combined with its temperature, they bring about the specific functions of the herb. If more tastes and temperature of herbs are combined, the range of applications is extended. The specific combination of temperature and tastes may lead to the following functions.

Pungent-hot herbs can strongly disperse Cold and Dampness, warm the Yang and activate the Qi

Heat can warm Cold and possesses the ability to move; pungency has a moving and dispersing ability, and it may accelerate the action of hot herbs. Therefore a hot-pungent herb can strongly expel Cold and Dampness, warm the Yang and activate the Qi. For instance, Ma Huang (*Ephedrae herba*)* can activate

the Lung-Qi, and strengthen the dispersing and descending function of the Lung; Fu Zi (*Aconiti radix lateralis preparata*)* can warm the Kidney-Yang and Gan Jiang (*Zingiberis rhizoma*) can warm the Spleen-Yang and both of them can expel Cold. As Cold may freeze water, a pungent-hot herb can also dissolve Damp-Cold.

Sweet-warm herbs can tonify the essential substances and their function in the body

Sweetness has a tonifying, moderating and harmonizing quality; warmth is the source and essential condition for growth, not only in nature but also in the human body. Therefore a sweet-warm herb can tonify the essential substances of the body as well as strengthening the functions of the internal organs. For instance, Huang Qi (*Astragali radix*) and Ren Shen (*Ginseng radix*) can tonify the Qi; Shu Di Huang (*Rehmanniae radix praeparata*) and Gou Qi Zi (*Lycii fructus*) can tonify the Essence and Blood.

Pungent-sweet-warm herbs can generate the Yang and strengthen the functions of the internal organs

Sweetness has a tonifying ability; warmth offers a condition of growth for the essential substances; pungency is able to spread and carry out the action from sweetness and warmth. Therefore, from a sweet-pungent-warm herb the Yang of the body and the functions of the internal organs can be generated. For instance, Dang Gui (*Angelicae sinensis radix*) can warm the body, tonify the Blood and promote the Blood circulation; Rou Gui (*Cinnamomi cassiae cortex*) and Ba Ji Tian (*Morindae radix*) can generate the Kidney-Yang.

Pungent-bitter herbs can disperse and descend the Qi and Blood

Since pungency moves outwards and upwards and bitterness moves downwards, a pungent-bitter herb can move the Qi in two directions simultaneously to activate the Qi movement and Blood circulation as well as water metabolism. For instance, Xing Ren (*Armeniacae semen*) can regulate the Lung-Qi to relieve coughing; Ban Xia (*Pinelliae rhizoma*) can regulate the Stomach-Qi and treat nausea and poor appetite; Lian Qiao (*Forsythiae fructus*) can regulate the Qi in the chest and relieve irritability; Xiang Fu

(*Cyperi rhizoma*) can circulate the Liver-Qi and treat Liver-Qi stagnation; Chi Shao Yao (*Paeoniae radix rubra*), Mu Dan Pi (*Moutan cortex*) and Yan Hu Suo (*Corydalidis rhizoma*) can promote Blood circulation and treat Blood stagnation.

Pungent-bitter-warm herbs can dry Dampness

Bitterness has drying properties, and pungency and warmth can disperse Dampness. Pungent-bitter-warm herbs rather than pungent-hot herbs are often used to dry Dampness, because Dampness is a Yin, sticky pathogenic factor that results in a lingering pathological process and it cannot be removed quickly. The action of pungent-bitter-warm herbs is more steady and constant and is more suitable for this situation than a quickly moving pungent-hot herb. For example, Qiang Huo (*Notopterygii rhizoma*) and Cang Zhu (*Atractylodis rhizoma*) can expel Wind-Damp-Cold pathogenic factors; Hou Po (*Magnoliae cortex*) and Chen Pi (*Citri reticulatae pericarpium*) can dry Dampness in the Middle Jiao and transform Phlegm in the Lung as well as promote Qi movement.

Sweet-cold herbs can generate Yin

Since sweetness can tonify the substantial aspect of the body, and Cold can clear Heat and protect the Yin, a sweet-cold herb is able to nourish the Yin of the body and is commonly used for different kinds of Yin deficiency syndromes. For instance, Mai Men Dong (*Ophiopogonis radix*) can generate the Heart-Yin and Stomach-Yin; Lu Gen (*Phragmitis rhizoma*) and Bai He (*Lilii bulbus*) can nourish the Lung-Yin; Yu Zhu (*Polygonati odorati rhizoma*) can nourish the Stomach-Yin; Bai Shao Yao (*Paeoniae radix lactiflora*) can nourish the Liver-Yin; Sang Shen (*Mori fructus*) can nourish the Kidney-Yin.

Sweet-bitter-cold herbs can clear Heat and generate Yin and Body Fluids

Since sweetness has a tonifying ability, and bitterness and Cold can clear Heat and direct it to descend, sweet-bitter-cold herbs can reduce Fire and nourish the Yin. They are used for syndromes of Yin deficiency with Excessive-Heat and when the Heat has consumed the Yin of the body. For instance, Sheng Di Huang (*Rehmanniae radix*) can reduce Heat from the Heart, Liver and Kidney and

nourish the Yin of the three organs; Tian Men Dong (*Asparagi radix*) can reduce Fire from the Lung and Kidney and nourish the Yin there; Sang Ye (*Mori folium*) can clear Lung-Heat and moisten the Dryness there; Ju Hua (*Chrysanthemi flos*) can clear Liver-Heat, nourish the Yin and brighten the eyes.

Sour-cold herbs can generate and stabilize the Yin

Sourness can hold and stabilize the essential substances of the body and Cold can clear Heat and protect the Yin. A sour-cold substance can thus generate and stabilize the Yin of the body. For instance, Bai Shao Yao (*Paeoniae radix lactiflora*) and Han Lian Cao (*Ecliptae herba*) are able to clear Heat and nourish and stabilize the Liver-Yin; Tian Hua Fen (*Trichosanthis radix*), also called Gua Lou Gen, can clear Heat and nourish the Lung-Yin and Stomach-Yin.

Bitter-cold herbs can clear Heat, reduce Fire and eliminate Damp-Heat

Bitterness and Cold both have a clearing ability and both move downwards; Cold can clear Heat and bitterness enhances this action. Therefore a bitter-cold combination is widely found in herbs that clear Excessive-Heat, reduce Fire, relieve Heat toxicity and drain downward. Since bitterness can dry Dampness and Cold can reduce Heat, a bitter-cold herb can also clear and dry Damp-Heat. Bitter-cold herbs are especially used in situations where strong Excessive-Fire flares up and must be reduced strongly and quickly in order to stop the development of the disease. For instance, Huang Lian (*Coptidis rhizoma*), Huang Qin (*Scutellariae radix*) and Huang Bai (*Phellodendri cortex*) can clear Heat and dry Dampness in the Upper Jiao, Middle Jiao and Lower Jiao respectively; Long Dan Cao (*Gentianae radix*) can reduce Liver-Fire and eliminate Damp-Heat from the Liver meridian; Da Huang (*Rhei rhizoma*) can reduce Heat and promote bowel movement; Zhi Zi (*Gardeniae fructus*) can drain Damp-Heat and promote urination. Bitter-cold herbs are usually not used for a long period of time as they can injure the Yin and Qi, especially that of the Stomach. They strongly suppress Fire downwards, but this action works against the up-flaring nature of Fire and therefore may cause constraint of Fire and lead to the development of a chronic hidden Fire syndrome.

Pungent-cold herbs can disperse and reduce constraint of Fire

Since pungency has a moving and dispersing ability, and Cold can clear Heat, a pungent-cold herb can disperse and clear Heat which is caused by accumulation of Qi, Blood, Dampness or food. Following the nature of Fire, which always flares upwards and outwards, pungency disperses Heat, separates the strength of Heat and Cold, clears Heat and reduces Fire. Pungent-cold herbs can clear Heat completely. For instance, Shi Gao (*Gypsum*) can disperse and reduce the Heat from the Lung and Stomach; Ci Shi (*Magnetitum*) can disperse Heat from the Heart and direct it to descend; Xia Ku Cao (*Prunellae spica*) can disperse and clear Liver-Fire; Lian Qiao (*Forsythiae fructus*) can disperse and clear Heat in the chest; Bo He (*Menthae herba*) and Man Jing Zi (*Viticis fructus*) can clear Heat in the head; Yu Xing Cao (*Houttuyniae herba cum radice*) and Bai Jiang Cao (*Patriniae herba*) can treat abscesses and relieve Heat toxicity; Mu Dan Pi (*Moutan cortex*) and Chi Shao Yao (*Paeoniae radix rubra*) can disperse and remove congealed Blood and promote Blood circulation.

Pungent-bitter-cold herbs can clear Heat in a moving state

Pungent-bitter-cold herbs have the strong points of both pungent-cold and bitter-cold herbs, which were analyzed earlier. They are very effective and strong in dispersing and clearing Heat and directing it to descend without the possibility of forming hidden Heat, the side-effect of bitter-cold herbs. For instance, Qian Hu (*Peucedani radix*) can clear Lung-Heat; Man Jing Zi (*Viticus fructus*) can expel Wind-Heat in the Upper Jiao; Niu Bang Zi (*Arctii fructus*) and Ye Ju Hua (*Chrysanthemi indici flos*) can reduce swelling and relieve toxicity; Yu Jin (*Curcumae radix*) and Yi Mu Cao (*Leonuri herba*) can clear Heat in the Blood and promote Blood circulation.

Salty-cold substances can clear heat and soften and eliminate hardness

Since Cold clears Heat and moves downward, and saltiness can soften hardness, salty-cold substances are often used to loosen Phlegm, soften stools and treat tumors. For instance, Hai Ge Ke (*Meretricis/Cyclinae concha*) and Hai Fu Shi (*Pumex*) can be used for Phlegm-Heat syndromes when the Phlegm is very thick and sticky; Mang Xiao (*Natrii sulfas*) is used to soften the stools and treat constipation; Hai Zao (*Sargassum*), Xuan Shen (*Scrophulariae radix*) and Mu Li (*Ostrea concha*) can soften hardness and treat tumors.

4 What are the applications of the concept that herbs enter meridians?

All herbs enter meridians; some enter one, some enter two or three, some even enter all the meridians. According to the meridian-entering concept, each herb works on its specific meridian as well as the organ which it enters. For instance, Ma Huang (*Ephedrae herba*)* enters the Lung and Bladder meridians, activates the dispersing function of the Lung-Qi and excites the movement of the Yang-Qi in the Bladder meridian, and therefore expels Wind-Cold in the superficial region of the body; Rou Gui (*Cinnamomi cassiae cortex*) enters the Kidney meridian and warms and tonifies the Kidney-Yang; Fu Zi (*Aconiti radix lateralis preparata*)* is so hot and pungent that it is able to enter all the meridians and expels Cold there; Zhi Gan Cao (*Glycyrrhizae radix preparata*) is sweet and moderate and also enters all the meridians and harmonizes their functions.

In most cases, each herb enters one main meridian and enters other meridians secondarily. For instance, Huang Qi (*Astragali radix*) mainly enters the Spleen meridian and enters the Lung meridian secondarily; Shu Di Huang (*Rehmanniae radix praeparata*) mainly enters the Kidney meridian and enters the Liver meridian secondarily; Dang Gui (*Angelicae sinensis radix*) mainly enters the Liver meridian and enters the Spleen meridian secondarily.

Although most of the herbs enter two or three meridians, their functions focus on only one meridian, through which the other functions are carried out in the secondary meridians. For instance, Huang Qi (*Astragali radix*) mainly enters the Spleen meridian, while it secondarily enters the Lung meridian. It can strongly tonify the Spleen-Qi, and strengthen the transportation and transformation function of the Spleen. When the Spleen-Qi is sufficient, it can generate and support the Lung-Qi as well as the Defensive Qi; however, the main function of Huang Qi is to tonify the Spleen. In clinical practice, Huang Qi treats poor appetite, lassitude and loose stools, as well as shortness of breath and a tendency to catch cold from a weak constitution.

In clinical practice, the concept of herbs entering specific meridians is very important for achieving good therapeutic results. Take treating headache as an example, how do you select the appropriate herbs? One method is to choose the herbs that enter the specific meridian which passes through the region of pain. For instance, Chuan Xiong (*Chuanxiong rhizoma*) enters the San Jiao (Triple Jiao) and Gall Bladder meridians and is particularly effective for treating headache on the sides of the head; Qiang Huo (*Notopterygii rhizoma*) enters the Bladder meridian and is effective for treating pain in the neck and occipital area; Bai Zhi (*Angelicae dahuricae radix*) enters the Stomach meridian and is effective for treating pain in the forehead; Wu Zhu Yu (*Evodiae fructus*) enters the Liver meridian and treats pain on the top of the head.

Some herbs especially enter one meridian and are used as envoy herbs. For instance, Jie Geng (*Platycodi radix*) enters the Lung meridian and is often used as an envoy to guide the other herbs into the Lung; it can also guide the Spleen-Qi upwards so that it enters the Lung to strengthen the Lung-Qi. Another example is Zhi Gan Cao (*Glycyrrhizae radix preparata*), which mainly enters the Spleen meridian. Because the Spleen is the source of Qi and Blood, the foundation of life, Zhi Gan Cao (*Glycyrrhizae radix preparata*) is considered as an agent that can enter all meridians and tonifies and harmonizes the functions of all the meridians and organs. For the same reason, it often plays a role of harmonizing the function of herbs which enter different meridians in one formula.

5 Do the taste and the color of herbs influence their function? What is the relationship between the taste of herbs and the internal organs, and what is the relationship between their color and the internal organs? What are the clinical applications?

According to the Five Elements theory, the colors and tastes of herbs particularly influence certain internal organs and meridians. This relationship suggests a method of selecting herbs to treat disorders of certain internal organs and meridians. In clinical practice, the therapeutic effects will be better if the combinations of the taste and the color as well as the function of herbs are considered. Furthermore, in this way, the formula is smaller and more efficient because each herb has multiple functions.

Herbs with a sour taste enter the Liver and Gall Bladder. Green in Chinese is called 'Qing' which also links with the Liver. For instance, Shan Zhu Yu (*Corni fructus*), Chi Shao Yao (*Paeoniae radix rubra*) and Bai Shao Yao (*Paeoniae radix lactiflora*) are sour and enter the Liver; Qing Pi (*Citri reticulatae viride pericarpium*), Qing Hao (*Artemisiae annuae herba*) and Qing Dai (*Indigo naturalis*) have a green color and they enter the Liver too.

Herbs with a bitter taste enter the Heart. Red in Chinese is called 'Hong', 'Chi', 'Dan' or 'Zhu' which link with the Heart. For instance, Huang Lian (*Coptidis rhizoma*) and Ku Zhu Ye (*Bambusae amarae folium*) are bitter in taste and enter the Heart; Dan Shen (*Salviae miltiorrhizae radix*), Chi Shao Yao (*Paeoniae radix rubra*) and Hong Hua (*Carthami flos*) are red in color and also enter the Heart and promote the Blood circulation.

Herbs with a sweet taste enter the Spleen. For instance, Gan Cao (*Glycyrrhizae radix*), Long Yan Rou (*Longanae arillus*) and Da Zao (*Jujubae fructus*) are sweet and enter the Spleen. Yellow in Chinese is called 'Huang' and it links with the Spleen. The color of many herbs can turn to yellow or brown when they are dry-fried or baked. They are easily digested and accepted by Stomach and Spleen. In this way, it is believed yellow enters the Spleen, such as Zhi Huang Qi (processed *Astragali radix*), Chao Bai Zhu (dry-fried *Atractylodis macrocephalae rhizoma*), Jiao Mai Ya (deep dry-fried *Hordei fructus germinatus*), Jiao Shen Qu (deep dry-fried *Massa medicata fermentata*) and Jiao Shan Zha (deep dry-fried *Crataegi fructus*).

Herbs that have a pungent taste enter the Lung. White in Chinese is called 'Bai' and it links with the Lung too. For instance, Ma Huang (*Ephedrae herba*)*, Bo He (*Menthae herba*) and Sheng Jiang (*Zingiberis rhizoma recens*) are pungent and enter the Lung meridian; Shi Gao (*Gypsum*), Chuan Bei Mu (*Fritillariae cirrhosae bulbus*), Yu Zhu (*Polygonati odorati rhizoma*) and Yin Er (*Tremellae*) are white in color and also enter the Lung.

Herbs with a salty taste enter the Kidney. Black in Chinese is called 'Hei', 'Xuan' or 'Wu' which links with the Kidney too. For instance, Rou Cong Rong (*Cistanchis herba*)** and Xuan Shen (*Scrophulariae radix*) are salty and enter the Kidney; Xuan Shen is also black in color, as is Hei Zhi Ma (*Sesami semen nigricum*) which enters the Kidney too.

It must be mentioned, however, that it is not always true that the five kinds of color of herbs must enter the correspondent organs. For instance, Huang Qin (*Scutellariae radix*) enters the Lung, Huang Lian (*Coptidis rhizoma*) enters the Heart, and Huang Bai (*Phellodendri cortex*) and Sheng Di Huang (*Rehmanniae radix*) enter the Kidney although they are all yellow in color.

This consideration of the characteristics of herbs is also applied to clinical practice in other ways. A small amount of herbs or food with a certain taste will benefit the corresponding organ while a large amount of a certain taste will damage the same organ. For instance, sweetness may strengthen the function of the Spleen, but an excess of sweet herbs or food may injure the transportation and transformation function of the Spleen; sourness can soften the Liver, but an excess of sour herbs or food may injure the Liver.

In order to enhance specific functions of herbs or let herbs enter specific meridians, herbs can be processed with vinegar, honey and salt. For instance, Chai Hu (*Bupleuri radix*) and Xiang Fu (*Cyperi rhizoma*) have a stronger effect in spreading the Liver-Qi after being processed by vinegar; Bai Zhu (*Atractylodis macrocephalae rhizoma*), Mai Ya (*Hordei fructus germinatus*), Shen Qu (*Massa medicata fermentata*) and Shan Zha (*Crataegi fructus*) are more effective in promoting digestion after they are dry-fried till they turn brown; Zhi Mu (*Anemarrhenae rhizoma*) and Huang Bai (*Phellodendri cortex*) are stronger in reducing Empty-Fire in the Kidney after they have been processed by salt.

6 What are the tendencies of action of the herbs in the body and what are the applications?

The tendency of action of a substance refers to the direction of movement of that substance in the body (e.g. upwards, downwards, outwards or inwards). This feature of a herb depends on several of its properties.

First of all, the temperature and the taste of a herb determine its tendency. The warm, hot, pungent and aromatic herbs tend to move upwards and outwards; the cold, cool, bitter, bland and salty herbs tend to move downwards; the sour and astringent herbs move inwards and the sweet herbs stay in their original place.

The tendency of action is also decided by the functions of the herbs. Generally speaking, herbs which tend to move upwards and outwards can be found in relation to functions such as releasing the Exterior, inducing vomiting, expelling Wind and Cold, dispersing Fire and Dampness, spreading the constraint of Qi, opening the orifices, unblocking the meridians and lifting the clear Yang. Herbs that tend to move downwards can be found in relation with functions such as clearing Fire, promoting bowel movement, promoting urination, directing the Liver-Yang or the Lung-Qi to descend, soothing the Stomach-Qi and calming the Spirit, as well as eliminating Phlegm, Blood stasis, food stagnation and parasites.

Another factor that decides the tendency of action is the nature of the herb. Generally speaking, flowers are light and tend to move upwards, whereas mineral substances are heavy and tend to move downwards. There are some exceptions, however; for instance, Xuan Fu Hua (*Inulae flos*) can direct the Lung-Qi to descend and eliminate Phlegm, and Shi Gao (*Gypsum*) can direct the Lung-Qi to descend and disperse Heat from the Lung.

In addition, processing can change action tendencies. Generally speaking, herbs processed by alcohol move upwards, those processed by ginger juice move outwards, those processed by vinegar move inwards and those processed by salt move downwards.

There are also herbs that move generally about the whole body without a special direction. For instance, Chuan Xiong (*Chuanxiong rhizoma*) can invigorate the Blood and promote Blood circulation; it moves in the four directions mentioned above. Xiang Fu (*Cyperi rhizoma*) can spread the Liver-Qi and also moves about the whole body.

The tendency of action of herbs is widely used in treatment to regulate Qi movement, Blood circulation and water metabolism, as well as that to eliminate accumulations of Qi, Blood, food, Phlegm and water.

Furthermore, the tendency of action of herbs is used to strengthen the functions of the internal organs and their cooperation. This tendency is especially important in the strategy of herbal combination as demonstrated by the following examples.

Regulating the Lung-Qi, eliminating Phlegm, reducing Fire, and regulating Qi in the Chest

Ma Huang (*Ephedrae herba*)* disperses and lifts the Lung-Qi; Xing Ren (*Armeniacae semen*) directs the Lung-Qi to descend and transforms Phlegm. They are used together to regulate the Lung-Qi.

Sang Ye (*Mori folium*) disperses Wind-Heat; Sang Bai Pi (*Mori cortex*) clears Heat and directs the Qi of the Lung to descend. They are used together to expel Wind-Heat from the Lung, bring down the Lung-Qi and relieve wheezing.

Jie Geng (*Platycodi radix*) lifts the Lung-Qi and Xing Ren (*Armeniacae semen*) directs the Lung-Qi to descend; both can eliminate Phlegm and stop cough. They are used together to regulate the function of the Lung and remove Phlegm.

Xi Xin (*Asari herba*)* disperses the Lung-Qi and Wu Wei Zi (*Schisandrae fructus*) stabilizes the Lung-Qi. They are used together to relieve Cold-type wheezing.

Ma Huang (*Ephedrae herba*) disperses Lung-Qi and disperses Heat from the Lung and Shi Gao (*Gypsum*) directs the Lung-Qi to descend and clears Heat from the Lung. They are used together to relieve Heat-type wheezing.

Zhi Zi (*Gardeniae fructus*) descends Heat in the chest and Dan Dou Chi (*Sojae semen praeparatum*) disperses Heat in the chest. They are used together to treat irritability due to constraint of Qi and Heat in the chest.

Regulating the Qi in the Middle Jiao and promoting digestion

Bai Zhu (*Atractylodis macrocephalae rhizoma*) strengthens the Spleen-Qi and promotes transportation and transformation of the Spleen in the Middle Jiao; Zhi Shi (*Aurantii fructus immaturus*) directs the Qi to descend in the intestines and removes the accumulation of food, Phlegm and Qi. They are used together to promote digestion.

Huang Lian (*Coptidis rhizoma*) descends Stomach-Fire and Sheng Ma (*Cimicifugae rhizoma*) disperses Stomach-Fire. They are often used together to treat toothache.

Ban Xia (*Pinelliae rhizoma*) disperses stagnation of Stomach-Qi and accumulation of Phlegm; Huang Qin (*Scutellariae radix*) clears Heat that is caused by the accumulation in the Stomach. They are used together to regulate the Stomach and effectively treat nausea and poor appetite, especially under stress.

Zhi Ke (*Aurantii fructus*) enters the Lung and Stomach meridians, disperses the Qi and opens the chest; Zhi Shi (*Aurantii fructus immaturus*) directs the Qi to descend in the intestines. They are used together to treat distension in the chest and abdomen.

Regulating the intestines and promoting bowel movement

Da Huang (*Rhei rhizoma*) reduces Heat and purges accumulation in the intestines and Hou Po (*Magnoliae cortex*) disperses the Qi and directs it to descend. They are used together to treat constipation.

Da Huang (*Rhei rhizoma*) descends the Qi in the intestines and moves stools, and Jie Geng (*Platycodi radix*) ascends the Lung-Qi to accelerate the Qi's downward movement in the Large Intestine. They are used together to treat constipation and distension in the abdomen.

Associating the Heart and Kidney

Huang Lian (*Coptidis rhizoma*) reduces Excessive-Heat from the Heart; Rou Gui (*Cinnamomi cassiae cortex*) strengthens the Kidney-Yang and warms the vital Fire. They are used together to treat insomnia due to the disharmony of the Heart and Kidney according to the Five Elements theory.

Lifting the Yang and strengthening the Exterior

Huang Qi (*Astragali radix*) strengthens and stabilizes the Defensive Qi; Fang Feng (*Saposhnikoviae radix*) disperses Wind from the Exterior. They are used together to regulate the opening and closing of the pores, strengthen the body resistance and prevent cold infections.

Regulating the Liver-Qi

Chai Hu (*Bupleuri radix*) lifts and disperses the Liver-Qi; Bai Shao Yao (*Paeoniae radix lactiflora*) directs Heat downward and stabilizes the Yin of the Liver. They are used together to treat Liver-Qi stagnation.

Dang Gui (*Angelicae sinensis radix*) tonifies the Blood and promotes the Blood circulation of the Liver; Bai Shao Yao (*Paeoniae radix lactiflora*) nourishes the Blood and stabilizes the Yin of the Liver. They are used together to soften the Liver and treat Liver-Qi stagnation caused by Blood deficiency.

Dispersing and descending the constraint of Qi and Fire

Chai Hu (*Bupleuri radix*) lifts and disperses Liver-Qi; Xiang Fu (*Cyperi rhizoma*) promotes Liver-Qi movement. They are used together to treat Liver-Qi stagnation.

Chai Hu (*Bupleuri radix*) lifts and disperses Liver-Qi; Zhi Ke (*Aurantii fructus*) broadens the chest. They are used together to reduce tight sensations in the chest.

Long Dan Cao (*Gentianae radix*) strongly descends Heat and drains Fire from the Liver; Chai Hu (*Bupleuri radix*) lifts and disperses constrained Fire and Qi in the Liver. They are used for Excessive-Fire in the Liver.

Huang Lian (*Coptidis rhizoma*) directs Fire downwards from the Stomach; Sheng Ma (*Cimicifugae rhizoma*) lifts and disperses constrained Qi and Fire in the Stomach. They are used together to treat Excessive-Heat in the Stomach.

Shi Gao (*Gypsum*) descends Fire from the Spleen and Stomach; Fang Feng (*Saposhnikoviae radix*) disperses constrained Heat and Qi. They are used for eliminating hidden Fire in the Spleen.

Subduing the Liver-Yang

Dai Zhe Shi (*Haematitum*) and Shi Jue Ming (*Haliotidis concha*) direct the Liver-Yang to descend; Qing Hao (*Artemisiae annuae herba*) and Mai Ya (*Hordei fructus germinatus*) lift constrained Qi from the Middle Jiao. They are used together to harmonize Qi movement in the process of bringing down the Liver-Yang.

Calming the Spirit

Long Gu (*Mastodi fossilium ossis*) calms the Heart and Liver; Chai Hu (*Bupleuri radix*) lifts the Liver-Qi. They are used together to treat restlessness and insomnia.

Ren Shen (*Ginseng radix*) tonifies the Heart-Qi and Wu Wei Zi (*Schisandrae fructus*) stabilizes it. They are used together to treat restlessness and palpitations caused by Heart-Qi deficiency.

Harmonizing the Qi and Blood and treating disorders in certain regions of the body

Gui Zhi (*Cinnamomi cassiae ramulus*) disperses the Defensive Qi and Bai Shao Yao (*Paeoniae radix lactiflora*) nourishes the Nutritive Qi. They are used together to harmonize the Nutritive and Defensive levels.

Qiang Huo (*Notopterygii rhizoma*) tends to expel Wind-Damp-Cold from the upper body; Du Huo (*Angelicae pubescentis radix*) tends to expel Wind-Damp-Cold from the lower body. They are used together to treat Bi syndrome in the entire body.

There are also situations where special attention should be paid towards the tendency of action. For instance, herbs which move upwards are not suitable for use alone in cases of Liver-Yang rising, such as in hypertension, hot flushes in menopause or in patients with constipation; equally, downward-moving herbs are not suitable for use alone in diarrhea, heavy menstruation and pregnancy.

The tendency of action of herbs can also be used to reduce the side-effects of some herbs. For instance, the sweet Shu Di Huang (*Rehmanniae radix praeparata*) is too sticky to be digested, so the pungent Sha Ren (*Amomi xanthioidis fructus*) is often used at the same time to remove the stagnation; the hot Fu Zi (*Aconiti radix lateralis preparata*)* and the cold Da Huang (*Rhei rhizoma*) move too quickly, but the sweet Zhi Gan Cao (honey-fried *Glycyrrhizae radix preparata*) can moderate their harsh nature and reduce the speed.

7 What are the specific functions of the specific parts of a plant?

The commonly used herbs are usually the roots, leaves, barks, stems, flowers, fruits and seeds of the plants. Sometimes, different parts of plants give specific functions to the herbs. In TCM theory, similes and allegories are used to explain the links between plants and the human body. The details are as follows.

- The peel of fruits and the bark of plants (in Chinese called 'Pi') enter the superficial layer of the human body. For instance, Chen Pi (*Citri reticulatae pericarpium*), Sheng Jiang Pi (*Zingiberis rhizoma recens cortex*), Da Fu Pi (*Arecae pericarpium*), Fu Ling Pi (*Poriae cocos cortex*) and Sang Bai Pi (*Mori cortex*) can eliminate Dampness in the superficial layer of the body and treat edema.
- The twigs of tree (in Chinese called 'Zhi') enter the limbs and the meridians. For instance, Gui

Zhi (*Cinnamomi cassiae ramulus*) can warm the meridians, promote the movement of Yang-Qi in the meridians and treat cold limbs; Sang Zhi (*Mori ramulus*) can expel Wind-Dampness from the meridians, relax tendons and treat Bi syndrome; Gou Teng (*Uncariae ramulus cum uncis*) can reduce Heat from the Liver, extinguish Wind and control convulsions.

• The vines (in Chinese called 'Teng') enter the collaterals. For instance, Ji Xue Teng (*Spatholobi caulis et radix*) can tonify the Blood, promote the Blood circulation and relieve pain, numbness of the limbs and tingling sensations in the muscles; Ye Jiao Teng (*Polygoni multiflori caulis*) can tonify the Blood, relieve uneasy feelings in the body due to Blood deficiency and improve sleep; Hai Feng Teng (*Piperis caulis*) and Luo Shi Teng (*Trachelospermi caulis*) can expel Wind-Dampness from the collaterals and treat Bi syndrome.

• The sprout enters the Heart and promotes the function of the internal organs. For instance, Lian Zi Xin (*Nelumbinis plumula*) clears Heat from the Heart; Mai Ya (*Hordei fructus germinatus*) generates and lifts clear Qi of the Spleen and Stomach, thus it can promote digestion.

• Some seeds (in Chinese called 'Zi' or 'Ren') enter the Kidney. For instance, Jiu Cai Zi (*Allii tuberosi semen*), Tu Si Zi (*Cuscutae semen*), Fu Pen Zi (*Rubi fructus*), Yi Zhi Ren (*Alpiniae oxyphyllae fructus*) and Sha Yuan Zi (*Astragali complanati semen*) can tonify the Kidney-Essence and strengthen the Kidney-Yang.

There are also the following regular patterns.

• Most of the flowers (in Chinese called 'Hua') are light in weight and nature and have an ascending tendency. For instance, Ju Hua (*Chrysanthemi flos*) and Mi Meng Hua (*Buddlejae flos*) can expel Wind-Heat from the Liver meridian and benefit the vision; He Huan Hua (*Albiziae flos*) calms the Mind and disperses constrained Qi in the chest, so is often used for depression; Jin Yin Hua (*Lonicerae flos*) can disperse and clear Heat from the Upper Jiao; Hou Po Hua (*Magnoliae officinalis flos*) can disperse stagnation of Qi, spread the accumulation of water in the Middle Jiao and promote digestion.

• Many seeds or fruits are heavy in weight and nature and have a descending tendency. For instance, Xing Ren (*Armeniacae semen*), Ting Li Zi (*Lepidii/Descurainiae semen*) and Su Zi (*Perillae fructus*) can direct the Lung-Qi to descend and treat wheezing and cough; Zhi Shi (*Aurantii fructus immaturus*), Bing Lang (*Arecae semen*) and Sha Ren (*Amomi xanthioidis fructus*) can bring down Qi in the Large Intestine and promote bowel movement.

• Many seeds contain lipids and can moisten the intestine and treat constipation. For instance, Huo Ma Ren (*Cannabis semen*), Yu Li Ren (*Pruni semen*), Xing Ren (*Armeniacae semen*), Tao Ren (*Persicae semen*) and Hei Zhi Ma (*Sesami semen nigricum*) can moisten the intestines and promote bowel movement.

• Mineral substances are heavy in weight and nature and have a descending tendency. For instance, Zhen Zhu Mu (*Concha margaritifera usta*) and Ci Shi (*Magnetitum*) can calm the Mind; Long Gu (*Mastodi fossilium ossis*), Mu Li (*Ostrea concha*) and Shi Jue Ming (*Haliotidis concha*) can direct the Liver-Yang to descend; Dai Zhe Shi (*Haematitum*) can subdue rebellious Stomach-Qi.

This relationship holds not only between humans and plants, but also between human and animal products. For instance, Chan Tui (*Cicadae periostracum*) can treat skin disorders; Sang Piao Xiao (*Mantidis oötheca*) can tonify the Kidney; worms and snakes are able to unblock the collaterals as they have the habit of drilling holes, for instance Di Long (*Pheretima*), Jiang Can (*Bombyx batrycatus*), Bai Hua She (*Agkistrodon acutus*)* and Wu Shao She (*Zaocys*).

8 What are the proper dosages when prescribing herbs?

The exact dosage of each herb is usually given in textbooks of Chinese herbal medicine. Nowadays, herb weights are given in metric units (grams or milligrams) instead of in traditional Chinese weights (*Liang*, *Qian* and *Fen*). The dosage of a single herb mentioned in books is always the dosage for 1 day. The dosages of the herbs in a formula are more complicated and they are not always for 1 day. In addition, the herbs are weighed according to different systems in different dynasties, so it is important to read the preparation of the formula carefully, as well as possess some knowledge of the classic in which the formula was recorded.

Here we discuss only the dosage of single herbs. To achieve the therapeutic results, it is important not only to choose the proper herbs, but also to use the proper dosage. For a junior practitioner, it is not so easy to remember the dosage of each herb, so it is necessary to find an easy way to memorize them.

Generally speaking, in Chinese texts the common dosage of most crude herbs is about 3–9 grams orally per day, which is divided into two or three portions and used during the course of the day. However, in the West it is generally not practical to prescribe the crude herbs for oral use since it takes too much time every day to prepare the decoction and the smell is not always pleasant. Concentrated herb powders produced in Taiwan and Hong Kong are thus more commonly used. It should be noted that the strength of the concentrated powder is six times stronger than that of the crude herbs, thus the given dosage of most single powdered herbs is 0.5–1.5 grams per day. According to my own experience, however, the correct dosage is generally somewhat lower, at 0.2–0.5 grams.

Although the dosage range of most herbs can be remembered in this way, there are some exceptions. In the exceptions mentioned in the following paragraphs, the dosage of the herbs should be memorized individually.

Poisonous herbs

Some poisonous herbs can be dangerous for patients if they are overdosed. The dosage of these herbs should be remembered by heart. As the toxic dose varies for each individual, the therapeutic range is small and only experienced doctors must prescribe these herbs.

The commonly used poisonous herbs are Fu Zi (*Aconiti radix lateralis preparata*)*, Wu Tou (*Aconiti radix*)*, Xi Xin (*Asari herba*)*, Ma Huang (*Ephedrae herba*)*, Yang Jin Hua (*Flos Daturae*)*, Lei Gong Teng (*Tripterygii wilfordii caulis*)*, Wu Gong (*Scolopendra*)*, Quan Xie (*Scorpio*)*, Bai Hua She (*Agkistrodon acutus*)*, Mang Chong (*Tabanus*)*, Zhe Chong (*Eupolyphaga seu opisthoplatia*)*, Nao Yang Hua (*Rhododendron molle flos*)*, Tian Xian Zi (*Hyoscyamus niger semen*)*, Shan Dou Gen (*Sopho-

rae tonkinensis radix*)*, Sheng Ban Xia (*Pinelliae rhizoma*), Tian Nan Xing (*Arisaematis rhizoma*), Bai Fu Zi (*Typhonii rhizoma praeparatum*)*, Wei Ling Xian (*Clematidis radix*), Xian Mao (*Curculinginis rhizoma*), Cang Er Zi (*Xanthii fructus*), Wu Zhu Yu (*Evodiae fructus*), Hua Jiao (*Zanthoxyli fructus*) and Yuan Zhi (*Polygalae radix*).

Poisonous substances that are used for special pathological situations, but are not often used, are Ku Lian Pi (*Meliae cortex*), He Shi (*Carpesii fructus*), Gua Di (*Pedicellus cucumeris*), Li Lu (*Veratri nigri radix et rhizoma*), Chang Shan (*Dichroae febrifugae radix*), Gan Sui (*Euphorbiae kansui radix*)*, Da Ji (*Knoxiae radix*)*, Yuan Hua (*Genkwa flos*)*, Shang Lu (*Phytolaccae radix*)*, Qian Niu Zi (*Pharbitidis semen*)*, Ba Dou (*Crotonis fructus*)* and Zhu Sha (*Cinnabaris*)*

Minerals

Mineral substances can be used at 30 grams per day in traditional decoctions. These include Shi Gao (*Gypsum*), Ci Shi (*Magnetitum*), Long Gu (*Mastodi fossilium ossis*), Mu Li (*Ostrea concha*), Zhen Zhu Mu (*Concha margaritifera usta*), Shi Jue Ming (*Haliotidis concha*) and Wa Leng Zi (*Arcae concha*). If the concentrated powder is prescribed, the dosage should be about 1–2 grams.

Light herbs

Herbs that are light in weight should be used in a lower dosage: 0.5–3 grams for crude herbs and 0.1–0.5 grams for concentrated powder, such as Tong Cao (*Tetrapanacis medulla*), Deng Xin Cao (*Junci medulla*), Ma Bo (*Lasiosphaera*) and Chan Tui (*Cicadae periostracum*).

The dosage of single herbs can be varied within the normal dosage range in the following conditions:

- Bland herbs, which promote urination and leach out Dampness, can be used in relatively large dosage; these include Fu Ling (*Poria*), Yi Yi Ren (*Coicis semen*), Che Qian Zi (*Plantaginis semen*) and Hua Shi (*Talcum*).
- Tonifying herbs can be used in relatively large dosage; these include Huang Qi (*Astragali radix*), Shu Di Huang (*Rehmanniae radix praeparata*), Mai Men Dong (*Ophiopogonis radix*) and Bai He (*Lilii bulbus*).

- Aromatic herbs that open the orifices, expel Wind-Heat or Wind-Cold and promote Qi movement should be used in relatively small dosage; these include Bing Pian (*Borneol*), Su He Xiang (*Styrax*), Bo He (*Menthae herba*), Chai Hu (*Bupleuri radix*), Xin Yi (*Magnoliae flos*), Bai Zhi (*Angelicae dahuricae radix*), Mu Xiang (*Aucklandiae radix*)** and Sha Ren (*Amomi xanthioidis fructus*).
- Herbs that are used alone should be in relatively large dosage, whereas in a formula the dosage should be smaller. For instance, Pu Gong Ying (*Taraxaci herba*) can be used by itself at 15 grams per day to treat carbuncle, but at only 6 grams in a formula with other herbs for treating carbuncle.
- The dosage should be varied according to the constitution and the age of the patient. For acute diseases, if the patient is young, or the constitution is quite good, the dosage of the herbs that expel exogenous pathogenic factors should be large. For chronic diseases, or if the patient is old and weak, the dosage of the herbs that expel the pathogenic factors should be smaller. The tonifying herbs should be started with a smaller dosage, then the dosage should be increased gradually because their cloying nature may cause indigestion.
- The dosage should be varied during the course of treatment. For acute diseases, or in the active stage of chronic diseases, the dosage should be high. When the situation is under control, the dosage should be reduced. Herbs that open the orifices, or induce sweating, diarrhea or vomiting, are used only once. Afterwards, the dosage must be adjusted according to the condition of the patient.

There are also herbs that should not be used at a high dosage for more than 4 weeks. These include herbs that disperse the Lung-Qi, disperse Wind, Cold and Dampness, strongly reduce Heat-toxin, drain downward, break up Qi stagnation, remove congealed Blood, remove food stagnation, calm the Mind and subdue the Liver-Yang. These herbs are usually used to treat asthma, rheumatic or rheumatoid arthritis, acute infections, tumors, emotional disturbance, insomnia or hot flushes and night sweats in menopause. In chronic disease, after intensive treatment for 1–4 weeks, these herbs should be used in a lower dosage to keep the condition stable; meanwhile, herbs that tonify or harmonize the functions of internal organs should be used if necessary. The intensive treatment can be repeated according to the disease and the condition of the patient.

Some gentle tonifying herbs can be used for months or even years in low dosage for the purpose of keeping the condition stable, strengthening the body resistance or maintaining good health. In this case, if the treatment course is long, it is better to have breaks. The best time for the break is summer because Summer-Heat or Damp-Heat may weaken the function of the Spleen and the herbs may place extra burden on the Spleen and cause digestive problems.

- The dosage should also be varied according to season and climate. In summer or in tropical countries, herbs that expel Wind and Cold and disperse the Lung-Qi should not be used in high dosage because the pores are not tightly closed. However, in winter or extremely northerly latitudes, herbs that expel Wind, Cold and Dampness and induce sweating should be used in high dosage.

9 What is the proper dosage for children?

Children have special physiological and pathological characteristics, which are quite different from those of adults. As their internal organs, muscles and bones are delicate and their physiological functions are not fully developed, children become ill more easily than adults, and diseases also develop quickly. However, as the body and the emotions of children are less impaired from chronic diseases, stress and medicine than those of adults, the reaction to herbal treatment is quicker and so children recover sooner from diseases than do adults. Therefore, for children, the treatment course is shorter than for adults and it should be stopped when the pathogenic factors are eliminated.

The dosage for children is varied according to age:

- infants: 1/10 of the adult dosage
- infants–1 year old: 1/6 of the adult dosage
- 1–2 years old: 1/4 of the adult dosage
- 2–4 years old: 1/3 of the adult dosage
- 4–6 years old: 1/2 of the adult dosage
- 6–14 years old: 2/3 of the adult dosage.

(The dosage of adults mentioned here is the average dosage for adults. The dosage of children is for children with a normal weight and length for that age. The dosage can be varied within the normal range according to the disease and constitution as well as the experience of the practitioner.)

10 How is a herbal decoction prepared?

The commonly used form of Chinese herbal medicine is the decoction. The preparation of the decoction directly influences the therapeutic result. In the traditional way, the herbal decoction should be prepared every day during the treatment course. The procedure is as follows.

1. Put the dry, crude herbs in an earthenware or stainless steel pot, pour cold water in the pot until the water is 3–4 cm above the herbs, and let the dry, crude herbs soak in the water for at least 1 hour.
2. Afterwards, place the pot on the fire, heating with a strong flame. When the liquid is boiling, turn the heat down to gentle, cook the herbs for 20 minutes and then strain the decoction from the pot. (Note, however, that herbs that expel Wind-Cold or Wind-Heat should be cooked for 10 minutes less and tonifying herbs should be cooked for 10 minutes longer each time.)
3. Pour another 200 ml of cold water onto the herbs in the pot and cook for a further 20 minutes, strain this decoction and then mix the two decoctions together; the total liquid should be about 200–250 ml.
4. Finally, divide the decoction into two or three portions, and drink each portion warmed over the course of the day in two or three lots.

Because some herbs have different qualities, there are also some special procedures for preparation.

Decocting first. Some substances are heavy and do not easily release the inactive ingredients into the decoction; these should be cooked for 30 minutes before adding the other herbs. Most are mineral substances, such as Ci Shi (*Magnetitum*), Long Gu (*Mastodi fossilium ossis*), Mu Li (*Ostrea concha*), Shi Jue Ming (*Haliotidis concha*) and Shi Gao (*Gypsum*). Some toxic herbs should also be cooked

longer to reduce their toxicity—for instance Fu Zi (*Aconiti radix lateralis preparata*)* and Wu Tou (*Aconiti radix*)*.

Decocting later. Some aromatic or pungent herbs have active ingredients that will be destroyed by long cooking and these should be added to the pot 5 minutes before the end of cooking. Examples are Bo He (*Menthae herba*), Qing Hao (*Artemisiae annuae herba*), Huo Xiang (*Agastachis herba*) and Xiang Ru (*Moslae herba*). Also, in order to increase certain actions, some herbs are cooked for less time than normal. For instance, Da Huang (*Rhei rhizoma*) can be cooked for a shorter time to increase its purgative action.

Some rare, expensive herbs, such as Ren Shen (Ginseng radix) should be prepared separately. Herbs that are traditionally used in powder form should be added to the prepared decoction without cooking; an example is San Qi (*Notoginseng radix*) powder. Gels and syrups such as E Jiao (*Asini corii colla*), Yi Tang (*Maltose*) and honey, as well as egg yolks, should also be dissolved in the prepared decoction without cooking.

11 What is the usual way to take herbal medicine?

The patient should pay attention to the method of taking herbal medicine to ensure the therapeutic result.

Herbal medicine should always be taken warm. If the herbal medicine is a decoction it should be taken when warm; herbal medicines that expel Wind-Cold are better taken hot. If the medicine is a concentrated herbal powder, it should be dissolved in boiling water and taken after it has cooled a little. Pills, tablets or capsules should be taken with warm water. There are some exceptions, however, such as if the patient suffers from an Excessive-Heat syndrome, in which the Heat is so strong that the person cannot tolerate warm drinks and the reaction to drinking warm decoctions is vomiting. In this condition, herbal medicine can be used when it is cool.

Another situation is when a patient has a Cold syndrome and cannot tolerate herbs that are warm in nature because of the obvious conflicts between the natures; then the decoction can be taken when it is cool.

The frequency of taking herbal medicine is varied according to the disease and the condition of the patient. Usually, herbal medicine is taken three times a day: in the morning, afternoon and evening. However, in acute and critical conditions, the herbal medicine should be taken every 4 hours, even during the night. For chronic diseases, it can be taken twice a day: in the morning and evening. When the condition of the patient improves, the herbal medicine can be used once a day, every other day, or even twice a week to stabilize the condition of the patient. The frequency should also be adjusted for herbs that induce sweating or for purgative herbs according to the condition of the patient and the effects of the herbs. Medicine to eliminate parasites is taken only once a day for a maximum of 3 days. Herbs to reduce swelling, pain or irritation in the throat should be kept in the mouth and throat as long as possible. The patient should be instructed to sip the liquid slowly and to finish a cup of the herbal tea in 2 or 3 hours.

The timing of taking herbal medicine is also varied according to the disease and the condition of the patient. Usually, the medicines are taken 1 hour before or after the meal on a rather empty stomach because then the body can absorb the herbs properly. There are some exceptions, though. Tonifying herbs are better taken 1 hour before a meal; medicines which promote digestion and strengthen the Stomach, or herbs that irritate the Stomach, should be taken directly after the meal; medicines which drain downwards or eliminate parasites should be taken in the morning on an empty stomach; herbs which calm the Mind and improve sleep should be taken before the patient goes to bed; herbs which control the attack of diseases such as asthma and malaria should be used 1 to 2 hours before the attack.

12 How should children be given herbal medicine?

As herbal medicine is administrated in rather small dosage and the diet of children is often simple compared with that of an adult, the method of giving herbal medicine to children also differs from that for adults.

For infants, the herbal powder can be tipped on the nipple while the baby is breast feeding or bottle feeding.

For children under 5 years, the herbal powder can be given mixed with milk, yogurt, lemonade or water. There is no strict time regulation of taking

medicine between the meals, but the frequency is the same as in adults. If the herbal medicine is a pill or tablet, it should be first dissolved in a little water. For children under 5 years of age, it is forbidden to prescribe pills, tablets or capsules because children of this age cannot swallow them properly, especially when they are nervous, ill or reluctant to take the medicine.

For children older than 5 years, the method of taking the medicine is somewhere in between the usual method for adults and that for smaller children because they can understand why they should take the medicine and so can cooperate better.

Of course, herbs prescribed for children should not be too strong in taste or smell. After the herbs are taken, favorite drinks can then be given as refreshment.

13 What are the contraindications and cautions when using Chinese herbal medicine?

In order to ensure the therapeutic effects of Chinese herbal medicine and the safety of the patients, it is important to know the contraindications of using Chinese herbal medicine so as to avoid mistakes and accidents.

The contraindications of Chinese herbal medicine can be divided into contraindications of particular syndromes, caution about herb combinations, caution during pregnancy and caution about diet.

Contraindications of particular syndromes

Some herbs should not to be used in certain syndromes. Apart from herbs that gently harmonize the functions of the internal organs, most herbs have specific actions and can be used in only certain pathological conditions. It is very important to learn contraindications by heart. The contraindications of each herb are usually mentioned after the functions of individual herbs in most textbooks as well as in the introductions to each chapter. However, there are some general principles, as follows.

- When treating Cold syndromes, herbs with a cold nature should not be used; equally, hot herbs should not be used in Heat syndromes. When the Qi, Yang or Fire and Wind are ascending in a pathological condition (e.g. in hypertension), herbs that move upwards and outwards should not be used; if the Qi and Yang are sinking (e.g. in diarrhea), herbs that move downwards should not be used. However, these contraindications apply only to the use of single herbs; they may be used in certain herb combinations, or formulas in some conditions. For instance, Ma Huang (*Ephedrae herba*)* is a pungent and hot herb, it can strongly disperse the Lung-Qi, expel Wind-Cold and is able to treat Exterior syndrome and asthma. It is forbidden to use it in patients suffering from Wind-Heat syndrome; it is also forbidden to be used alone for patients with shortness of breath due to Heat in the Lung so the Lung-Qi is not able to descend (e.g. in asthma, asthmatic bronchitis or pneumonia). However, in the latter condition it can be used with Shi Gao (*Gypsum*), which is cold and able to direct the Lung-Qi to descend and clear the Heat. In this case, the two substances are used in a ratio of 1 (Ma Huang) to 4 (Shi Gao), so overall the combination has a cooling and descending action.

- If there is an Exterior syndrome then sweet, cloying, tonifying herbs and sour or astringent herbs should not be used because they will keep the pathogenic factors in the body and reduce the strength of the herbs that expel the exogenous pathogenic factors. This mistake is called 'closing the door and keeping your enemy in'. This contraindication applies to single herbs as well as to the main actions of herbal combinations. If the body resistance of the patient is too weak, a small amount of herbs that strengthen the body resistance and tonify the Qi can be used in combination with a larger amount of herbs that expel the exogenous pathogenic factors, in order to assist the herbs that expel exogenous pathogenic factors.
- If the patient sweats easily during the course of an Exterior syndrome, this suggests that the pores are open at that moment, therefore herbs that induce sweating and expel exogenous pathogenic factors should not be used at that time because they are too strong and may cause overdispersion of the Qi and Body Fluids. For instance, if a patient with asthma catches a cold and the asthma is worsening and also the patient's Defensive Qi is weak, although the

syndrome is caused directly by Wind-Cold the patient may sweat and feel dry in the mouth, so Ma Huang (*Ephedrae herba*) cannot be used alone in this condition. However, it can be used with Shi Gao (*Gypsum*) but the dosage of Shi Gao must be much higher than that of Ma Huang.

- Before tonifying herbs and astringent herbs are applied, the body should be comparatively clean; that is, there should be no accumulations of Phlegm, water, food, Fire, Qi and Blood, because most of the sweet tonifying and the astringent or sour herbs may retain the pathogenic factors in the body and complicate the syndrome. The correct procedure is first to remove pathogenic factors, and especially the substantial pathogenic factors, and then start treatment with tonifying herbs. There are some exceptions, however. If accumulations are caused by deficiency of Qi, Blood, Yin or Yang, it is impossible to remove these pathogenic factors completely at first. In this case, tonifying herbs should be added in combination with the reducing herbs. The ratio between the two sorts of herbs must also be varied depending on the change of strength in the pathogenic factors and the person's resistance.
- If the Stomach of the patient is weak or sensitive, then harsh herbs should not be chosen, such as very hot or very cold herbs or herbs with strong tastes. In TCM, the Stomach and Spleen are regarded as the foundation of life, not only in physiology but also in pathology. 'If there is only one percent Stomach-Qi, there is still one percent chance of recovery of the patient' is a saying found in many classics. Restoring the Stomach to a good condition is considered as the first step in achieving different therapeutic results. In other words, protecting and strengthening the transportation and transformation functions of the Stomach and Spleen will allow the herbs to be absorbed by the body.

Cautions about herb combinations

There are three groups of herbs that are forbidden to be used together, otherwise toxicity and side-effects may occur.

1. Gan Cao (*Glycyrrhizae radix*) may not be used with Gan Sui (*Euphorbiae kansui*

radix)*, Da Jĭ (Knoxiae radix)*, Yuan Hua (Genkwa flos)* or Hai Zao (Sargassum).

2. Wu Tou (Aconiti radix)* may not be used with Chuan Bei Mu (Fritillariae cirrhosae bulbus), Zhe Bei Mu (Fritillariae thunbergii bulbus), Gua Lou (Trichosanthis fructus), Ban Xia (Pinelliae rhizoma), Bai Lian (Ampelopsitis radix) or Bai Ji (Bletillae tuber).

3. Li Lu (Veratri nigri radix et rhizoma) may not be used with Ren Shen (Ginseng radix), Bei Sha Shen (Glehniae radix), Nan Sha Shen (Adenophorae radix), Ku Shen (Sophorae flavescentis radix), Xuan Shen (Scrophulariae radix), Dan Shen (Salviae miltiorrhizae radix), Xi Xin (Asari herba)*, Bai Shao Yao (Paeoniae radix lactiflora) or Chi Shao Yao (Paeoniae radix rubra).

As Gan Cao (Glycyrrhizae radix) and Wu Tou (Aconiti radix)* are very commonly used, the first two groups of the herbs should be learnt by heart.

There are also nine pairs of herbs that are traditionally forbidden to be used together. It is believed that such combination can minimize or even neutralize the therapeutic effects:

- Liu Huang (Sulfur)* antagonizes Po Xiao (Glauberis sal)
- Shui Yin (Hydrargyrum)* antagonizes Pi Shuang (Arsenicum)*
- Lang Du (Euphorbiae fischerianae radix)* antagonizes Mi Tuo Seng (Lithargyrum)*
- Ba Dou (Crotonis fructus)* antagonizes Qian Niu Zi (Pharbitidis semen)*
- Wu Tou (Aconiti radix)* antagonizes Xi Jiao (Rhinoceri cornu)**
- Ya Xiao (Nitrum) antagonizes San Leng (Sparganii rhizoma)
- Ding Xiang (Caryophylli flos) antagonizes Yu Jin (Curcumae radix)
- Ren Shen (Ginseng radix) antagonizes Wu Ling Zhi (Trogopterori faeces)
- Rou Gui (Cinnamomi cassiae cortex) antagonizes Chi Shi Zhi (Halloysitum rubrum).

Among these nine pairs, the first five are rarely used in clinical practice because their functions are so different that they can hardly be combined to treat one syndrome and some of them are very poisonous so they are also hardly used nowadays. However, the last four pairs would possibly be combined to treat one syndrome, so these must be memorized by heart.

Cautions during pregnancy

During pregnancy, herbs can influence physiological changes in both the pregnant woman and the fetus, especially during the first 3 months. Generally speaking, it is better to keep the pregnancy as natural as possible, and try to avoid all kinds of treatment if they are not really necessary at that moment. According to the strength and characteristics of the herbs, there are some herbs which are forbidden to be used during pregnancy and others that should be used with caution.

Herbs that are forbidden include poisonous or harsh herbs which are used for breaking up congealed Blood and draining downwards, such as Ba Dou (Crotonis fructus)*, Qian Niu Zi (Pharbitidis semen)*, Da Jĭ (Knoxiae radix)*, Shang Lu (Phytolaccae radix)*, Ban Mao (Mylabris)*, She Xiang (Moschus)**, San Leng (Sparganii rhizoma), E Zhu (Curcumae rhizoma), Mang Chong (Tabanus)* and Shui Zhi (Hirudo).

If it is really necessary, some herbs can be used during the pregnancy, such as in conditions of tumor, bleeding due to stagnation of Blood, severe deficiency of Qi and Blood and severe internal coldness, where if the pathological situation is not treated it may injure the woman and the fetus; however, the dosage and treatment course must both be controlled carefully. Herbs that are to be used with caution include all the substances that promote Qi movement and Blood circulation, especially in the Lower Jiao, and herbs that remove the obstruction of food and Phlegm, promote bowel movement and promote urination and have pungent or lubricating properties; examples include Tao Ren (Persicae semen), Hong Hua (Carthami flos), Da Huang (Rhei rhizoma), Zhi Shi (Aurantii fructus immaturus), Fu Zi (Aconiti radix lateralis preparata)*, Gan Jiang (Zingiberis rhizoma), Rou Gui (Cinnamomi cassiae cortex), Dong Kui Zi (Malvae semen), Hua Shi (Talcum), Fu Ling (Poria) and Ze Xie (Alismatis rhizoma).

Cautions about diet

Caution about diet means, on the one hand, that certain kinds of food should not be taken in certain syndromes or diseases and, on the other hand, that certain kinds of food should not be taken when certain herbs are used.

Generally speaking, during herbal treatment, all cold, raw, heavy and spicy food should be avoided. It is wise to suggest that patients drink light tea instead of coffee, do not take fresh drinks and fruits directly from the refrigerator, and eat lightly cooked vegetables rather than salads.

If heavy food is eaten, it is better to take some tea or orange juice afterwards to remove the fat, or to take semiskimmed milk and to take less candy, sugar, chocolate and alcohol.

For Cold syndromes, raw and cold food should be avoided; for Heat syndromes or syndromes of Liver-Yang rising, spicy and heavy food, coffee and alcohol should be avoided. For syndromes of Damp-Phlegm or Damp-Heat accumulation, sweet, heavy food, milk products, nuts and alcohol should be avoided. For skin disorders or wounds characterized by itching, weeping and redness, seafood, spicy food and alcohol should be avoided.

For some herbs mentioned in the classics, certain foods are contraindicated. For all of the substances that tonify the Blood, strong tea should be avoided. Dan Shen (*Salviae miltiorrhizae radix*) and Fu Ling (*Poria*) are contraindicated with vinegar; Sheng Di Huang (*Rehmanniae radix*), Shu Di Huang (*Rehmanniae radix praeparata*) and He Shou Wu (*Polygoni multiflori radix*) are contraindicated with onion, garlic and radish; Gan Cao (*Glycyrrhizae radix*), Huang Lian (*Coptidis rhizoma*), Jie Geng (*Platycodi radix*) and Wu Mei (*Mume fructus*) are contraindicated with pork; Tu Fu Ling (*Smilacis glabrae rhizoma*) and Shi Jun Zi (*Quisqualis fructus*) are contraindicated with tea; Chang Shan (*Dichroae febrifugae radix*) is contraindicated with onion.

14 Which herbs can be used as substitutes for substances that are banned or unavailable?

Traditional Chinese herbal medicine has a long history, which dates back 5000 years to the beginning of the Chinese civilization. It is the result of people's effort to utilize nature for survival and is developed on the basis of long-term observation, study and practice under the guidance of ancient philosophy.

However, as the relationship between humans and nature has changed with time, some ingredients in TCM have become unavailable or protected and banned by legislation. Traditional herbal medicine must accommodate such change. Beside the usage of cultivated herbs and synthetic ingredients in the clinical practice, one can also use herbs with similar actions as substitutes. However, one must always bear in mind that, due to the specific function and characteristic of each herb, the therapeutic result of the substituted herb will never be completely the same as the original one.

The suggested substitutes are as follows:

- Xi Jiao (*Rhinoceri cornu*)** can be replaced by Shui Niu Jiao (*Bubali cornu*). It can be also replaced by Da Qing Ye (*Isatidis folium*) and Sheng Ma (*Cimicifugae rhizoma*) at a ratio of 10:1.
- Hu Gu (*Tigris os*)** can be replaced by Qian Nian Jian (*Homalomenae rhizoma*) and the bones of cat, pig or ox.
- Ling Yang Jiao (*Antelopis cornu*)** can be replaced by Shan Yang Jiao (*Naemorhedis cornu*). It can also be replaced by Shi Jue Ming (*Haliotidis concha*) and Qing Dai (*Indigo naturalis*) with a small amount of Chai Hu (*Bupleuri radix*).
- Lu Rong (*Cervi cornu*)** can be replaced by the combination of Ba Ji Tian (*Morindae radix*) and Rou Gui (*Cinnamomi cassiae cortex*). It will also be helpful if venison is included in the patient's diet.
- Gui Ban (*Testudinis carapax*)** can be replaced by the combination of Shu Di Huang (*Rehmanniae radix praeparata*) and Shan Zhu Yu (*Corni fructus*). Meat and bone-marrow are also recommended in the patient's diet.
- Bie Jia (*Trionycis carapax*)** can be replaced by Shu Di Huang (*Rehmanniae radix praeparata*) and Sheng Di Huang (*Rehmanniae radix*) with Mu Dan Pi (*Moutan cortex*).
- She Xiang (*Moschus*)** and Niu Huang (*Bovis calculus*)** should be replaced by synthetic ones.
- Tian Ma (*Gastrodiae rhizoma*)** can be replaced by Gou Teng (*Uncariae ramulus cum uncis*), Man Jing Zi (*Viticis fructus*), Ju Hua (*Chrysanthemi flos*) or Bai Ji Li (*Tribuli fructus*) to pacify the Liver and extinguish

Liver-Wind, or combined with Xia Ku Cao
(*Prunellae spica*), Di Long (*Pheretima*) and
Jiang Can (*Bombyx batrycatus*) to eliminate
Wind-Phlegm.

- Shi Hu (*Dendrobii caulis*)** can be replaced
by the combination of Sheng Di Huang
(*Rehmanniae radix*) and Shu Di Huang
(*Rehmanniae radix praeparata*).
- Gou Ji (*Cibotii rhizoma*)** can be replaced
by Gu Sui Bu (*Drynariae rhizoma*).
- Bai Ji (*Bletillae tuber*)** can be replaced by
Zi Zhu Cao (*Callicarpae folium*).
- Guang Mu Xiang (*Aucklandiae radix*)** can
be replaced by Chuan Mu Xiang (*Vladimirae
radix*), Qing Pi (*Citri reticulatae viride
pericarpium*) or Sha Ren (*Amomi xanthioidis
fructus*).
- Hou Po (*Magnoliae cortex*) can be replaced
by Zi Su Geng (*Perillae caulis et flos*) and
Chuan Mu Xiang (*Vladimirae radix*) to
regulate Qi and reduce distension. To direct
Qi downward and remove dampness and
food stagnation it can be replaced by Cang
Zhu (*Atractylodis rhizoma*), Zhi Shi
(*Aurantii fructus immaturus*) and Ban Xia
(*Pinelliae rhizoma*).
- The use of Zhu Sha (*Cinnabaris*)* is
forbidden. It can be replaced by Long Chi
(*Mastodi fossilia dentis*) and Zhen Zhu
(*Margarita usta*) with Huang Lian (*Coptidis
rhizoma*) to calm the Mind.
- Guan Mu Tong (*Hocquartiae manshurensis
caulis*)* is a poisonous herb and its use is
forbidden. It should be replaced by Chuan
Mu Tong (*Clematidis armandii caulis*) with
careful control of both the Chinese name
and the Latin name, or it can be substituted
by Zhi Zi (*Gardeniae fructus*) or Tong Cao
(*Tetrapanacis medulla*) with Huang Lian
(*Coptidis rhizoma*) or Long Dan Cao
(*Gentianae radix*).

15 What attention should be paid to some common names of herbs in Traditional Chinese Medicine?

Traditional Chinese herbal medicine has a long
history of discovering plants which can be used for
medical purposes. The accumulation of the knowledge and experience increases with time. In this
development, some plants that have a similar appear-
ance share the same common names. Although there
are differentiating names to the plants, people still
often use only the common names, which can bring
confusion—even danger—in the practice as some of
the herbs are toxic. Thus practitioners should pay
special attention to the differentiating names and
also check the Latin names to ensure that the correct
herb is prescribed before applying them in practice.
The most commonly used herbs with common
names and differentiating names are as follows:

- Chuan Bei Mu (*Fritillariae cirrhosae bulbus*)
and Zhe Bei Mu (*Fritillariae thunbergii
bulbus*)
- Chuan Niu Xi (*Cyathulae radix*) and Huai
Niu Xi (*Achyranthis bidentatae radix*)
- Nan Sha Shen (*Adenophorae radix*) and Bei
Sha Shen (*Glehniae radix*)
- Nan Wu Jia Pi (*Acanthopanacis cortex*) and
Bei Wu Jia Pi (*Periploca sepium bunge*)
- Han Fang Ji (*Stephaniae tetrandrae radix*)
and Mu Fang Ji (*Aristolochiae fangchi
radix*)*
- Guan Mu Tong (*Aristolochia manshurensis
caulis*)* and Chuan Mu Tong (*Clematidis
armandii caulis*)
- Qing Mu Xiang (*Aristolochia debilis*)*,
Chuan Mu Xiang (*Vladimirae radix*), Guang
Mu Xiang (*Aucklandiae radix*)** and Mu
Xiang (*Aucklandiae radix*)**.

PART **2**

Comparisons and characteristics of the commonly used Chinese herbal medicines

常用中药的比较与特性

PART 2

Chapter Two

Herbs that release the Exterior

解表药

1 What is Exterior syndrome? How should one treat Exterior syndrome? What are the characteristics of the herbs that release the Exterior?

The term Exterior syndrome indicates, in a broad sense, that the pathogenic change is in the superficial layer of the body. The main characteristic of this change is the conflict between the six exogenous pathogenic factors and the body's resistance, which is represented mainly by the Defensive Qi in the superficial layer of the body. An Exterior syndrome also includes further pathogenic changes of the associated organs, meridians, Qi and Blood.

The Lung is an important organ in Exterior syndrome because it governs the Exterior by dispersing the Defensive Qi to the superficial layer of the body. Moreover, Wind-Heat and Dryness can directly disturb the function of the Lung because they can invade the body through the nose, and not the superficial level.

The main symptoms can be divided into two groups. On the one hand, chills, fever and aversion to cold or wind are present. These are the manifestations in the superficial layer of the body caused by the conflict between pathogenic factors and the Defensive Qi. On the other hand, headache, general pain, thirst, blocked nose, cough and sore throat may be present; these are manifestations caused by disharmony of the circulation of the Qi and Blood in the Bladder meridian and dysfunction of the Lung-Qi.

The purpose of treatment is to expel the exogenous pathogenic factors, and to restore the normal functioning and harmony of all the organs, meridians, Qi and Blood. Methods that can stimulate or strengthen the function of the Defensive Qi or disperse the Lung-Qi and therefore eliminate the pathogenic factors are often used. Other methods, such as promoting Qi and Blood circulation, or regulating the Large Intestine in order to regulate the Lung-Qi, can also be used as assistant procedures in the whole treatment strategy.

Herbs that release the Exterior have the functions of expelling Wind-Cold or Wind-Heat. They are used in conditions where the pathogenic Wind-Cold or Wind-Heat invades the superficial layer of the body. They have the following properties.

Pungent or pungent and warm

Most of the herbs in this category possess a pungent property. As pungency has a dispersing capacity, the pungent herbs are able to activate Qi movement, open the pores and subcutaneous layer, connect the Exterior with the Interior, disperse the Lung-Qi, harmonize the Nutritive and Defensive systems and therefore expel Wind. Moreover, many of the herbs are pungent and warm in nature. Their functions of activating the Yang and Qi and opening the pores are represented by their induction of sweating in different degrees. Through sweating, Wind and other exogenous pathogenic factors can be eliminated from the superficial layer of the body, therefore stopping the progress of the disease in its primary stage.

Aromatic

Many of the herbs in this category are aromatic, which gives them the ability to open the orifices, penetrate turbidity, spread the pure Qi and transform Dampness. They are therefore used to treat headache, dizziness, nasal obstruction and loss of the sense of smell.

Light in weight and gentle in nature

Many herbs in this category are light in weight and gentle in nature. They mainly enter the Lung and the Bladder meridians, so they are suitable for treating the external pathogenic syndromes that mainly affect those layers and meridians. As wind characteristically attacks the upper body, which includes the head, the Lung, the Upper Jiao and the superficial layer of the body, these herbs are often used to treat symptoms such as headache, dizziness, nasal obstruction, runny nose, itchy and painful eyes, cough with or without production, sore throat and general body pain. Many are also used to treat allergies such as hay fever and asthma, as well as many kinds of skin diseases.

2 What precautions should be observed in the usage of herbs that release the Exterior?

First of all, since herbs that release the Exterior are pungent and their tendencies of action are ascending and dispersing, especially with the herbs that can cause sweating, overdose may disperse the Qi too much, consume the Yin of the body and cause other complications. In patients who are deficient in Yin or Qi owing to their constitution, chronic disease, stress or dietary habit, these herbs should be used with caution. Furthermore, as pungency also has the property of movement, these herbs should also be used with caution in bleeding conditions or in pregnancy.

Secondly, the dosage of herbs should be adjusted to suit the condition of the individual, the syndrome and the season. For elderly people, children, people with a weak constitution and for mild syndromes, in a gentle climate and in the summer, the dosage should be reduced. For adults with a strong constitution and for severe syndromes, in a cold winter or a cold place, the dosage should be increased. If sweating must be induced, the dosage is adjusted according to the syndrome. A mild sweat over the whole body is required. Heavy sweating must be avoided because it can only weaken the Qi and Yin.

In the third place, as eliminating Wind-Cold or Wind-Heat is not generally difficult, these herbs should not be used for a long period of time. A dosage of 3 days is recommended to treat Exterior syndrome. If the exogenous pathogenic factors have not been removed completely, then another 3-day dosage can be prescribed. With regard to herbs that may cause heavy sweating, the dosage and treatment course should be adjusted according to the reaction of the patient after each use.

3 Ma Huang (*Ephedrae herba*)* and Gui Zhi (*Cinnamomi cassiae ramulus*) can both expel Wind-Cold to treat Exterior Wind-Cold syndrome. What are the differences between their actions and characteristics? What are the cautions regarding their use?

Ma Huang and Gui Zhi can expel Wind-Cold and treat Exterior Wind-Cold syndrome. Compared with Gui Zhi, Ma Huang is stronger in inducing sweating and expelling Wind-Cold from the surface of the body. This is because Ma Huang is very pungent and warm, and its speed of movement and strength are stronger than Gui Zhi. When Wind-Cold attacks the body surface, the pores are closed by Cold, which is characteristically contracting, so the Defensive Qi is not able to spread over the surface of the body. In consequence, the patient feels chilly because the surface of the body is not warmed up by the Yang and Qi. The blockage of Defensive Qi inside may then produce Heat and the patient may have a fever. Because Cold initially injures the Yang-Qi in the Greater Yang (*Tai Yang*) meridian, this stops the Qi circulating freely, and the patient feels pain and stiffness in the back of the body. Due to dysfunction of the dispersion of Lung-Qi, there are also cough and shortness of breath. Ma Huang enters the Lung meridian, disperses the Lung-Qi, enters the Bladder meridian, activates the

Defensive Qi, opens the pores, causes sweating and expels Wind and Cold so that the Exterior can be released. This herb is considered as the strongest one for causing sweating. It is the first-line choice where Wind-Cold is severe and the patient has severe chills and fever without sweating, such as in upper respiratory tract infection, cold infections, influenza, acute bronchitis, pneumonia and asthma.

Gui Zhi can also treat Wind-Cold syndrome. Here the therapeutic result is achieved by warming the Blood, promoting Blood circulation, opening up the meridians and activating the Yang-Qi to expel Wind and Cold. Compared with Ma Huang, Gui Zhi is not so warm and pungent, but sweet. It enters the Heart meridian primarily, and the Lung and Bladder meridians secondarily. The warm nature of this herb can reduce Cold in the Blood. Pungency and warmth may also activate the Blood circulation and open up the meridians. The sweetness moderates the warmth and pungency so that the medicinal action may be balanced. As it enters the Lung and Bladder meridians, it can activate the Yang-Qi to eliminate Wind and Cold in the Exterior layer. When the pathogenic Cold is not so severe, the pores are not closed so tightly, which manifests as slight sweating or a milder cold sensation and less pain in the back of the body, Gui Zhi can be used alone. It is especially useful for patients with Exterior syndromes against the background of a Yang-deficient constitution, Bi syndrome or Cold in the Blood, such as in elderly people, patients with chronic bronchitis, pulmonary emphysema, rheumatism or Raynaud's disease.

In clinical practice, Ma Huang and Gui Zhi are often used together to treat severe Wind-Cold syndrome, as they work on different aspects—for instance, the former enters the Qi level, the latter enters the Blood level; the former induces sweating and eliminates Wind-Cold by a short, quick and strong action, the latter promotes the Blood circulation, warms it, stops pain and activates the Yang-Qi in the Blood, thereby expelling Wind-Cold. When they are used together, the therapeutic effects are enhanced.

Although there are differences between Ma Huang and Gui Zhi, they both belong to quite warm and pungent herbs in the herbal group of expelling Wind-Cold. The dosage should be carefully managed. Age, constitution and the present state of health should also be considered. Generally speaking, after taking these herbs, if the patient does not sweat, the dose should be increased within the normal dosage range. If the patient becomes sweaty and the chills and fever are less severe, Ma Huang and Gui Zhi should not be used again. Some herbs with a gentler action can be substituted, such as Jing Jie (*Schizonepetae herba*) and Fang Feng (*Saposhnikoviae radix*). If, after a while, the chills and fever return, Ma Huang and Gui Zhi should be used again but in a smaller dosage as the Wind and Cold have already been partially expelled.

Moreover, as the tendency of action of these two herbs is upward and outward, in the following conditions they should not be used or used with caution: patients suffering from acute infection of the nose and throat where there is internal Heat or Heat due to Deficiency in the body, patients suffering from hypertension which indicates a tendency to Liver-Yang rising, or women suffering from menopausal syndrome with hot flushes and night sweats, and people with a Yang constitution or with heart disease, because these herbs can increase the contraction of the cardiac muscle and increase oxygen consumption, which makes the heart overwork.

4 What are the differences between the actions of Ma Huang (*Ephedrae herba*)*, Zhi Ma Huang (honey-roasted *Ephedrae herba*) and Ma Huang Gen (*Ephedrae radix*)?

Ma Huang is also called Sheng Ma Huang. 'Sheng' means 'raw'. Sheng Ma Huang is very pungent and warm. It is a very strong herb used to expel Wind and Cold to release Exterior Wind-Cold syndrome. As Sheng Ma Huang is pungent and hot, the dosage should be controlled and it should not be used over a long period of time. Overdose may cause heavy sweating, which injures the Yin, Body Fluids and Qi. It should be used with caution, especially in patients with a weak constitution and Deficiency syndrome. As its actions have an upward and outward tendency, Ma Huang should not be used or used with caution in cases of hypertension and heart disease.

Zhi Ma Huang is gentler in action compared with Sheng Ma Huang, because roasting with honey moderates the pungent taste. Zhi Ma Huang acquires the nature of honey, which is sweet and moistening, so its dispersing action is not as strong and quick as that of Sheng Ma Huang. It is often used to disperse the Lung-Qi and cause it to descend, to moisten the Lung and stop wheezing. In clinical practice, it is often used for treating asthma, bronchitis, pneumonia and acute nephritis.

Ma Huang Gen has completely different characteristics from both Sheng Ma Huang and Zhi Ma Huang. It is neutral, sweet and astringent, and enters the Lung meridian. It is excellent for stopping sweating. It can be used for treating spontaneous sweating and night sweating. It treats only the symptoms however, so it is often combined with other herbs that treat the cause of sweating. In addition, it should not be used in the syndrome of Phlegm accumulation or Exterior syndrome because it has an astringent property, which can retain Phlegm, close the pores and retain the pathogenic factors within the body.

5 What are the characteristic functions of Gui Zhi (*Cinnamomi cassiae ramulus*)?

'Twig of plants enters the limbs of human body': such similes and allegories were often used in ancient times in Chinese medicine to explain the complicated links between the human and the natural environment. Gui Zhi is an example of this. This herb is the twig of the plant and has a warm, pungent and sweet nature. Besides expelling Wind and Cold to treat Exterior syndrome, Gui Zhi is often used to treat Bi syndrome. In this case, it can relieve pain and cold sensations in the affected limbs or joints. The therapeutic effects are achieved by warming and strengthening the Heart-Yang, promoting the Blood circulation, spreading the Yang-Qi and unblocking the meridians, especially in the limbs. This is why it is often used in Bi syndrome caused by blockage of the circulation of Qi and Blood by Wind, Dampness or Cold; examples are rheumatic fever, rheumatoid arthritis, rheumatic heart disease, Raynaud's disease and the early and mid phases of vasculitis.

In chronic diseases, when internal Cold blocks the meridians, a small amount (about 10 m) of Gui Zhi alcohol drink is also a preferred formulation for daily use in the diet. Soaking 15 grams of Gui Zhi in a liter of alcohol (about 40% alcohol) made from cereals for 6 weeks yields Gui Zhi alcohol drink. Alcohol is pungent and warm, so is considered to

have the functions of invigorating the Blood and unblocking the meridians. The functions of Gui Zhi and alcohol therefore enhance each other. It is commonly used for chronic Bi syndrome.

As Gui Zhi is pungent and warm, it should be used with caution if there is any deficiency of Yin with Empty-Fire or Liver-Yang rising in the syndrome or in the treatment of Heat-type Bi syndrome.

6 Jing Jie (*Schizonepetae herba*) and Fang Feng (*Saposhnikoviae radix*) are often used for Exterior Wind-Cold syndrome. What are the differences between using Ma Huang (*Ephedrae herba*) and Gui Zhi (*Cinnamomi cassiae ramulus*)?

Jing Jie and Fang Feng are both pungent and warm. However, they are far gentler than Ma Huang and Gui Zhi. They can expel Wind and Cold and are commonly used for mild Exterior Wind-Cold syndrome. In regions with temperate climates, where Wind and Cold do not close the pores tightly, they are more often applied than Ma Huang and Gui Zhi for cold infections, influenza, certain stages of infectious childhood diseases and some skin diseases in which Exterior syndromes are involved. Meanwhile, they are also often used with pungent-cold herbs in syndromes where Wind-Heat is mixed with Wind-Cold. The patient may have symptoms such as chills, fever, thirst, sore throat and general pain. These two herbs are more often used in combination with cold herbs than Ma Huang and Gui Zhi.

Comparing Jing Jie with Fang Feng, Jing Jie is lighter and more dispersing. It is pungent but not strong, slightly warm but not dry. It is especially good at expelling Wind, no matter whether it is Wind-Cold or Wind-Heat. Moreover, it can expel Wind from the Blood so is often used in skin disorders when there is itching caused by Wind invasion, for instance in eczema, urticaria and food allergy. It is also used for infectious childhood diseases with Exterior syndrome and skin eruptions, such as measles, rubella, scarlet fever, chickenpox and so on.

Fang Feng is sweet, pungent and warm and enters the Bladder, Lung and Spleen meridians. As its sweet taste moderates the pungent taste, it is less strong in dispersing Wind on the surface of the body than Jing Jie. However, as it is warmer than Jing Jie and enters the Spleen meridian, it is especially good at expelling Dampness and Cold in the layers below the body surface, such as the subcutaneous region and muscles, which are controlled by the Spleen. When the patient feels pain and heaviness of the muscles, Fang Feng is more suitable than Jing Jie. This is also the reason that Fang Feng is more often used in Bi syndromes.

Although both herbs are gentle, they do have a pungent and warm nature, so both should be used with caution in patients without Wind invasion or in Yin deficiency with Empty-Heat.

7 What are the differences between the actions of Jing Jie (*Schizonepetae herba*), Jing Jie Sui (*Schizonepetae flos*), Chao Jin Jie (dry-fried *Schizonepetae herba*) and Jing Jie Tan (the charcoal of *Schizonepetae herba*)?

Generally speaking, Jing Jie Sui is more thin-pungent than Jing Jie as it is the bud, which is believed to be lighter in nature. It has a quicker and lighter action in expelling Wind. It is used at the very beginning of Wind-Cold syndrome or Wind-Heat syndrome.

Comparing raw with roasted Jing Jie, raw Jing Jie is more pungent. It is used for Exterior Wind-Cold syndrome when sweating is not present, which means that the pores are closed. It can open the pores, cause mild sweating and expel Wind and Cold. Roasted Jing Jie is less pungent because processing has reduced the taste. If the pores are open, sweating is present, or the patient has an aversion to wind instead of cold; this indicates that it is not necessary to open the pores, so roasted Jing Jie is then more suitable.

Jing Jie Tan is able to stop bleeding and it is used in bleeding conditions. When Jing Jie is roasted to charcoal, its pungent property is reduced, but an astringent property emerges. It can stabilize the

Blood and stop bleeding. Meanwhile, it can also expel Wind and calm the Blood, therefore stopping bleeding.

8 Why is Xiang Ru (*Moslae herba*) called Summer Ma Huang (*Ephedrae herba*)?

'*Xiang*' means 'aroma', 'fragrance'; '*Ru*' means 'gentle'. As the name explains, this herb is pungent and slightly warm with an aromatic smell. It enters the Spleen, Stomach and Lung meridians. Xiang Ru can, on the one hand, disperse Wind and Cold, induce sweating and release the Exterior; on the other hand, it transforms Dampness and harmonizes the Spleen and Stomach. The functions are similar to that of Ma Huang, but gentler. It is often used in summer when the weather is warm, the Wind-Cold is not so strong, the pores are not closed so tightly as in winter and the mild Wind-Cold attacks the body and causes an Exterior Wind-Cold syndrome. Meanwhile, Xiang Ru is used to treat abdominal pain, vomiting and diarrhea in summer, if overconsumption of cold drinks has injured the Stomach and Spleen, such as in acute gastritis.

Like Ma Huang, Xiang Ru can also direct the Lung-Qi to descend and relieve wheezing, transform Dampness and reduce edema, but its actions are too gentle, so it is rarely used alone.

Because Xiang Ru has similar actions to Ma Huang, and is more suitable for use in the summer, it is called 'Summer Ma Huang'.

9 Xi Xin (*Asari herba*)* is a commonly used herb for Exterior syndrome and Bi syndrome. What are its characteristics? What caution should be applied in clinical practice?

In Chinese, '*Xi*' means 'fine', 'thin'; '*Xin*' means 'pungent'. As described in the name, Xi Xin is a very pungent and hot herb with an aromatic smell. Its temperature and taste are as strong as Ma Huang

(*Ephedrae herba*)* and Gui Zhi (*Cinnamomi cassiae ramulus*). However, Ma Huang and Gui Zhi enter the Bladder meridian and are often used to induce sweating. Xi Xin does not enter the Bladder meridian, but rather the Kidney meridian, which is why it has no function in inducing sweating. It is very effective in eliminating Cold and Wind in very deep layers of the body, such as the bones and tendons. Because of its strong aromatic smell, pungent taste and hot nature, it can easily penetrate into the deep layers. Meanwhile, entering the Kidney meridian makes it easy to reach the bones and tendons. It has the characteristic of searching out and eliminating Wind, Cold and Dampness, even if they are in the 'corners' or 'chinks' of the deep layers of the body, so it is often described as a 'detector' or 'policeman' in the body.

Because of this characteristic, it is often used in clinical practice in Exterior Wind-Cold syndromes if there is Kidney-Yang deficiency—for instance in elderly people, patients suffering from chronic diseases with internal Cold and patients with Bi syndrome. In these people, Wind and Cold may invade the body more deeply than usual, or the development can be very acute, the patient feels severe pain in the whole body and the pulse is deep and tight instead of superficial and tight.

Because of the same characteristic, this herb is also often used to stop pain and treat Bi syndrome when Wind, Cold and Dampness remain in the deep layers of the body and the Kidney-Yang is weak. In this case, patients not only have pain and a cold sensation in the affected joints, but also feel pain in the bones. They have difficulty with walking or cannot stand for long, and feel very stiff and painful in the tendons, especially in the lower body, feel cold in the extremities and are also afraid of cold. In winter or humid weather all these symptoms worsen.

Xi Xin can also be used for various stubborn pains, such as migraine, trigeminal neuralgia and toothache. This is because this herb is hot, has a very strong aromatic smell and pungent taste. It possesses a penetrating power, removes obstructions and its speed is very high. It can treat pain which is caused by stagnation of Qi and Blood.

Because of the same characteristic, it is also often used for opening the orifices. It enters the Lung meridian, and is effective in opening the nose, removing nasal obstruction, stopping a runny nose, transforming Dampness and pus and improving the sense of smell. In clinical practice, it is often used for treating sinusitis, acute and chronic rhinitis and allergic rhinitis.

The side-effects of Xi Xin can be shown in clinical practice when it is used improperly. Because it is very hot and pungent, it easily injures the Yin, Blood and Body Fluids and weakens the Qi. It should not be used, or used with caution, in patients suffering from Bi syndrome or Exterior Wind-Cold syndrome complicated with Excessive-Heat or Empty-Heat, or weakness of Yin, Blood and Body Fluids.

The dosage of Xi Xin should also be controlled carefully within the range of 1–3 grams per day for crude herbs. If the concentrated herbal powder is used, this dosage should be reduced to 0.1–0.5 grams per day. Overdose may cause numbness in the throat and tongue, stifling in the chest and even death due to paralysis of the diaphragm. Modern research indicates that this herb should be used with particular caution in patients with renal problems as it has nephrotoxic effects. Moreover it is incompatible with Li Lu (*Veratri nigri radix et rhizoma*).

10 Sheng Jiang (*Zingiberis rhizoma recens*), Sheng Jiang Zhi (*Zingiberis rhizoma recens succus*), Wei Jiang (roasted *Zingiberis rhizoma recens*) and Sheng Jiang Pi (*Zingiberis rhizoma recens cortex*) are all products of the same herb. What are the differences between their actions?

Sheng Jiang is pungent and slightly warm, and enters the Lung, Spleen and Stomach meridians. It can disperse Cold and Wind, but its action is not strong. It is used only for mild Exterior Wind-Cold syndrome. However, as it enters the Spleen and Stomach meridians, it has some other excellent functions. It can warm the Middle Jiao, soothe the Stomach-Qi and alleviate nausea and vomiting. Because it is so effective in stopping vomiting, it is considered as the first-line choice for treating nausea. This herb is also a good choice if a patient suffers from a Wind-Cold syndrome, has fever, chills, blocked nose and headache, and in the meantime the Stomach-Qi fails to descend, so nausea and vomiting are present—such as in abdominal influenza or acute gastritis.

As Sheng Jiang enters the Lung and Stomach meridians, and is warm and pungent, it can dissolve Phlegm in the Lung and stop a cough. It can be used in patients with chronic bronchitis or asthma and in the meantime who are being attacked by Wind-Cold once more. Sheng Jiang is also suitable for conditions of water accumulation in the Stomach when overconsumption of cold drinks has injured the Stomach and Spleen. The manifestations include fullness in the upper abdomen, poor appetite, nausea and vomiting, such as in acute gastritis.

Sheng Jiang can also reduce the toxicity of Ban Xia (*Pinelliae rhizoma*) so it is often used to process Ban Xia. After processing, Ban Xia is then called Jiang Ban Xia or Zhi Ban Xia (processed *Pinelliae rhizoma*).

In Chinese kitchens, Sheng Jiang is often used not only for the taste of the dishes, but also for promoting digestion. It soothes the Stomach-Qi, improves the appetite, and reduces or prevents the toxicity of seafood if it is not fresh. The warm nature of Sheng Jiang can also reduce the cold nature of seafood, so the latter is more easily digested and healthy.

If Sheng Jiang is smashed and the juice squeezed out, the result is Sheng Jiang Zhi. This is pungent and slightly warm. Its function is more or less the same as Sheng Jiang, but stronger and quicker. It is therefore used in acute conditions, such as severe nausea, vomiting and coma due to Phlegm covering the orifices. In this situation, the normal dose is 3–10 drops of Sheng Jiang Zhi in warm water.

If Sheng Jiang is cleaned with water, then covered with a moistened soft paper and placed near the fireplace, but not above the fire, after a while the paper turns brown and the Sheng Jiang is roasted; it is then called Wei Jiang. It is warm and pungent, but after this processing its pungent taste and the dispersing function are weaker than those of Sheng Jiang and Sheng Jiang Zhi. Meanwhile, the temperature has been increased and the harmonizing function is obtained. It is good at warming the Spleen and Stomach and is used for nausea, vomiting, abdominal pain and diarrhea caused by Cold invasion of the Middle Jiao.

Sheng Jiang Pi is the peel of Sheng Jiang. It is the only product of Jiang that is cold in temperature. It is also pungent and enters the Spleen meridian. It can regulate water metabolism, promote urination and leach out Dampness. As the herb is quite gentle, it is used especially for edema in pregnant women.

For severe edema, it must be used with other herbs that have stronger actions.

11 Qiang Huo (*Notopterygii rhizoma*), Bai Zhi (*Angelicae dahuricae radix*), Chuan Xiong (*Chuanxiong rhizoma*) and Gao Ben (*Ligustici sinensis radix*) are often used for treating headache. What are the differences between their actions?

Headache is a symptom as well as a syndrome. Besides the treatment of the causes according to the differentiation of syndromes, some specific herbs that are very effective for alleviating headache as a symptom are often used in treatment.

All of these four herbs can alleviate headache. They are warm, pungent and aromatic. Warmth and pungency can activate Qi movement, pungency and aroma can penetrate the accumulation of Dampness, Qi and Blood, therefore dispersing the accumulation. Warmth and pungency can also dry Dampness and unblock the meridians, so relieving pain. They are very effective in the treatment of headache caused by invasion of exogenous pathogenic factors and disturbance of the Qi movement and Blood circulation. They can also be used for headache due to stagnation of Qi and Blood in the dysfunction of internal organs.

The four herbs also have their individual characteristics in their action because they enter different meridians. Qiang Huo enters the Bladder meridian and treats pain in the occiput especially; Bai Zhi enters the Stomach meridian and is especially effective for relieving pain in the forehead; Chuan Xiong enters the San Jiao and Gall Bladder meridians and treats headache on the sides of the head; Gao Ben enters the Bladder meridian, so can reach the top of the head and alleviate the pain there.

As many meridians pass through the head, headache is often caused by blockage of one or more meridians, such as in migraine, headache due to stress, spondylosis and sinusitis. These herbs are often used together according to the location of the pain. Since they focus on the symptoms rather than the syndrome, they should be used as only one part of the complete treatment of the syndrome.

12 Ge Gen (*Puerariae radix*), Sheng Ma (*Cimicifugae rhizoma*) and Chai Hu (*Bupleuri radix*) are all commonly used herbs for dispersing and lifting the Yang-Qi. What are the differences between them?

Ge Gen, Sheng Ma and Chai Hu all have the functions of releasing the Exterior, and dispersing and lifting the Yang-Qi. However, there are some differences between their actions because they enter different meridians and work in different regions of the body.

Ge Gen enters the Spleen and Stomach meridians. It is pungent, but sweet and neutral. Pungency can disperse the Yang-Qi, but the sweet and neutral properties make the dispersing action gentler. Generally speaking, Ge Gen is gentle and light in its action. It can gently disperse and lift the pure Yang and Qi, especially from the Spleen and Stomach. It is used for Exterior syndromes when the exogenous pathogenic factors have passed through the superficial layer of the body and entered the subcutaneous region and the muscles, which are considered to be governed by the Spleen and Stomach. The corresponding manifestations are rashes and fever. Ge Gen can gently disperse the Qi from this region and expel the exogenous pathogenic factors to vent rashes. It is used to hasten recovery from measles when the expression of the rash is incomplete.

Ge Gen can treat diarrhea due to weakness of the Spleen-Qi and sinking of the Yang. In this situation, dry-fried Ge Gen is the preferred choice because a warm property has been acquired from the processing, so it is more effective for lifting the Yang and Qi in the Middle Jiao. It can treat diarrhea due to Damp-Heat in the intestines or due to sunken Spleen-Yang when it is used with other herbs to treat the cause of the disorder.

As Ge Gen enters the Stomach meridian of foot Bright Yang (*Yang Ming*) and lifts the pure Yang-Qi, it can treat Wasting and Thirsty syndrome, which is termed diabetes in Western medicine. This disease is caused by Dryness in the Stomach, while the Spleen-Qi is too weak to spread the Body Fluids. The patient may suffer from excessive thirst, and a dry mouth and throat. Ge Gen is able to lift the Yang-Qi from the Middle Jiao to assist the spreading of the Body Fluids and alleviate Dryness.

Sheng Ma enters the Spleen, Stomach, Large Intestine and Lung meridians. It is sweet, pungent and slightly cold. Compared with Ge Gen, it has the particular effect of clearing Heat and dispersing it from these meridians. It disperses Wind-Heat and treats headache in the forehead where the Bright Yang meridian passes through; it also clears and disperses Heat in the Stomach, Large Intestine and Spleen, and treats ulcers in the cheeks, tongue and gums. Compared with Ge Gen, it has a stronger action of lifting the Yang-Qi in cases of prolapse of the stomach, uterus and rectum, and diarrhea. As Sheng Ma is slightly cold in nature, it should be used together with some warm herbs to tonify the Spleen if the Spleen-Qi is weak.

Chai Hu enters the Liver and Gall Bladder meridians. It is pungent, neutral and aromatic. It possesses a dispersing and ascending capability. Chai Hu is particularly effective in spreading the Qi in the Lesser Yang (Shao Yang) meridians. It can disperse Wind-Heat if the exogenous pathogenic factors stay at the Lesser Yang level. The symptoms of them are alternating chills and fever, a dry throat and bitter taste in the mouth, and fullness in the chest and hypochondriac region. As Chai Hu enters the Liver and Gall Bladder meridians, it can spread the Liver-Qi effectively. It is the most commonly used herb to treat stress, irritability, resentment, depression and other mental and emotional disorders due to stagnation of the Liver-Qi.

Chai Hu has similar functions to Sheng Ma, like lifting sunken Yang-Qi to treat prolapse of internal organs and tissues. The two are often used together to enhance the effect of each other.

These three herbs should be used with caution in clinical practice. As they all have dispersing and ascending abilities, the dosages should be well controlled. According to both theory and experience, *small amounts of herbs may lead to a dispersing action whereas large amounts can actually lead to a descending and purging action*, so the dosages of the three herbs should be less in their usual dosage than other herbs. If the concentrated herbal powder is prescribed, 0.3–0.5 grams is the daily dosage. In addition, these herbs should be used with caution in patients suffering from uprising of Yang or flaring up of Fire.

13 Bai Zhi (*Angelicae dahuricae radix*), Xin Yi (*Magnoliae flos*) and Cang Er Zi (*Xanthii fructus*) are often used together to treat rhinitis and sinusitis. What are the differences between them?

All of these three herbs enter the Lung meridian. They are warm and pungent, expel Wind-Cold, open the obstruction of the nose and stop pain; they are often prescribed together.

Bai Zhi enters not only the Lung meridian, but also the Stomach meridian. It is pungent with a rich aromatic smell, and so possesses a strongly ascending property. It is often used to treat disorders in the area of the head through which the Bright Yang meridians pass. This is why this herb is often used for rhinitis and sinusitis. Moreover, it possesses a strong aromatic smell, which is believed to be able to penetrate turbidity, transform Phlegm and pus, dry Dampness and reduce swelling. It is appropriate for sinusitis, especially if there is a green nasal discharge that has a foul smell and the patient feels a sensation of fullness in the sinuses. Meanwhile, some herbs which are bitter and cold in nature should also be used simultaneously to clear Heat and dry Dampness.

Xin Yi is pungent, warm and aromatic, but more moderate in action and lighter in nature than Bai Zhi. It is particularly effective for opening the nose, and gently dispersing and lifting the pure Qi in the facial area. It is often used in cases of nasal obstruction, and loss of, or reduced, sense of smell, such as in atrophic rhinitis, pachyntic rhinitis and allergic rhinitis. Xin Yi is able to lift the pure Yang to the top of the head, so it can stop pain and can be used for ethmoidal sinusitis, frontal sinusitis and sphenoiditis.

Cang Er Zi is bitter and warm and enters the Lung meridian. It is effective for drying Dampness. Its warm and bitter nature gives it a spreading ability, so it can spread the Qi and expel Wind. It has a similar function to that of Bai Zhi in transforming Dampness and treating profuse nasal discharge. However, its aromatic smell is less strong than that of Bai Zhi, so it has a lesser ability to transform turbidity and pus. However, it is used particularly when there are large amounts of clear nasal discharge and itchiness of the nasal passage, which is considered as Wind invasion.

Cang Er Zi also has a wider application range than Bai Zhi and Xin Yi. It can treat headache due to Wind-Dampness. It has a drying nature but is not harsh, so it is also used in some skin diseases where the skin lesions are characterized by itching and weeping.

As in rhinitis or sinusitis, these symptoms often exist simultaneously with nasal obstruction, a reduced sense of smell, a feeling of fullness in the nose or sinuses, an itchy nasal passage, profuse discharge and headache, so the three herbs are often used together.

14 Bo He (*Menthae herba*), Chan Tui (*Cicadae periostracum*), Niu Bang Zi (*Arctii fructus*), Jiang Can (*Bombyx batrycatus*) and Jing Jie (*Schizonepetae herba*) are able to expel Wind and alleviate itching, and are commonly used for different skin diseases. What are the differences between them?

Itching, in skin disorders, is considered in TCM to be an invasion of Wind in the Exterior or the Blood level. The Lung is believed to be the directly corresponding organ in skin disorders as it governs the superficial layer of the body. Any factor which directly or indirectly disturbs the function of the Lung may induce or aggravate skin disorders.

All of these five herbs enter the Lung meridian. Only Jing Jie is pungent and slightly warm; the rest are pungent and cold. Apart from the action of releasing the Exterior, they can expel Wind and alleviate itching, so are often used in various itchy skin disorders, such as eczema, urticaria and different types of dermatitis and pruritus. Sometimes the itching is so pronounced that these herbs have to be used together. However, these herbs all have their own characteristics and could be used in different types of itching.

Bo He is pungent and cold and enters the Lung and Liver meridians. It not only treats itchy rashes due to Wind-Heat in the Exterior, but also clears Heat and benefits the throat. It is particularly appropriate for use in the acute phase of a chronic skin disorder, when Wind-Heat invades the body, and fever, chills, itching and a dry throat are present. It can also be used for infectious diseases in children, which are often accompanied by skin manifestations due to Heat in the Lung and Liver meridians (e.g. rubella, measles, chickenpox and scarlet fever).

Chan Tui is the sloughed skin of the cicada. It is very light in weight, salty and slightly cold. Its light, ascending property gives it a gentle dispersing action, and it can expel Wind-Heat in the Lung. Saltiness enters the Blood, and saltiness and Cold may clear Heat in the Blood and extinguish Wind, sweetness and Cold can generate the Body Fluids, moisten Dryness and calm Wind, while the slough (skin), enters the skin of humans according to the concept of Chinese herbal medicine. Therefore, Chan Tui can alleviate itching caused by external Wind and treat itchy skin diseases such as urticaria, eczema, pruritus and neurodermatitis.

Chan Tui also enters the Liver meridian. As saltiness enters the Blood and Cold can clear Heat, saltiness and Cold may cool the Blood and clear Heat in the Heart and Liver, calm the Mind and control spasm. It is effective for treating irritability, restless sleep, and even convulsions due to Heat in the Liver meridian in children. If a child suffers from skin disease and there is Heat in the Liver, Chan Tui is a good choice. It is also an appropriate choice in adults when skin disorders worsen under stress and in elderly people when there is deficiency of Body Fluids and Dryness of the Blood, which generate Wind and cause itching over all the body, especially during sleep.

Niu Bang Zi is pungent, bitter and cold, and enters the Spleen and Stomach meridians. Pungency can disperse Wind; bitterness and Cold can drain Heat. It is rich in plant oils so can moisten the intestines and promote bowel movement. It is the coldest of these herbs and is able to remove Heat-toxin. For skin problems, this herb is more appropriate for red skin lesions which are not only itchy, but also slightly painful with a burning sensation, and where the skin problem worsens when there is also constipation, which suggests that Heat from the Bright Yang meridians may be affecting the Lung.

Jiang Can is pungent, salty and neutral. It enters the Lung and Liver meridians. Pungency can disperse Wind so it is good at relieving itching in skin conditions. Jiang Can is able to dissolve Phlegm and also calms the Mind. It is preferred for treating patients who have fever, itchy skin rashes, irritability and restless sleep—for instance in some infectious childhood diseases.

Jing Jie is an excellent herb in TCM for treating disorders caused by Wind. It is a gentle herb, warm but without a drying property and is particularly effective for expelling Wind. Jing Jie is pungent, slightly warm and enters the Lung and Liver meridians. It can disperse Wind-Heat from the Blood level to stop itching. It can be chosen for different kinds of skin disease due to Wind-Heat in the Lung or Heat in the Blood. It is often used together with Jin Yin Hua (*Lonicerae flos*) and Lian Qiao (*Forsythiae fructus*) for red skin lesions. Its powder can be applied topically to stop itching.

15 Bo He (*Menthae herba*), Ju Hua (*Chrysanthemi indici flos*), Sang Ye (*Mori folium*) and Chai Hu (*Bupleuri radix*) have similar functions of expelling and dispersing Wind-Heat in the Upper Jiao. What are the differences between them?

All of these four herbs possess light, ascending and dispersing properties. They are used to expel Wind, disperse Heat and treat Exterior Wind-Heat syndrome.

Of these herbs, Bo He is the coldest. It primarily enters the Lung meridian and secondarily enters the Liver meridian. Pungency may disperse Heat; coolness may reduce Heat; lightness in weight and nature can disperse Heat in the Upper Jiao and the aromatic smell can open the orifices. Thus Bo He is excellent for Exterior Wind-Heat syndrome when the head is affected—for instance in patients suffering from headache, sore and red eyes and a sore throat. These complaints are often seen in cold infections, bronchitis, sinusitis, influenza and pruritic rash in infectious childhood diseases. Apart from this, because Bo He enters the Liver meridian it is effective for spreading the Liver-Qi and clearing Heat and so is used for Liver-Qi stagnation with flaring up of Liver-Heat. The manifestations of this condition include headache, dizziness, poor concentration, a bitter taste in the mouth and a feeling of fullness in the chest and hypochondrium. These symptoms can be seen in hypertension, hepatitis, premenstrual syndrome, depression and other mental disorders.

Ju Hua is sweet, bitter and slightly cold, and enters the Lung, Liver, Kidney and Gall Bladder meridians. Sweetness and Cold can generate Yin; bitterness and Cold can reduce Heat. As it particularly enters the Liver meridian, can calm the Liver and benefit the eyes, it is used for treating acute inflammation of the eyes. It can also be used for dizziness, blurred vision, dryness of the eyes due to deficiency of Liver-Yin and Kidney-Yin, stagnation of Liver-Qi and uprising of Liver-Yang, and in conditions such as eye strain, hypertension, glaucoma and retinal bleeding.

Sang Ye is bitter, sweet and cold and it enters the Lung meridian. It is gentle and light, and possesses both dispersing and ascending properties. It can disperse Wind and Heat as it is collected in late autumn (the season of the Lung according to the Five Elements theory) and after frost, so it receives its cool property from nature. Sweetness and coolness may generate Body Fluids and clear Heat which lasts from summer. It is used for cough without production, and dryness of the throat that is caused by Dry-Heat injuring the Lung-Yin. This herb is also good for treating those symptoms that are present after febrile disease when the Heat has disappeared but the Yin has been consumed—for instance after pneumonia or acute bronchitis.

Because Sang Ye also enters the Liver meridian, it can be used for treating cough caused by Liver-Fire attacking the Lung. It is good at clearing Lung-Fire and pacifying the Liver. It is particularly suitable for treating paroxysmal cough without production, thirst, and a dry mouth and throat, and concomitant depression, hypochondriac distension and irritability, such as seen in chronic bronchitis, pulmonary tuberculosis and diabetes.

Chai Hu is pungent, bitter and neutral; it enters the Liver and Gall Bladder meridians. Pungency and lightness lead to ascending and spreading actions, so it is particularly effective for spreading the Liver-Qi and lifting the clear Qi at the Lesser Yang level. Bitterness may lead the Qi or Heat downwards, which is why it is very often used for venting Wind-Heat in the Upper Jiao and at the Lesser Yang level, although it is not cold. It can treat conditions with alternating chills and fever, a dry throat, a bitter taste in the mouth, dizziness and irritability. Since the

Liver is an important organ in the Qi movement of the whole body, stagnation of the Liver-Qi may lead to disturbance of Qi in the whole body and bring about emotional and physical disorders such as tightness in the chest and hypochondria, irritability, depression, irregular menstruation, heartburn, nausea, vomiting and reduced appetite. Chai Hu is the most important and commonly used herb for spreading the Liver-Qi. In clinical practice, it is used for treating hepatitis, cholecystitis, cholelithiasis, gastritis, gastric ulcer, gastroneurosis, asthma, depression, neurosis, premenstrual syndrome and other mental disorders.

16 How many kinds of Ju Hua (*Chrysanthemi indici flos*) are used for medical purposes and how does one choose the correct one in practice?

There are several kinds of Ju Hua and Ju Hua products that have various properties according to the growing habitat, the color and the processing procedure. Huang Ju Hua, the yellow flower, is sometimes called Hang Ju Hua, as it comes from Hang Zhou. Bai Ju Hua, the white flower, is also called Gan Ju Hua, which means sweet Ju Hua. It is also sometimes called Chu Ju Hua because the white Ju Hua growing in Chu county is considered to have the best quality. There is also. Ye Ju Hua, the wild Ju Hua, is a third kind of Ju Hua also used in clinical practice. Generally speaking, Ju Hua is sweet, bitter and slightly cold. It has the functions of clearing Heat in the Upper Jiao, pacifying the Liver and benefiting the eyes.

Huang Ju Hua especially enters the Lung meridian. It is more effective for expelling Wind-Heat in the Upper Jiao and is often used in cold infections, feverish sensations in the head and headache. It can also be used for acute infection of the eyes, such as acute conjunctivitis, which in TCM is considered to be Wind-Heat disturbing the Upper Jiao. In this condition, as well as oral use, the steam from Ju Hua decoction can be used for painful and itchy eyes. The method is simple: pour the hot decoction into a glass, and bring the affected eye close to the glass for 2–3 minutes. Care should be taken not to burn the eye. Moreover, the cool decoction can be used externally to wash the affected eye.

Bai Ju Hua is sweeter and cooler, and can slightly generate Yin and clear Heat. Because it enters the Liver meridian, it is more effective in cooling and pacifying the Liver and benefiting the eyes. It is used for dizziness, blurred vision, dry eyes and a tired feeling in the eyes, which are caused by Yin deficiency or Yin deficiency with uprising of the Liver-Yang. For patients with a Yin-deficient condition as well as eye problems as mentioned above, Bai Ju Hua is a good choice. Ju Hua tea is also recommended for daily use in this condition.

Ye Ju Hua is bitter and neutral. It can reduce Heat and remove Heat-toxin. It is used for all types of boils, furuncles and carbuncles with localized erythema, swelling, heat and pain. This herb can also be used topically: the smashed fresh Ju Hua can be applied to the affected region as a compress to reduce swelling and pain—for instance in mumps.

17 Besides treating cold infections or influenza, are there other uses for the herbs in the category of releasing the Exterior?

Cold infections are often not treated and most people recover in 1 or 2 weeks without medical intervention. It may take longer to recover from influenza. Herbs that release the Exterior are often used in cold or influenza infections as they can alleviate the symptoms and shorten the duration of morbidity. This is especially useful and important for elderly people, children, patients with chronic diseases and people with a weak constitution.

Herbs in the category of releasing the Exterior can be used, in clinical practice, in many other conditions if the disorders link with the superficial layer of the body, or if the disorders have the same pathological changes in the body as those of the Exterior syndromes. Examples include the following.

Alleviation of pain

As pungency and warmth have dispersing and moving properties, most of these herbs that are warm and pungent can disperse Wind, Cold and Dampness. They are often used for Bi syndrome due to invasion of exogenous pathogenic Wind, Dampness and Cold. The commonly used herbs are Gui Zhi (*Cinnamomi cassiae ramulus*), Qiang Huo (*Not-*

opterygii rhizoma), Qin Jiao (*Gentianae macrophyllae radix*), Xi Xin (*Asari herba*)* and Fang Feng (*Saposhnikoviae radix*). Some herbs are very effective for treating certain kinds of pain. For example, Xi Xin is very good for treating toothache; Bai Zhi (*Angelicae dahuricae radix*) is effective for treating headache due to sinusitis; Qiang Huo can relax the muscles in the neck and treat pain in the occiput, neck and upper back; Zi Su Ye (*Perillae folium*) can alleviate abdominal pain in abdominal influenza; Gui Zhi can warm the Blood, promote Blood circulation and relieve general pain.

Dispersal of the Lung-Qi and treatment of asthma

Most of the herbs that release the Exterior enter the Lung meridian. Because the Lung governs the superficial level of the body, dispersal of the Lung-Qi may assist in expelling Exterior pathogenic factors. In addition, these herbs are also often used to treat asthma, which is caused by dysfunction of dispersing and descending of the Lung-Qi. The commonly used herbs are Ma Huang (*Ephedrae herba*)*, Xi Xin (*Asari herba*)* and Sheng Jiang (*Zingiberis rhizoma recens*).

Regulation of water metabolism and treatment of edema

As most of the herbs that release the Exterior enter the Lung and Bladder meridians, which are important in water metabolism, they can also disperse the Lung-Qi, regulate the water passages and treat edema due to dysfunction of the Lung. For instance, Ma Huang (*Ephedrae herba*)* and Fang Feng (*Saposhnikoviae radix*) can be used in Wind-Water syndrome. In this syndrome, the patient suddenly has edema on the face as a result of Wind disturbing the Lung and blocking the upper part of the water passage. This can be seen in acute nephritis, premenstrual syndrome and menopausal syndrome.

Expelling of Wind, clearing of Heat and treatment of skin diseases

Exterior syndromes are located on the surface of the body, where skin diseases are also located. The pungent and cold herbs can disperse Wind to relieve itching; these include Chan Tui (*Cicadae periostracum*), Jing Jie (*Schizonepetae herba*), Bo He (*Menthae herba*), Niu Bang Zi (*Arctii fructus*) and Fang Feng

(*Saposhnikoviae radix*). Some cold herbs such as Ju Hua (*Chrysanthemi indici flos*), Niu Bang Zi (*Arctii fructus*) and Bo He (*Menthae herba*) may reduce Heat and calm reddish skin lesions. Herbs entering the Lung meridian may regulate the function of the Lung to regulate the condition of the skin.

Treatment of infection or allergic reactions of the ears, nose, throat and eyes

The pungent and cold herbs that expel Wind-Heat are light in weight and nature. They enter the Upper Jiao and can disperse Wind-Heat in the head, so can be used for acute or chronic infections and allergic rhinitis as well as some types of food allergies, which in TCM are considered to be Wind-Heat disturbance in the Upper Jiao. Herbs that can be used include Bo He, Ju Hua, Niu Bang Zi, Xin Yi (*Magnoliae flos*), Fang Feng and Jing Jie.

Treatment of initial stages of infectious childhood diseases

Many infectious childhood diseases, especially those with skin rashes such as chickenpox, scarlet fever and rubella, belong to the category of Wind-Heat attacking the Lung. The treatment in the initial stage is focused on expelling Wind, clearing Heat and regulating the Lung-Qi. Herbs such as Bo He, Ju Hua, Chan Tui and Niu Bang Zi are often used.

Treatment of acute infections, infectious diseases or inflammation

For some acute infections, such as pneumonia or acute bronchitis, if caused by a virus then treatment with antibiotics is ineffective because the fever is still there and the infection continues. In such conditions, herbs that expel Wind-Heat combined with other herbs can bring a better result. In TCM there is a saying: no matter how high the fever is, *if there is one percent chill, there is one percent Exterior syndrome*. Antibiotics are considered in TCM to be bitter and cold substances; therefore their action tendency is downward and they can only clear the Heat. This action may bring about the side-effects of constrained Fire, so the result of treatment is not completely satisfactory. Herbs used in this condition not only clear Heat but also disperse it and at the same time expel other exogenous pathogenic factors. They match the pathogenic changes and the nature of Heat so are better in reducing fever and controlling the infections.

Comparisons of strength and temperature in herbs that release the Exterior

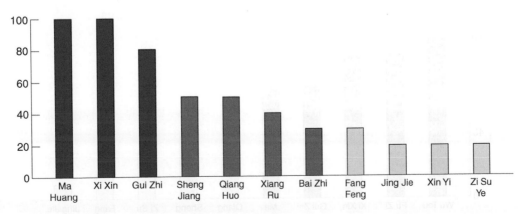

Fig. 2.1 • Comparison of the temperature of the warm herbs.
Ma Huang (*Ephedrae herba*)*, Xi Xin (*Asari herba*)*, Gui Zhi (*Cinnamomi cassiae ramulus*), Sheng Jiang (*Zingiberis rhizoma recens*), Qiang Huo (*Notopterygii rhizoma*), Xiang Ru (*Moslae herba*), Bai Zhi (*Angelicae dahuricae radix*), Fang Feng (*Saposhnikoviae radix*), Jing Jie (*Schizonepetae herba*), Xin Yi (*Magnoliae flos*), Zi Su Ye (*Perillae folium*).

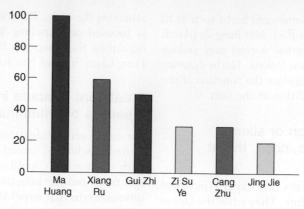

Fig. 2.2 • **Comparison of the herbs that induce sweating.**
Ma Huang (*Ephedrae herba*)*, Xiang Ru (*Moslae herba*), Gui Zhi (*Cinnamomi cassiae ramulus*), Zi Su Ye (*Perillae folium*),
Cang Zhu (*Atractylodis rhizoma*), Jing Jie (*Schizonepetae herba*).

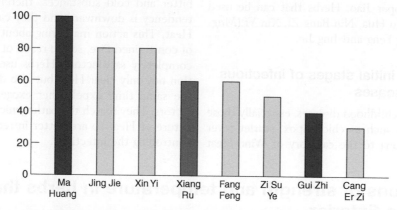

Fig. 2.3 • **Comparison of the light and dispersing features of the warm herbs.**
Ma Huang (*Ephedrae herba*)*, Jing Jie (*Schizonepetae herba*), Xin Yi (*Magnoliae flos*), Xiang Ru (*Moslae herba*), Fang Feng
(*Saposhnikoviae radix*), Zi Su Ye (*Perillae folium*), Gui Zhi (*Cinnamomi cassiae ramulus*), Cang Er Zi (*Xanthii fructus*).

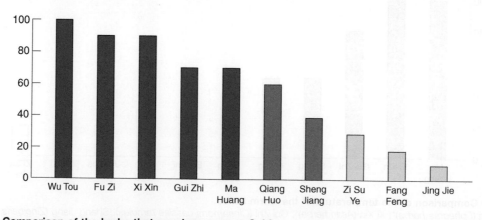

Fig. 2.4 • **Comparison of the herbs that expel exogenous Cold.**
Wu Tou (*Aconiti radix*)*, Fu Zi (*Aconiti radix lateralis preparata*)*, Xi Xin (*Asari herba*)*, Gui Zhi (*Cinnamomi cassiae ramulus*),
Ma Huang (*Ephedrae herba*)*, Qiang Huo (*Notopterygii rhizoma*), Sheng Jiang (*Zingiberis rhizoma recens*), Zi Su Ye (*Perillae folium*), Fang Feng (*Saposhnikoviae radix*), Jing Jie (*Schizonepetae herba*).

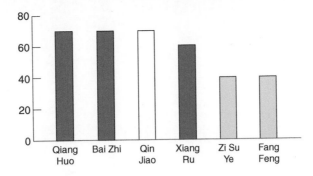

Fig. 2.5 • Comparison of the herbs that expel exogenous Dampness.
Qiang Huo (*Notopterygii rhizoma*), Bai Zhi (*Angelicae dahuricae radix*), Qin Jiao (*Gentianae macrophyllae radix*), Xiang Ru (*Moslae herba*), Zi Su Ye (*Perillae folium*), Fang Feng (*Saposhnikoviae radix*).

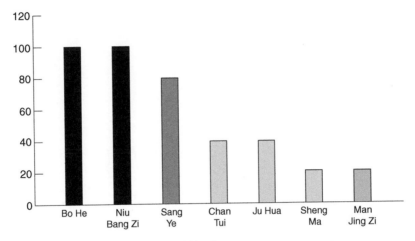

Fig. 2.6 • Comparison of the temperature of the cold herbs.
Bo He (*Menthae herba*), Niu Bang Zi (*Arctii fructus*), Sang Ye (*Mori folium*), Chan Tui (*Cicadae periostracum*), Ju Hua (*Chrysanthemi indici flos*), Sheng Ma (*Cimicifugae rhizoma*), Man Jing Zi (*Viticis fructus*).

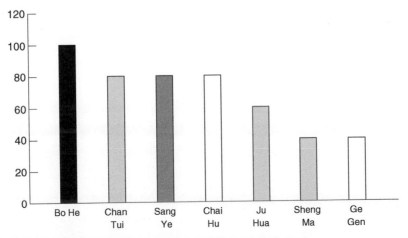

Fig. 2.7 • Comparison of the light and dispersing features of the cold herbs.
Bo He (*Menthae herba*), Chan Tui (*Cicadae periostracum*), Sang Ye (*Mori folium*), Chai Hu (*Bupleuri radix*), Ju Hua (*Chrysanthemi indici flos*), Sheng Ma (*Cimicifugae rhizoma*), Ge Gen (*Puerariae radix*).

Chapter **Three**

3

Herbs that clear Heat

清热药

1 What are the characteristics of herbs that clear internal Heat? What precautions should be observed when they are used?

According to the characteristics of internal Heat and the principle of treatment that *Heat syndrome should be treated by Cold*, all the herbs that clear Heat are cold in temperature. Because of their other properties, the individual herbs also have specific functions. The characteristics are as follows.

Pungent and cold

Pungency has a dispersing action; Cold may clear Heat. The former moves upwards and outwards, the latter moves inwards and downwards. In herbs that clear Heat, their cold property is stronger than their pungent property, therefore the main direction of the herb is downward. Herbs with both pungent and cold properties can more easily clear Heat than herbs with only a cold property. Because pathogenic Heat has a tendency to ascend and the cold herb has a tendency to descend, there is a severe conflict between the Cold and Heat. Cold herbs are able to suppress pathogenic Heat in very high dosage, so the Heat has to move downwards. But constrained Heat does not agree with Cold herbs and it hides itself in the body. As soon as the patient stops taking the cold herbs, the Heat spreads again. In clinical practice, some chronic infections, such as persistent sinusitis, bronchitis, gastroenteritis, dysentery, hepatitis and urinary tract infection, are the result of using high dosages of cold herbs or antibiotics.

Pungent-cold herbs are able to clear Heat completely without the possibility of producing constrained Heat or hidden Fire and are more suitable for this pathological situation. As pungency can disperse and lift Fire, it can divide the strength of Heat and reduce the conflict between the cold herbs and the Heat pathogenic factor. Thus pungency can assist the cold property of herbs to reduce Fire when the Fire shows itself clearly. These are especially effective for treating intensive Heat, constrained Heat and Fire blazing upwards. They are also used when there is Blood stagnation caused by Heat. Examples include Shi Gao (*Gypsum*), Xia Ku Cao (*Prunellae spica*) and Mu Dan Pi (*Moutan cortex*).

Sweet and cold

Sweetness possesses tonifying and harmonizing abilities. Cold can clear Heat so that it may protect the Body Fluids and Yin. Sweet and cold herbs are effective for reducing Heat and protecting the Body Fluids as well as increasing them when they have been injured by Heat, and for relieving thirst. They are used when Heat is in the Qi and Nutritive levels in acute febrile diseases. The herbs Shi Gao (*Gypsum*), Lu Gen (*Phragmitis rhizoma*), Sheng Di Huang (*Rehmanniae radix*) and Tian Hua Fen (*Trichosanthis radix*) possess these properties.

Salty and cold

Saltiness possesses purging and softening actions. It enters the Kidney and the Blood. The salty-cold herbs may reduce Heat and descend Fire, protect the Blood and Yin, and increase the Body Fluids and Yin which have been consumed by Heat. Their effect of directing Heat downwards is stronger than that of pungent-cold herbs or sweet-cold herbs. They mainly treat the syndrome of Heat in the Nutritive and Blood levels in acute febrile diseases. Herbs such as Qing Dai (*Indigo naturalis*) and Xuan Shen (*Scrophulariae radix*) are the commonly used ones.

Bitter and cold

Bitter substances have a draining ability and a dry nature. Bitter-cold herbs are able to direct Heat or Damp-Heat downwards, reduce Fire and relieve Fire-toxin. Bitter-cold substances treat syndromes of Excess-Heat in the internal organs and in the Qi level, and are used for acute infectious diseases, sores, boils, carbuncles and skin disorders. Examples include Huang Lian (*Coptidis rhizoma*), Huang Qin (*Scutellariae radix*), Huang Bai (*Phellodendri cortex*), Zhi Zi (*Gardeniae fructus*) and Long Dan Cao (*Gentianae radix*).

Generally speaking, to treat Excessive-Heat, herbs with pungent-cold, bitter-cold and sweet-cold properties should be used, and especially those herbs that enter the Lung and Stomach, Liver and Heart meridians. If the pathogenic Heat is not very strong but the Body Fluids have been injured, then sweet-cold and salty-cold herbs that enter the Liver and Kidney meridians are often chosen.

What precautions should be observed in the use of these herbs?

Most of the herbs that clear Heat are bitter and cold. They can quickly and strongly clear Heat and reduce Fire in the related organs and places. However, these herbs cannot be used for a long period of time with high dosage, otherwise they may cause a *hidden Heat syndrome*, the common side-effect of bitter-cold herbs. Because pathogenic Heat

has a tendency of ascending and the cold herb has a tendency of descending, a severe conflict between the nature of Cold and Heat develops. Cold herbs are able to suppress pathogenic Heat when their dosages are very high, and the Heat thus has to move downwards; however, as Heat does not agree with the cold nature of the herbs, it withdraws and becomes constrained and hides itself in the body. As soon as the patient stops using the cold herbs, the constrained Heat is free from suppression and it spreads again. In clinical practice, some chronic infections, such as sinusitis, bronchitis, gastroenteritis and urinary tract infection, are the result of using high dosage of cold herbs or antibiotics. Therefore, a small amount of aromatic or pungent herbs that follow the nature of Fire and disperse constrained Fire should be used with the bitter and cold herbs in order to clear the Heat completely.

Generally speaking, cold herbs, and especially bitter-cold herbs, can easily injure the Yang and produce Dampness, so they should not be used for too long and at a large dosage. Bitter-cold herbs may also easily injure the Stomach and may cause stomach cramps and pain, so a proper dosage and a proper course should be arranged carefully. Also, patients with a weak constitution, or suffering from Cold in the Middle Jiao, or weakness of the stomach and intestines, should not use cold herbs in too great a quantity or for too long.

2 What kind of diseases can be treated by the herbs that clear Heat? How should one choose the herbs in clinical practice?

Herbs that clear Heat are used for treating internal Heat syndrome. They are cold in nature and able to reduce Heat, relieve Fire-toxin, cool the Blood and generate the Body Fluids. They can be used for various internal Heat syndromes, which can be differentiated according to the affected internal organs and the Defensive, Qi, Nutritive and Blood levels. Internal Excessive-Heat often develops from exogenous pathogenic Heat, although it also could be the result of other pathological processes in the body. However, no matter what the reasons are, when the Heat and its location are found, specific herbs can be used. The internal Excessive-Heat can be seen and the proper herbs thus can be chosen as follows.

Heat in the Heart and Small Intestine

If heat stays in the Heart and its meridian, the main manifestations are fever, thirst, a dry mouth, bitter taste in the mouth, restlessness, irritability and insomnia. The tongue body is red with a yellow, thin coating. The pulse is rapid and forceful. Herbs that are bitter and cold, or sweet and cold, and enter the Heart meridian are often chosen, such as Huang Lian (*Coptidis rhizoma*), Zhu Ye Juan Xin (*Bambusae viride folium*), Lian Zi Xin (*Nelumbinis plumula*) and Sheng Di Huang (*Rehmanniae radix*).

If the urine is also dark with a foul smell, and urination is accompanied by urgent and painful sensations, this indicates that the Small Intestine, the internally–externally related organ, is also disturbed by Heat. Herbs that are bitter and cold, and promote urination and clear Heat, such as Dan Zhu Ye (*Lophatheri herba*) and Zhi Zi (*Gardeniae fructus*), should be added.

In TCM, many kinds of sores, boils and carbuncles, which are characterized by warmth, swelling, redness and pain, are regarded as the result of a disturbance of the Heart-Fire. Herbs that are cold and bitter and enter the Heart meridian should be used—for instance, Jin Yin Hua (*Lonicerae flos*), Lian Qiao (*Forsythiae fructus*) and Pu Gong Ying (*Taraxaci herba*).

Heat in the Liver and Gall Bladder

If Heat stays in the Liver and its meridian, the symptoms of the patient will include irritability, red and dry eyes, hypochondriac pain and distension, dream-disturbed sleep, insomnia, headache, dizziness and tinnitus. The tongue body is red or red on the border and the coating is yellow. The pulse is wiry, rapid and forceful. Herbs that are bitter and cold and enter the Liver and Heart meridians, such as Huang Lian (*Coptidis rhizoma*), Long Dan Cao (*Gentianae radix*) and Xia Ku Cao (*Prunellae spica*), are selected.

If a female patient also complains that her menstruation is ahead of the expected time and is considerably heavy, this indicates that Heat has disturbed the Blood, and Mu Dan Pi (*Moutan cortex*) and Chi Shao Yao (*Paeoniae radix rubra*), which are cold and enter the Blood, should be added.

As the Liver opens into the eyes, Liver-Heat or Fire may cause disorders of the eyes, such as dry, red, painful eyes and blurred vision. Herbs that are sweet and cool and enter the Liver meridian are particularly effective in reducing Liver-Fire and benefiting the eyes, such as Qing Xiang Zi (*Celosiae semen*), Xia Ku Cao, Jue Ming Zi (*Cassiae semen*) and Mi Meng Hua (*Buddlejae flos*).

If Damp-Heat accumulates in the Liver meridian, it may bring about symptoms such as swelling of the external genitals or itching in the vagina, eczema, and turbid and foul smelling leukorrhea and urine. Bitter-cold herbs such as Long Dan Cao, Ku Shen (*Sophorae flavescentis radix*) and Zhi Zi (*Gardeniae fructus*) should be used.

If Damp-Heat accumulates in the Liver and Gall Bladder meridians and obstructs the movement of Qi and water, patients may feel a sense of tightness in the chest, stickiness in the mouth and distension in the hypochondriac region. If Damp-Heat disturbs the secretion of bile then jaundice may appear. Bitter-cold herbs with a fragrant smell, which are able to penetrate turbidity, should be used—for example, Qing Hao (*Artemisiae annuae herba*) and Chang Shan (*Dichroae febrifugae radix*).

Heat in the Spleen and Stomach

The Spleen and Stomach are in the Middle Jiao. They are responsible for receiving the food and transforming it into Essence, Qi and Blood. Because of its physiological characteristics and functions, the Stomach is considered as a Yang organ which easily generates Heat, and pathogenic Heat easily accumulates here too. The Spleen is regarded as a Yin organ and it is easily injured by Cold; if the Spleen fails to transport water, then water may accumulate in the Middle Jiao and generate Heat, and bring about Damp-Heat here too.

A Stomach-Heat syndrome is characterized by severe thirst, a dry mouth, preference for cold drinks, a tendency to be hungry, toothache, facial swelling, foul breath, a red tongue body with a yellow coating and a flooding, rapid pulse. Pungent, sweet and cold substances that can disperse the intensive Heat and direct it downwards should be chosen—for example, Shi Gao (*Gypsum*). Salty, bitter, sweet and cold herbs, which can clear Heat and generate the Body Fluids, are also a good choice—for instance, Zhi Mu (*Anemarrhenae rhizoma*), Huang Lian and Sheng Di Huang. If there is bleeding (e.g. hematemesis, bloody stools or purpura), herbs that enter the Blood level and are cold in nature should be used to cool the Blood—for example, Mu Dan Pi, Chi Shao Yao, Zi Cao (*Arnebiae/Lithospermi radix*) and Sheng Di Huang.

If Damp-Heat accumulates in the Middle Jiao, the patient may suffer from distension in the stomach and abdomen, loose stools or difficult bowel movements, a reduced appetite and eczema or other itching and weeping skin disorders. Bitter and cold herbs should be used to dry Dampness and clear Heat, such as Ku Shen, Bai Xian Pi (*Dictamni cortex*) and Bai Tou Weng (*Pulsatilla radix*).

Heat in the Lung and Large Intestine

The Lung is, in TCM, considered a delicate organ. Heat or Cold easily injures it. If Heat invades the Lung and disturbs its dispersing and descending functions, the patient may have a cough, shortness of breath, wheezing, dryness of the nasal passage and of the lips, and some patients chiefly have skin disease. To clear Heat and to restore the normal function of the Lung, sweet, pungent, bitter, salty and cold substances are suggested, such as Shi Gao, Zhi Mu, Huang Qin (*Scutellariae radix*) and Lu Gen (*Phragmitis rhizoma*).

If Heat disturbs the function of the Large Intestine, the main disorders are abnormal bowel movements and pain in the abdomen. Herbs that regulate bowel movement and clear Heat should be chosen—for instance, Huang Qin, Bai Tou Weng, Qin Pi (*Fraxini cortex*) and Ma Chi Xian (*Portulacae herba*).

The throat is the gateway of the Lung and the Heat in the Lung may also influence the throat. In clinical practice, many cases of swollen throat, sensations of obstruction in the throat, hoarseness and sore throat are caused by Heat in the Lung. Herbs such as Shan Dou Gen (*Sophorae tonkinensis radix*), She Gan (*Belamcandae rhizoma*) and Ma Bo (*Lasiosphaera*) are particularly suitable for this situation. Because they enter the Lung meridian and are pungent, bitter and cold, they are able to clear Heat, relieve Heat-toxin in the throat and disperse constrained Heat, Phlegm and Qi in the throat.

Heat in the Kidney and Bladder

The Kidney is an organ that stores the Essence and is believed never to have a real Excessive syndrome during pathogenic processes. However, sometimes Empty-Heat in the Kidney can be very strong and may further consume the Essence and the Yin of the Kidney. The symptoms are night sweating, 'bone steaming' (a type of fever due to deficiency of Yin, which may not always show when taking temperatures, as though the heat is spreading from the inside of the bone to the outside of the skin), low-grade fever, bleeding gums, spermatorrhea and hypersexuality. Treatment should be given to nourish the Kidney-Yin and at the same time reduce Empty-Fire. Bitter, salty, sweet and cold herbs are often used—for instance Zhi Mu, Huang Bai (*Phellodendri cortex*), Di Gu Pi (*Lycii cortex*) and Sheng Di Huang.

The Bladder stores the urine, but the Kidney controls the opening and closing of the Bladder. If Heat invades the Lower Jiao or the Bladder, then turbid, scanty urine and difficult and painful urination may appear. Herbs that are bitter and cold and enter the Bladder and Small Intestine meridians should be used to clear the Heat and dry Dampness, or to promote urination, thereby eliminating Damp-Heat; these include Huang Bai, Zhi Mu, Dan Zhu Ye and Long Dan Cao.

Apart from treating internal Heat syndromes of the internal organs, herbs that clear Heat can be used for treating acute febrile diseases and pestilence. Acute febrile diseases are caused by pathogenic Heat invasion in different seasons. These pathogenic changes are characterized by a relatively acute onset, predominance of Heat in the initial stages, and damage of the Body Fluids and Yin. In clinical practice, this is seen in acute infections caused by bacteria, viruses or other pathogenic microorganisms, such as pneumonia, bronchitis, gastroenteritis and dysentery. Pestilence is a kind of virulent infectious disease caused by Heat-toxin—for instance, epidemic cerebrospinal meningitis and poliomyelitis. Acute febrile diseases develop in the body following the four levels—that is, Defensive (*Wei*), Qi, Nutritive (*Ying*) and Blood (*Xue*).

Heat in the Defensive level

This is the initial stage of an acute febrile disease. The clinical manifestations are fever, slight aversion to wind and cold, headache, general aching in the body, a slight thirst and sweating, a red tip and border to the tongue, and a superficial and rapid pulse. Treatment must be given to expel Warm pathogenic factor and clear Heat. Herbs that are pungent, cool, or bitter and cold but fragrant and have dispersing properties should be used; these include Chai Hu (*Bupleuri radix*), Ju Hua (*Chrysanthemi flos*), Bo He (*Menthae herba*), Jin Yin Hua and Lian Qiao.

Heat in the Qi level

This is the mid phase of febrile disease. The clinical manifestations are high fever without chills, perspiration, a dry mouth and thirst, red face, shortness of breath, scanty urine, a red tongue body with a yellow coating, and a rapid, forceful pulse. These symptoms indicate that the Heat is increasing inside the body, and it may injure the Body Fluids. Treatment should use sweet, salty, pungent and cold herbs to clear the Heat, reduce Fire, protect the Body Fluids and vent the Heat to the Defensive level and eliminate it. Herbs such as Shi Gao, Zhi Mu, Jin Yin Hua, Lian Qiao, Zhu Ye and Lu Gen (*Phragmitis rhizoma*) are often used.

Heat in the Nutritive level

This is the later and critical stage of an acute febrile disease. The clinical manifestations are fever that worsens at night, severe irritability, restlessness, delirium and indistinct erythema and purpura. The tongue body is deep red without a coating; the pulse is thready and rapid. The symptoms indicate that the Heat is very intensive, has disturbed the Mind and Blood circulation, and has injured the Body Fluids and Yin. Herbs that are sweet, salty, bitter and cold are used to reduce the Fire and increase the Body Fluids and Yin, such as Sheng Di Huang, Mai Men Dong (*Ophiopogonis radix*), Dan Shen (*Salviae miltiorrhizae radix*) and Xuan Shen (*Scrophulariae radix*). At the same time, herbs that can bring the Heat to the Qi level should be used. Because the Heat comes from outside, no matter how deep it has invaded the body, it must be eliminated from the inside to the outside. The commonly used herbs are Jin Yin Hua, Lian Qiao and Zhu Ye.

Heat in the Blood level

This is the most critical stage of an acute febrile disease. The clinical manifestations are fever which is higher during the night, restlessness, obvious purpura, hematemesis, epistaxis, blood in the stools, occasional coma, delirium, convulsions, a deep red or purple tongue without coating and a thready, rapid pulse. The symptoms indicate that Heat-toxin has already entered the Blood, consumed it, disturbed its circulation and caused bleeding. At this point, treatment should be focused on cooling the Blood and dispersing the congealed Blood in time. Herbs that are cold in nature, enter the Blood level and are pungent or with dispersing ability, should be used; these include Mu Dan Pi, Sheng Di Huang, Chi Shao Yao and Dan Shen.

During the recovery stage of a febrile disease, the pathogenic factors are no longer so strong, but the Qi and Yin of the body have also been severely consumed. The main symptoms are fever which starts in the night and disappears in the morning, or a lingering low-grade fever, tiredness, poor appetite, shortness of breath, a red tongue with thin coating or without coating, and a weak, thready, rapid pulse. Herbs that are sweet and cold and enter the Kidney, Stomach or Lung meridians are used to reduce the Deficient-Heat from the Yin level, such as Yin Chai Hu (*Stellariae radix*), Di Gu Pi and Bai Wei (*Cynanchi atrati radix*).

3 What are the characteristics of Shi Gao (*Gypsum*)? Why is it often used with Zhi Mu (*Anemarrhenae rhizoma*)? What are the differences between their actions?

Shi Gao is the most important substance to clear internal Heat, especially Heat in the Qi level. As it is a mineral substance and is heavy in weight, it is considered to have a descending tendency. It is pungent, sweet and very cold, and enters the Lung and Stomach meridians. Shi Gao can clear Heat in these meridians and organs directly and strongly. It is often used to treat Heat in the Lung when the patient has a high fever, thirst, irritability, shortness of breath, profuse sweating, a very red tongue and a forceful, rapid pulse. This syndrome can be found in pneumonia, acute bronchitis or some infectious childhood diseases. It can also be used in headache and toothache in the region where the Stomach meridian passes through.

Shi Gao can quickly and directly clear Heat in the Stomach; it also powerfully clears Heat in the other parts of the body. It is used in acute infectious disease, epidemic cerebrospinal meningitis, epidemic encephalitis B, measles and scarlet fever in children. It can also be used for disorders such as asthma, cerebrovascular accident when the Heat has spread through the Lung, Heart, Liver, Stomach and Large Intestine meridians.

Shi Gao can also be applied to clear Heat in the other organs and meridians. It is especially used when the Heat is so strong that it covers many meridians and organs. The Stomach meridian is the Bright Yang meridian where there is an abundance of Yang and Heat. That is because the Stomach is responsible for receiving, 'ripening', digesting and transporting food. The whole process produces a large amount of heat; therefore the organ and meridians are called the 'Sea of Yang and Heat'. Moreover, the Stomach meridian connects with many other meridians; if Heat has spread through the whole body, then clearing Heat in the Bright Yang meridian may reduce Heat in the other meridians. This is a clearing-Heat strategy.

Shi Gao has another feature compared with the other herbs which clear Excessive-Heat. Most of those herbs are bitter and cold. Because bitterness has the tendency to move downwards, and Cold, of course, can clear Heat, they can quickly and strongly clear Heat and reduce Fire in the right situation. But these herbs cannot be used for a long period of time; with a high dosage or long period of time of usage, the bitter-cold herbs may cause a hidden Heat syndrome, which is a common side-effect of bitter-cold herbs. Moreover, bitterness possesses a drying property, so may injure the Yin of the body, which has already been injured by Excessive-Heat. Bitter and cold substances may injure the Stomach-Qi and Yang and disturb the digestion, especially in patients with weakness in the Middle Jiao. Shi Gao has a strong point compared with these herbs: it is very cold, but sweet. The combination of cold and sweetness may generate the Body Fluids and benefit the Yin of the body. Shi Gao can strongly clear Heat, but without the side-effect of injuring the Stomach-Yang. Moreover, Shi Gao also has a pungent property, so it not only clears Heat and reduces Fire but also disperses the Heat. This feature is closer to the

ascending nature of Fire so that it does not cause constrained Fire or hidden Heat. In addition, the pungent property of Shi Gao can vent Heat from the Qi level to the Defensive level in acute febrile diseases and is more effective for Excess conditions.

Zhi Mu is bitter and cold and enters the Lung, Stomach and Kidney meridians. Although it is cold and bitter, it is moist in nature. This is the difference from the other herbs that are bitter, cold and with drying properties. It can clear Heat, reduce Fire, moisten the Dryness and generate Yin. Because it can generate the Kidney-Yin, it is particularly used for Heat in the Qi, Nutritive and Blood levels. Shi Gao and Zhi Mu are often used together, as this enhances the effect of clearing Heat.

4 What are the differences between Sheng Shi Gao (raw *Gypsum*) and Duan Shi Gao (calcined *Gypsum*)?

Shi Gao is a kind of mineral substance which contains calcium sulfate. After being mined, cleaned and smashed, the product is called Sheng Shi Gao. Sheng Shi Gao is sweet, very cold and pungent, and enters the Lung and Stomach meridians. It can strongly clear Excessive-Heat in the Lung and can be used for febrile diseases which manifest with high fever, intense thirst, irritability, profuse sweating, shortness of breath and cough. At the same time, it can clear Stomach-Fire and can therefore treat headache, toothache, mouth ulcers, a foul smell in the mouth and burning in the Stomach.

After Shi Gao is calcined by strong fire, it is called Duan Shi Gao. Its cold and pungent properties are reduced by this process, while it obtains an astringent property and is effective in drying Dampness. This fine powder can be applied topically to treat skin diseases or wounds that are weeping, and is also used if the healing process is slow, such as in eczema, burns and ulcerated sores.

5 Why is Shi Gao (*Gypsum*) the first-line choice when Excessive-Heat spreads through the entire body?

The syndrome of Excessive-Heat spreading throughout the entire body is often seen in acute febrile diseases which manifest as high fever without chills, profuse sweating, anxiety, thirst, irritability, even unconsciousness and delirium. The patient has a very red tongue with dry yellow coating and a rapid, forceful pulse. This syndrome can be seen in some infectious diseases and inflammations in Western medicine. At this stage, the Heat is so strong that it is hard to tell which organ is not disturbed by the Heat. The treatment must be given in time to reduce Heat quickly and protect the Yin and Body Fluids in order to stop the process of the disease. The Stomach meridian of foot Bright Yang has an abundance of Qi and Blood from the digestion and transportation of food. It also easily produces Heat from all these activities; that is why the Bright Yang meridian and organ are regarded as the 'Sea of Food' and the 'Sea of the Yang and Heat'.

One of the strategies for clearing Heat from the entire body is to clear Heat from the Bright Yang meridian and organ. After that it will be much easier to reduce the Heat from the other organs and meridians. As Shi Gao enters the Stomach meridian and is very cold in nature, it can rapidly and strongly clear Heat from the Bright Yang organ and meridian in order to reduce Heat elsewhere. Since it is sweet and cold, it can also generate the Yin and Body Fluids to supplement the consumed fluids and to prevent their further consumption. Moreover, it is also pungent, so can disperse Heat and direct it downwards; therefore it can clear Heat without the possibility of forming hidden Fire. For these reasons, Shi Gao is an excellent substance for treating internal Excessive-Heat.

6 What are the differences in clearing Liver-Heat between the herbs Zhi Zi (*Gardeniae fructus*), Xia Ku Cao (*Prunellae spica*), Long Dan Cao (*Gentianae radix*) and Chuan Lian Zi (*Toosendan fructus*)?

All four of these herbs are bitter and cold, are very effective for draining Liver-Fire and are often used for Excessive Liver-Heat syndrome. However, there are differences between their actions.

Zhi Zi is bitter and cold, and does not enter the Liver meridian, but enters the Heart, San Jiao and Lung meridians. Its bitter and cold nature gives it a descending action, and it is able to clear Heat and to reduce Fire from the Upper Jiao, especially from the Heart. As the Liver and Heart have a mother–son relationship according to the Five Elements theory, Liver-Fire can very easily and quickly transport the Heat into the Heart. Treatment aimed at reducing Heart-Fire in order to reduce Liver-Fire is very effective and has become a commonly used strategy. For this reason, Zhi Zi can not only reduce Heart-Fire and treat restlessness, insomnia, a bitter taste in the mouth and a warm sensation in the chest, but also reduces Liver-Fire indirectly and treats irritability and dream-disturbed sleep. Besides clearing Heart-Fire and Liver-Fire, this herb has the function of promoting urination, reducing Fire and regulating the San Jiao water passage. It is also used for painful urinary dysfunction due to Damp-Heat in the Lower Jiao, as well as jaundice due to Damp-Heat in the Liver and Gall Bladder when bile is obstructed by Damp-Heat, such as in acute hepatitis and acute cholelithiasis.

Xia Ku Cao is bitter, cold and pungent, and enters the Liver meridian. Cold and bitterness can reduce Liver-Fire; pungency may disperse stagnant Qi and constrained Heat. Compared with the other herbs, which are cold and bitter with a drying property, it has a gentle action of nourishing the Liver-Blood. As the Liver opens into the eyes, Liver-Fire may in turn lead to disorders of the eyes. Xia Ku Cao is particularly effective for treating painful and dry eyes, a distending sensation of the eyes that worsens at night or in stressful situations due to weakness of blood, and stagnation of Liver-Qi with Liver-Fire, such as in hypertension or glaucoma. As Xia Ku Cao is pungent and has a dispersing tendency, it is quite different from the other bitter-cold herbs, which have only a descending action. It is effective for dissipating lumps and nodules which are caused by stagnation of Liver-Qi and accumulation of Phlegm and Heat, such as galactocele, scrofula, lipoma and goiter. A cream made from this herb can be applied topically in these diseases.

Long Dan Cao is very bitter and cold and enters the Liver, Gall Bladder and Bladder meridians. Its functions are twofold: it clears Liver-Fire from the upper body and eliminates Damp-Heat from the lower body. As Fire always flares up, the symptoms are headache, dizziness, red, painful and swollen eyes, insomnia and irritability. In clinical practice, the herb is very useful for treating hypertension, eczema, acute conjunctivitis, nerve deafness and nerve tinnitus which worsen under stressful conditions. Long Dan Cao can eliminate Damp-Heat from the Liver meridian and the Lower Jiao. As Dampness often accumulates in the lower body, the symptoms are itching in the genital area, a swollen scrotum, and turbid, foul-smelling urine or leukorrhea. Long Dan Cao can be used for herpes zoster, urinary tract infections, vaginitis, scrotal hydrocele and scrotitis. It is a strong herb that can clear Heat and Damp-Heat in the Liver rapidly, but it should not be used for a long period of time as it is too cold and bitter. Overdose may cause diarrhea and an uncomfortable sensation in the stomach and intestines. Patients with Spleen deficiency should use this herb with caution.

Chuan Lian Zi is bitter and cold and enters the Liver, Small Intestine and Bladder meridians. Like Long Dan Cao, it is very bitter and cold. It not only clears Heat in the Liver, but also drains stagnant Liver-Qi and constrained Fire; therefore it can relieve pain, especially distending pain in the hypochondriac region and sides of the lower abdomen. As the draining action is very strong, this herb is used only for pain caused by intensive Liver-Fire with Qi stagnation. In addition, this bitter-cold herb should not be used for a long period of time because it may irritate the Stomach and injure the Stomach-Yin and Stomach-Yang. Chuan Lian Zi contains toxic substances and overdose may lead to liver damage, even death; therefore the dosage should be controlled carefully.

7 What are the characteristics of the herbs that clear Liver-Heat and benefit the eyes?

As the Liver opens into the eyes, disorders of the Liver may cause disorders of the eyes. For instance, emotional disturbance and stress cause Liver-Qi stagnation, which can change into Liver-Heat or Fire; exogenous pathogenic Wind-Heat may disturb the Qi movement in the Liver and Gall Bladder meridians of the head and cause disorders of the eyes; if the Liver-Yin and Liver-Blood are insufficient, they may fail to nourish the eyes, and cause dryness of the eyes and blurred vision. Deficiency of the Liver-Yin and Kidney-Yin may cause Liver-Yang rising, which leads to pain and distension of the eyes, blurred vision and headache.

Most of the herbs that are able to cool the Liver and benefit the eyes are cold in nature and enter the Liver meridian. They can reduce Liver-Fire or constrained Heat of the Liver, expel Wind-Heat in the head (especially from the eyes) and direct the Liver-Yang to descend; therefore they treat different kinds of disorders of the eyes. In clinical practice, Qing Xiang Zi (*Celosiae semen*), Mi Meng Hua (*Buddlejae flos*), Jue Ming Zi (*Cassiae semen*), Xia Ku Cao (*Prunellae spica*), Man Jing Zi (*Viticis fructus*) and Shi Jue Ming (*Haliotidis concha*) are often used. Although they are often used together to enhance the effects, there are some differences between their functions.

Qing Xiang Zi and Mi Meng Hua are sweet and cool in nature. They both enter the Liver meridian. They are able to clear Excessive Liver-Heat or Wind-Heat to treat red, painful, swollen eyes, excessive tearing and photophobia. These complaints can be seen in hay fever, acute infectious conjunctivitis or influenza. If you compare the functions of these two herbs, Mi Meng Hua can gently nourish the Yin and Blood and is able to treat blurred vision; Qing Xiang Zi is able to reduce Fire directly, so its function is stronger than Mi Meng Hua in treating Excessive-Fire.

Jue Ming Zi is bitter, sweet, salty and cool. It enters the Liver and Kidney meridians. Compared with Qing Xiang Zi and Mi Meng Hua, it has a stronger action in clearing Liver-Heat and reducing Liver-Fire. As it is also able to nourish the Kidney-Yin and Liver-Yin, it is also used for the syndrome of Liver-Yin deficiency with Liver-Yang rising, which manifests as asthenopia, dry, painful eyes and blurred vision. These disorders can be found in hypertension and glaucoma.

Xia Ku Cao is pungent, bitter and cold. It enters the Liver meridian. Compared with the three herbs mentioned above, it is the strongest one for reducing Fire and clearing Heat. Meanwhile it can also nourish the Yin of the Liver. It is especially useful for pain in the eyes which worsens at night. It is also often used to treat hypertension if combined with other herbs that spread the Liver-Qi and descend the Liver-Yang.

Man Jing Zi is bitter, pungent and cold. It enters the Liver, Stomach and Bladder meridians. It has a similar function to Qing Xiang Zi and Mi Meng Hua in clearing Wind-Heat, but it is stronger in expelling Wind because it has a pungent nature. It is used only for treating syndromes that are caused by Excess and exogenous pathogenic factors. Because it also has the function of drying Dampness, it can also be used for pain, itching of the eyes and increased secretion in meibomitis, hordeolum and blepharitis.

Shi Jue Ming is salty, slightly cold and enters the Liver and Kidney meridians. It has no function in expelling Wind-Heat in the head, but can strongly clear Heat from the Liver and direct the Liver-Yang to descend because it is a cold, mineral substance. It can treat headache, dizziness, red eyes, photophobia and pterygium in hypertension, glaucoma and cataract.

8 What are the differences in the function of cooling the Blood between Mu Dan Pi (*Moutan cortex*) and Chi Shao Yao (*Paeoniae radix rubra*)?

Mu Dan Pi and Chi Shao Yao are both cold in nature. They are very often used for cooling the Blood and treating Heat in the Blood. Moreover, both of them are also able to promote Blood circulation and they are often chosen because they have fewer side-effects than other cold herbs of making congealed Blood in the process of cooling the Blood. However, there are some differences between these two herbs.

Mu Dan Pi is bitter, pungent and slightly cold, enters the Liver meridian and the Blood level primarily and the Heart and Kidney meridians secondarily. Bitterness and Cold can clear Heat; pungency can disperse stagnation. The characteristic of this herb is that it can treat both Excessive-Heat and Empty-Heat in the Blood. Excessive-Heat in the Blood is often manifested in febrile diseases as symptoms of fever, irritability, bleeding, irregular menstruation, menorrhagia and polymenorrhea. Empty-Heat in the Blood is caused by deficiency of Kidney-Yin and Liver-Yin, and manifests as menorrhagia, polymenorrhea, hot flushes during the menopause, 'bone steaming' and a warm feeling in the chest and on the palms and soles of the feet.

Chi Shao Yao is bitter and cold, and enters the Liver meridian and the Blood. Compared with Mu Dan Pi, it is especially effective in clearing Excessive-Heat in the Blood, but it does not reduce Empty-Heat, so it is only used for Excessive syndromes. At the same time, compared with Mu Dan Pi, it is stronger in promoting the Blood circulation

and removing congealed Blood, so is very effective in alleviating pain and reducing swelling. This herb is thus used more for bleeding conditions in febrile diseases or dysmenorrhea which is caused by Excessive-Heat in the Blood. It is also used for treating pain and swelling in cases of trauma, strain and fracture. Chi Shao Yao is one of the commonly used herbs for applying topically to relieve pain and reduce swelling. In addition, as it enters the Liver meridian, it can also be used for red and swollen eyes and pain in the hypochondriac region due to Heat accumulation in the Blood.

9 What are the differences between Chi Shao Yao (*Paeoniae radix rubra*) and Bai Shao Yao (*Paeoniae radix lactiflora*)?

Chi Shao Yao and Bai Shao Yao come from similar plants. Both are cold in nature and enter the Blood and the Liver meridian. Because Chi Shao Yao is cold and bitter, it is able to reduce Liver-Heat as well as Heat in the Blood. It has a dispersing property, can invigorate the Blood and remove congealed Blood, and is therefore often used for treating pain due to Blood stagnation.

Compared with Chi Shao Yao, Bai Shao Yao is less cold but bitter, so it can clear Liver-Heat or Heat in the Blood, but its function is weaker than that of Chi Shao Yao. One difference is its sour taste, which results in an astringent property. Cold and sourness may generate and stabilize the Yin. As it enters the Liver meridian, it particularly nourishes the Liver-Yin and Blood. It is an appropriate herb when there is Yin deficiency with slight Empty-Heat in the Blood. In this situation, the main symptoms are dizziness, dry and burning eyes, irritability, hypochondriac pain and distension. Like Chi Shao Yao, Bai Shao Yao can also alleviate pain, but it alleviates pain caused by Liver-Yin and Blood deficiency, in which the muscles and tendons lose their nourishment. This pain is cramping in nature, such as in abdominal pain and cramp after diarrhea, menstruation, labor or cramp of the muscles of the limbs. Moreover, as Bai Shao Yao has a sour taste, it may stabilize the Yin and Body Fluids and inhibit sweating, so is used for spontaneous sweating and night sweating.

10 What are the differences between and characteristics of Sheng Di Huang (*Rehmanniae radix*) and Xuan Shen (*Scrophulariae radix*) in the function of clearing Heat?

Sheng Di Huang and Xuan Shen are both cold in nature. They have similar functions in clearing Heat, especially when the Heat has consumed the Yin of the body. Both of them are often used for treating internal Heat syndromes with Yin deficiency. However, there are differences between their functions.

Sheng Di Huang is sweet, bitter and cold and moist in nature. It enters the Heart, Liver and Kidney meridians. Bitterness and Cold can clear Heat, and sweetness and Cold may generate the Yin of the body. It can directly clear Excessive-Heat in the Heart and Liver and therefore calm the Mind, and relieve irritability, restlessness, thirst and sensations of warmth in the chest. It is often used in febrile diseases. Sheng Di Huang can also be used for Empty-Heat due to deficiency of Heart-Yin, Liver-Yin or Kidney-Yin. The manifestations are insomnia, restlessness, irritability, a dry throat and 'bone-steaming' disorder.

As this herb enters the Heart and Liver meridians, it can also enter the Blood. It is particularly effective in clearing Heat from the Blood, cooling the Blood and stopping bleeding. This is why Sheng Di Huang is an important herb for clearing Heat not only in the Qi level, but also in the Nutritive and Blood levels. It can generate the Yin to prevent the consumption of Yin from Heat.

Xuan Shen is bitter, cold and salty, and enters the Kidney meridian. It can clear Heat and reduce Fire. Unlike Sheng Di Huang, it is not sweet and has no function in generating the Yin. As it does not enter the Liver and Heart meridians, it does not enter the Blood and has no function in cooling it. In clinical practice, Xuan Shen is often used instead of Sheng Di Huang to treat Excessive-Heat and Empty-Heat in the Heart, and to relieve thirst, a dry throat, sensation of warmth in the chest and irritability. This is because it has a characteristic of *lifting the Kidney Water (Yin) upwards to reduce the Fire of the Heart*. It is often used for Excessive-Heat and Empty-Heat in the Upper Jiao. However, its

function is not to nourish the Yin but to transport it so it is quite different from Sheng Di Huang. When a patient has Yin deficiency, especially Kidney-Yin deficiency, this herb should not be used over a long period of time, or it should only be used with herbs that tonify the Yin.

Xuan Shen also has some other characteristics. It is salty and able to soften hardness and is especially effective in relieving toxin. It is used for painful and swollen throat or eyes, chronic dry eczema, sores, scrofula and tumors.

However, Xuan Shen can have a toxic effect if it is used in overdose; 10–15 grams of crude herbs or 1–1.5 grams of concentrated herbal powder per day is a safe dosage.

11 What are the differences between the products of Di Huang (*Rehmanniae radix*)?

There are three kinds of product from the same plant. The part of the plant that is used is called Di Huang. As it is processed in different ways, the functions are different and the names are also different.

The first is Gan Di Huang, which is also called Sheng Di Huang. ('*Gan*' means 'dry' and '*Sheng*' means 'raw'.) It is the most commonly used form of Di Huang. The herb is processed by baking, and is then dried by wind or the sun until it turns black. Gan Di Huang is sweet, bitter and cold, and enters the Heart, Liver and Kidney meridians. Sweetness and Cold may generate the Yin and Body Fluids; as this herb is also moist in nature, it can nourish the Yin of the body. Bitterness and Cold can clear Heat, cool the Blood and stop bleeding. This herb is especially effective when internal Heat has injured the Yin and disturbed the Blood. For instance, this may occur in febrile disease with symptoms of fever, thirst, irritability, constipation, scanty urine, night sweating, flushes, menorrhagia, nose bleeding and hemoptysis.

Xian Di Huang is fresh Di Huang. It is collected in spring or autumn and is used directly after washing. It is juicy and fresh, sweet, bitter and very cold. The function is similar to the dried form but weaker in its effect of nourishing the Yin and stronger in clearing Heat. It is very effective in relieving irritability and thirst. This herb is used in clinical practice for diabetes.

When Sheng Di Huang is steamed, or alternatively, soaked in rice wine and dried in the sun until both its outside and inside have turned black and glossy, the product is called Shu Di Huang (*Rehmanniae radix praeparata*). Shu Di Huang is quite different from Sheng Di Huang. The main difference is that it is not cold but warm in nature and sweeter in taste. Sweetness and warmth can generate the Qi; sweetness and glossiness can tonify the Essence and Blood. As it enters the Kidney and Liver meridians, its main function is to tonify the Kidney-Essence and the Liver-Blood. It is a strong herb for treating dizziness, tinnitus, forgetfulness, weakness in the back and knees, and tiredness due to deficiency of the Kidney-Yin and Essence, Liver-Yin and Blood. Shu Di Huang is able to reduce Empty-Heat but its action is quite different from that of Gan Di Huang and Xian Di Huang. It is used in conditions where the Blood and the Kidney-Essence have been severely consumed and they are not able to control the Fire so the Empty-Fire blazes up. The symptoms are 'bone steaming', warmth in the palms and soles, fever in the afternoon or in the evening, hot flushes and night sweating. In addition, as it is not cold, it does not have the function of clearing Heat and cooling the Blood as with Sheng Di Huang and Xian Di Huang.

12 What are the characteristics of pathological change when Heat enters the Blood and what precautions should be observed when using herbs that cool the Blood and stop bleeding?

Herbs that cool the Blood are used for conditions where Heat enters the Blood. Heat in the Blood causes several specific pathological changes. First of all, Heat disturbs the Blood circulation so that the Blood moves recklessly and leaves its normal pathways; specific symptoms of this include bleeding, such as nose bleeding, hemoptysis, uterine bleeding, and blood in the urine and stools. Meanwhile, Heat may consume the Blood, making the Blood thicker and forming congealed Blood. When the Blood is disturbed by Heat it may also directly cause stagnation. In this situation, deep-red maculopapular or other types of rashes appear in infectious diseases

such as scarlet fever, epidemic meningitis and encephalitis, as well as in skin diseases such as eczema. If Heat enters the Blood, then the patient does not feel thirsty or rinses the mouth with water but has no desire to swallow it, although the tongue proper is red and the pulse is rapid. This indicates that the Heat is consuming the Blood instead of the Body Fluids.

In treating the syndrome of Heat in the Blood, an important principle is to cool the Blood and avoid Blood stasis. The Blood in a normal condition should circulate smoothly and quietly. Heat may force it to move faster, become unstable and, at the same time, the Heat may consume the Blood and cause Blood stagnation and bleeding. If cold herbs are used they may slow the Blood circulation but may also cause the Blood to stagnate. Therefore, to treat Heat in the Blood, herbs that enter the Blood and are cold-pungent-sweet or sour-cold in property are often used—for example, Sheng Di Huang (*Rehmanniae radix*), Chi Shao Yao (*Paeoniae radix rubra*), Mu Dan Pi (*Moutan cortex*) and Zi Cao (*Arnebiae/Lithospermi radix*). They have the function not only of cooling the Blood but also of promoting its circulation and preventing its stagnation. Some are pungent, which may disperse stasis; some are sweet, which may generate the Yin. They mainly enter the Heart and Liver meridians so that they can easily regulate the Blood circulation. These herbs are suitable for the pathogenic changes of Heat in the Blood.

To treat Heat in the Blood, cold and bitter herbs should not be used as they may dry the Blood. Herbs that enter the Qi level should not be used either because the pathological change is not in the Qi level. Very cold herbs should not be used for a long period of time or in a very large dosage, otherwise they may cause Blood stasis.

13 How many kinds of Zhu Ye (*Bambusae folium*) are used in Chinese herbal medicine? What are their differences?

Zhu Ye, in Chinese herbal medicine, can be divided into two kinds: the bitter form and the bland form.

The bitter form in Chinese is called Ku Zhu Ye (*Bambusae amarae folium*). It is pungent, sweet, slightly bitter and cold, and enters the Heart and Lung meridians. Pungency may disperse Heat;

bitterness and Cold may clear Heat. Ku Zhu Ye is very effective in reducing Heat in the chest and eliminating irritability. It is often used to treat febrile diseases when there is Heat in the Heart, Lung or chest.

The bland form is called Dan Zhu Ye (*Lophatheri herba*) in Chinese. It is less strong in clearing Heat than the bitter form but is good at promoting urination, thereby leaching out the Heat from the Heart and the Small Intestine. In clinical practice, it is used to treat urinary dysfunction which starts or worsens in stressful situations. It is also used to treat eczema due to Damp-Heat.

Zhu Ye Juan Xin (*Bambusae viride folium*) is the fine young leaf of bamboo. Early morning is the best time to collect it. As it contains the full energy of growing, it is considered to be the center, or heart, of the plant. Since according to TCM the heart of the plant may enter the Heart of a human, it is a very effective herb for clearing Heat in the Heart, especially in severe conditions when there is high fever, loss of consciousness and delirium.

14 What are the characteristics of Zhi Zi (*Gardeniae fructus*)? What are the differences between the shell, the seed and the deep-dry-fried Zhi Zi?

Zhi Zi is bitter and cold and enters the Heart, Lung and San Jiao meridians. Bitterness and Cold may clear Heat and descend Fire. Zhi Zi can gently and slowly direct Heat downwards from the Upper Jiao through the San Jiao passages to the Lower Jiao. It can also promote urination and leach out Heat from the Heart and Lung. It can be used for Heat accumulation in the chest, irritability, restlessness, sensations of tightness in the chest and insomnia. In febrile diseases there may also be fever.

As the San Jiao is the passage not only of Qi, but also of water, Zhi Zi enters the San Jiao meridian and regulates its function. As bitterness can dry Dampness and Cold can clear Heat, this herb can be used to treat Damp-Heat syndrome in the Upper Jiao, Middle Jiao and Lower Jiao—for example, jaundice due to Damp-Heat in the Middle Jiao and Qi constraint of the Liver and Gall Bladder; painful urinary dysfunction due to Damp-Heat in

the Lower Jiao which disturbs the function of the Bladder; infections of the eyes or eczema on the face and neck caused by Damp-Heat in the Upper Jiao.

Zhi Zi also has the function of cooling the Blood and relieving Heat-toxin. It can be used in different bleeding conditions, such as nose bleed, hematemesis and blood in the urine. It can also be applied topically for burns.

The different parts of Zhi Zi are considered to have different characteristics. Zhi Zi Pi, the shell, is believed to be especially effective for dispersing constrained Heat in the chest to treat sensations of warmth in the chest, restlessness, insomnia and palpitations. Zhi Zi Ren, the seed, is more effective in clearing Heat in the Heart to treat thirst, a dry mouth, ulcers on the tongue, constipation and scanty urine.

Zhi Zi can be processed in different ways. Sheng Zhi Zi, the raw form, has a stronger effect in clearing Heat; Jiao Zhi Zi, the deep-dry-fried form, is more effective for stopping bleeding caused by internal Heat.

As Zhi Zi is a herb with bitter and cold properties, the tendency of its action is downward. It may cause loose stools or diarrhea. It is suitable for use in patients who have constipation due to Heat in the intestines, but it is not suitable for those with Spleen-Qi deficiency with loose stools.

15 Dan Dou Chi (*Sojae semen praeparatum*) and Zhi Zi (*Gardeniae fructus*) can both treat Heat accumulation in the chest and release irritability. What are the differences between them?

Dan Dou Chi and Zhi Zi can both treat Heat accumulation in the chest and release irritability and sensations of warmth and tightness in the chest. In clinical practice, they are often used together. Although they treat the same syndrome, their approaches are different.

Dan Dou Chi is pungent, slightly warm and enters the Lung and Stomach meridians. Pungency and warmth give this herb dispersing, ascending and penetrating abilities. It is able to disperse and eliminate exogenous pathogenic factors, and to induce sweating gently; it therefore treats Exterior syndromes. It is often processed with the warm herbs such as Ma Huang (*Ephedrae herba*)*, Zi Su Ye (*Perillae folium*) or cold herbs such as Sang Ye (*Mori folium*) and Qing Hao (*Artemisiae annuae herba*). After it has acquired the warm or cold properties of these herbs, it is more suitable for treating Wind-Cold or Wind-Heat syndromes.

As Dan Dou Chi enters the Lung and Stomach meridians and has a dispersing and ascending character, it is able to disperse constrained Heat in the chest and treat tightness in the chest, restlessness, insomnia, depression or sensations of warmth in the chest. It has the function of dispersing constrained Heat rather than that of clearing Heat.

Zhi Zi is bitter and cold and enters the Heart, Lung and San Jiao meridians. Bitterness and Cold may clear Heat and direct it downwards through the San Jiao meridian, where the heat can be eliminated by urination. It is very effective for treating Heat in the chest, which manifests as irritability, restlessness, insomnia and anxiety. Unlike Dan Dou Chi, it eliminates irritability by clearing Heat, and directing it downwards.

Since both these herbs enter the Upper Jiao, and one disperses and lifts the constrained Qi and Heat, while the other clears Heat and directs it to descend, they are often used together to enhance their therapeutic effects. This combination is more suitable for the pathogenic condition of Heat in the chest.

16 Which parts of the plant Lian (*Nelumbinis*) can be used for medical purposes and what are their functions?

Almost every part of the plant Lian (*Nelumbinis*) is used in Chinese herbal medicine. Although they are all from one plant, the function of each of the different parts has its own specification.

The most commonly used part is Lian Zi (*Nelumbinis semen*). It is sweet, astringent and neutral. It enters the Spleen, Kidney and Heart meridians. As sweetness possesses a tonifying action, this herb is able to tonify the Spleen-Qi, Kidney-Qi and the Heart-Qi. Its astringent property may stabilize the Qi and also prevent leakage of the Essence and Body Fluids from these organs. It treats chronic diarrhea due to sinking of the Spleen-Qi, and premature

ejaculation and spermatorrhea due to the Kidney-Qi deficiency. It also treats restlessness, palpitation and anxiety due to recklessness and weakness of the Heart-Qi.

Lian Zi Xin (*Nelumbinis plumula*) is cold and bitter. 'Xin', in Chinese, means 'heart' or 'center'; 'Li Zi Xin' means 'the heart of Lian Zi'. As similes and allegories are used to explain the relationship between humans and nature in Chinese medicine, it is said that 'the heart of Lian Zi enters the Heart of the human'. It is therefore effective for clearing Heat in the Heart and calming the Mind. It is used to eliminate irritability, restlessness, convulsion and loss of consciousness.

Lian Xu (*Nelumbinis stamen*) has the same taste and temperature as Lian Zi. It also has similar functions as Lian Zi but is weaker in its effect of tonifying the Qi and is stronger in its action of controlling the leakage of Essence and Body Fluids. It is also able to stop bleeding because of its strongly astringent property.

Lian Fang (*Nelumbinis receptaculum*) is bitter, astringent and warm. It enters the Blood level and is able to stop bleeding and dissolve congealed Blood. The charcoal of Lian Fang is stronger in these actions; it is especially used for uterine bleeding and blood in the urine.

He Ye (*Nelumbinis folium*) is bitter, astringent and neutral. It has a light fragrant smell, which gives the herb dispersing, ascending and penetrating capabilities. It can clear Heat and transform turbid Dampness and is used to treat fever, headache, nausea and diarrhea. It can also lift the clear Qi from the Spleen and stop diarrhea and bleeding. Together with herbs that clear Heat, it is effective in treating bleeding due to Heat.

He Geng (*Nelumbinis ramulus*) is bitter and neutral. It can dry Dampness and promote Qi movement in the chest, and is used to treat tightness in the chest due to obstruction of the Qi.

Ou Jie (*Nelumbinis nodus rhizomatis*) has the same taste as Lian Zi but enters the Lung, Stomach and Liver meridians. It is especially effective for stabilizing the Blood and stopping bleeding, and is used for bleeding conditions caused by dysfunction of these organs.

In addition, this plant is not only used for medical purposes; its flower is the favorite of many people so it has become a commonly used name for girls in China; Lian Zi and Ou Jie are used as vegetables in the Chinese kitchen and He Ye can be cooked with rice so that the rice acquires its faint scent.

17 What are the characteristics of Huang Qin (*Scutellariae radix*), Huang Lian (*Coptidis rhizoma*) and Huang Bai (*Phellodendri cortex*)?

Huang Qin, Huang Lian and Huang Bai are together called 'San Huang', which means 'the three yellow'. This is not only because the color of the three herbs is yellow, but also because they are often used in combination in clinical practice as they accentuate the therapeutic actions of each other. All three are very bitter and cold and very effective in clearing internal Excessive-Heat. Since they enter different meridians, their actions are different too.

Huang Qin enters the Lung and Large Intestine meridians. It clears Heat, particularly in the Lung and Upper Jiao, and Damp-Heat in the intestines. It can be used for acute bronchitis, pneumonia, asthma, acute infections of the upper respiratory tract, tonsillitis and tracheitis. As the skin is related to the Lung, Huang Qin can be used for acute and subacute skin disorders, which manifest as red, itchy and weepy skin lesions. As the herb enters the Large Intestine meridian and is bitter and cold, it can dry Dampness and clear Heat. In clinical practice, it is often chosen for acute and chronic enteritis, colitis, Crohn's disease, intestinal parasitic diseases, imbalance in the intestinal flora and allergies.

Huang Lian enters the Heart and Stomach meridians. It can strongly reduce Fire in the Heart and Stomach, and treat irritability, restlessness, insomnia, thirst and a bitter taste in the mouth. Because of the mother–son relationship between the Liver and Heart, Huang Lian can be used for treating the syndrome of Liver-Fire rising. It can also be used to treat the syndrome when Liver-Fire attacks the Spleen and Stomach. In this condition, there may be symptoms such as hypochondriac pain and distension, a short temper, dream-disturbed sleep, burning in the stomach, acid regurgitation, poor appetite and nausea.

Huang Bai enters the Kidney and Bladder meridians. It can clear Heat and dry Dampness in the Lower Jiao and is an appropriate herb for treating urinary tract infection, cystitis, trichomonas vaginitis, monilial vaginitis, cervical erosion, pelvic parametritis, pruritus vulvae, scrotitis, penitis and spermatorrhea due to Damp-Heat in the Lower Jiao and disturbance of Empty-Fire of the Kidney.

As the three herbs enter different meridians and regions, they can be used together to treat syndromes in which the intensive Heat has spread through the entire body. When the three herbs are used in combination, the function of clearing Heat is stronger and works more rapidly, so can stop the development of the disease in time.

In addition, each of these herbs can be applied topically in lotions or pastes to clear Heat and dry Dampness. They are combined in a cream, which is called 'San Huang Gao' meaning 'three yellow cream'. This is very effective for treating different infections on the skin, such as eczema, folliculitis and cellulitis.

Although these three herbs are very effective in removing Damp-Heat, all of them are very cold and bitter, so can injure the Yin and Yang of the Stomach. Moreover, if used in large dosage they may cause hidden Heat syndrome or a syndrome of Heat complicated with Cold. Therefore, the practitioner should avoid using these three herbs for a long period of time, and especially not with a large dosage.

18 Why are herbs that clear Heat and dry Dampness often used for skin diseases? What are the characteristics of the commonly used herbs?

Although the pathological change is on the skin, most skin diseases are caused by internal Heat, Dampness, toxin or Wind. That is why herbs that clear Heat and dry Dampness are often used.

When the skin lesions are red, swollen and with sensations of warmth and burning or pain, this indicates that the Heat has entered the internal organs, disturbed the Blood circulation and caused Qi and Blood stagnation and Heat accumulation in the area. At this moment, Jin Yin Hua (*Lonicerae flos*) and Lian Qiao (*Forsythiae fructus*) can be used. These two herbs are cold in nature and are able to clear Heat and reduce Fire. Both also have dispersing properties so they can disperse stagnant Qi and constrained Fire and therefore reduce the sensation of warmth and burning pain of the skin lesions.

Shi Gao (*Gypsum*) is also often used in this situation as it enters the Lung and Stomach meridians. It is cold and pungent, and can clear and disperse

Heat. It is particularly appropriate for treating skin lesions that are very swollen and red, and have reached not only the skin, but also the subcutaneous layer and muscles, which belong to the region of the Spleen and the Stomach.

If infection exists, and there is purulent discharge from the skin lesions, herbs such as Pu Gong Ying (*Taraxaci herba*) and Di Ding (*Violae herba*) should be added because they can clear Heat and remove toxicity. If the skin lesions are very red, itchy and weepy, this indicates accumulation of Damp-Heat in the body. Herbs such as Ku Shen (*Sophorae flavescentis radix*), Bai Xian Pi (*Dictamni cortex*), Di Fu Zi (*Kochiae fructus*) and Huang Bai (*Phellodendri cortex*) can be used as these herbs are able to clear Heat and dry Dampness. They can also be applied topically to relieve itching and dry oozing.

Because many skin lesions are characterized by red, itch and oozing, such as in eczema and skin infections caused by viruses, bacteria, dermatophytes and parasites, herbs that clear Heat and dry Dampness are often used. Huang Lian (*Coptidis rhizoma*), Huang Qin (*Scutellariae radix*), Huang Bai (*Phellodendri cortex*), Zhi Zi (*Gardeniae fructus*) and Long Dan Cao (*Gentianae radix*) are strong herbs that clear Heat and dry Dampness. All are very cold and bitter. Huang Lian enters the Heart and Stomach meridians, Huang Qin enters the Lung and Large Intestine meridians, Huang Bai the Kidney meridians, Long Dan Cao the Liver meridian and Zhi Zi the San Jiao meridian. If the skin disorder is in the upper body, or worsens after the patient catches a cold, then Huang Qin should be used. If the skin disorder is in the middle of the trunk, or worsens in stressful situations, then Huang Lian and Long Dan Cao should be used. If the skin disorder worsens after eating the wrong food, then Huang Lian and Huang Qin are the appropriate choice. If the skin lesions are in the lower body, then Huang Bai and Zhi Zi should be used.

There are four herbs that are very effective for treating skin disorders caused by fungi, in which the pathological changes are also caused by Damp-Heat. They are Bai Xian Pi (*Dictamni cortex*), Ku Shen (*Sophorae flavescentis radix*), She Chuang Zi (*Cnidii fructus*) and Di Fu Zi (*Kochiae fructus*). As the skin lesions are on the surface of the body, the external treatment is also very important. All of these herbs can be used topically in lotions and pastes, or the fresh herbs smashed and just placed on the skin lesions. It should be mentioned that these herbs are very bitter and cold, and are dry in

nature, thus they can injure the Spleen and Stomach. They should not be used for a long period of time or in a large dosage.

19 What is Fire-toxin syndrome and what are the differences between Jin Yin Hua (*Lonicerae flos*) and Lian Qiao (*Forsythiae fructus*) in treating it?

Fire-toxin syndrome is characterized by localized redness, swelling, sensations of warmth or burning and pain. High fever and general pain may also be present. This syndrome appears in acute inflammations, such as carbuncles, furuncles and abscesses. In *The Yellow Emperor's Classic of Internal Medicine*, it is written 'Most of the sores which are painful, itchy and swollen are due to Fire'. In clinical practice, this syndrome is related to Fire of the Heart, Liver and Stomach. The Heart is a Fire organ and also easily receives Fire from the Liver, its mother organ. The Fire can be so strong that it may generate Fire-toxin. The Stomach is a Bright Yang organ and is responsible for receiving, ripening and transporting food. All these activities increase or produce Heat and can easily cause Fire-toxin syndrome in pathogenic conditions.

Jin Yin Hua enters the Heart, Liver and Stomach meridians and is sweet and cold. It is a strong herb for clearing Heat in these organs and meridians. Its sweet and cold properties may generate Body Fluids to prevent the consumption of Yin from internal Heat. As Jin Yin Hua is collected at the time that the flowers are still in bud in the early summer, this herb has a light fragrant smell, and dispersing and ascending actions. It may slightly disperse and lift Fire, especially constrained Fire, so this facilitates the main action of clearing Fire and directing it to descend.

Fresh Jin Yin Hua can be used topically, smashed and placed on the painful and swollen places. It can directly reduce swelling and pain and accelerate the recovery process. Because Jin Yin Hua has such characteristics, it is an appropriate herb for treating Fire-toxin syndrome, and is thus praised as 'the sublime herb to treat Fire-toxin'.

Lian Qiao is less cold than Jin Yin Hua but it has a bitter taste. It enters the Heart and Small Intestine meridians. Bitterness may bring down Fire from the Heart and Cold may clear Heat. It possesses strong dispersing and ascending properties and is especially effective in dispersing Heat in the Heart and relieving restlessness and sensations of warmth in the chest. Meanwhile, it is able to dissipate clumps and nodules caused by constraint of Heat, accumulation of food and Phlegm and stagnation of Blood. Its dispersing and dissipating actions are stronger than those of Jin Yin Hua. In addition, as it enters the Small Intestine meridian, it can also clear Heat there to treat painful urinary dysfunction.

As Jin Yin Hua and Lian Qiao have similar properties and actions, they are often used together in the treatment of Fire-toxin syndrome in order to strengthen the effect.

20 What are the differences between Da Qing Ye (*Isatidis folium*), Ban Lan Gen (*Isatidis/Baphicacanthis radix*) and Qing Dai (*Indigo naturalis*) for clearing Fire-toxin?

Da Qing Ye, Ban Lan Gen and Qing Dai are cold in nature; they have similar functions of clearing Heat, reducing Fire, cooling the Blood and removing toxicity. All are used to treat Fire-toxin syndrome. However, there are some differences between their actions.

Of the three herbs, Da Qing Ye is the coldest. It is also bitter and salty and enters the Heart and Stomach meridians. Saltiness enters the Blood, Cold can clear Heat and bitterness may descend Fire. The herb is particularly effective in reducing Fire in the Heart and Stomach. It is used for aphthous ulcers, acute pharyngitis, tonsillitis and carbuncles. As it is very cold, it is able to cool the Blood and reduce macules. It can be used for high fever, irritability, skin eruptions and changes of the consciousness. Da Qing Ye can also be applied topically in the affected area to reduce Heat-toxin.

Ban Lan Gen is less cold and enters the Heart and Kidney meridians. Its function and indications are similar to those of Da Qing Ye, but it is especially effective in treating severe facial erysipelas, a red and swollen throat in tonsillitis, scarlet fever and mumps.

Qing Dai enters the Liver meridian and is salty and cold. It can relieve toxicity and cool the Blood and is used for many kinds of skin disorders and inflammations due to Heat in the Blood. It can also be used topically. Qing Dai can also clear Heat from the Liver, eliminate irritability, reduce high fever, relieve convulsions in children and cough and hemoptysis due to Liver-Fire attacking the Lung.

In addition, these three herbs are often used together nowadays to treat hepatitis, encephalitis, mumps, myocarditis and influenza. In laboratory research and in clinical practice, these herbs are found to be effective against viruses and bacteria.

21 What kind of herbs can treat sore throat and benefit the throat?

There are several herbs that are especially effective for treating disorders of the throat. They are Shan Dou Gen (*Sophorae tonkinensis radix*), Ma Bo (*Lasiosphaera*), She Gan (*Belamcandae rhizoma*), Jie Geng (*Platycodi radix*) and Sheng Gan Cao (*Glycyrrhizae radix*). Generally speaking, all of these herbs are able to clear Heat, reduce swelling and relieve sore throat. They can be used for Fire-toxin syndrome in the throat, especially with the herbs that enter the Lung, Stomach and Kidney meridians.

Shan Dou Gen is bitter and cold and enters the Heart, Lung and Stomach meridians. It is a strong herb for clearing Heat and removing poison from the throat. It can be used for acute laryngopharyngitis, tonsillitis and hoarseness. Shan Dou Gen is also able to disperse Blood stasis and expel Phlegm so it can be used for severe chorditis and singers' nodes. Nowadays, combined with other herbs, it is used to treat tumors. Shan Dou Gen is a poisoning herb, thus it should be used for a short period of time and the dosage should be controlled carefully.

Ma Bo is pungent and neutral and enters the Lung meridian. Compared with Shan Dou Gen, it is less strong in reducing Fire, but it is stronger in dispersing constrained Heat and expelling Wind from the Lung, so it is able to treat swelling and pain in the throat, hoarseness and cough.

She Gan is bitter and cold and enters the Lung meridian. Its functions and indications are similar to that of Shan Dou Gen but it is less strong in relieving toxicity. It can also remove Phlegm and descend the Lung-Qi, so it is able to treat sore throat, swollen throat and cough due to Phlegm-Heat and obstruction in the throat.

Jie Geng is pungent, bitter and neutral and enters the Lung meridian. Pungency disperses stasis, and bitterness reduces stasis. It is light in weight and nature and moves upwards and outwards. It is effective for regulating the Lung-Qi, and reducing swelling and pain in the throat which is due not only to Fire-toxin, but also to Cold or Phlegm stasis. It is also a commonly used herb to remove Phlegm and treat cough.

Sheng Gan Cao is neutral and sweet. It has the function of reducing toxicity and harmonizing the Qi and Body Fluids in the throat in order to benefit the throat. Its sweet taste is especially appropriate for patients who do not like the strong tastes of the other herbs.

22 What kind of herbs can be used to treat internal abscesses and what are their characteristics?

Internal abscesses are a result of accumulation of Damp-Heat-toxin. There are several herbs that are effective for treating internal abscesses. They are Yi Yi Ren (*Coicis semen*), Lu Gen (*Phragmitis rhizoma*), Bai Jiang Cao (*Patriniae herba*), Yu Xing Cao (*Houttuyniae herba cum radice*), Ma Chi Xian (*Portulacae herba*) and Hong Teng (*Sargentodoxae caulis*). All these herbs are able to clear Heat, reduce toxicity and transform Dampness. They are used for either superficial sores or internal abscesses. However, there are differences between the actions of these herbs.

Yi Yi Ren, Lu Gen and Yu Xing Cao all enter the Lung meridian and are cold in nature. All can treat Lung abscesses. Besides its main function, Yi Yi Ren is very effective for transforming Dampness and pus; it is also used to treat tumors. Lu Gen is sweet and cold and is effective in reducing Heat, generating the Body Fluids and relieving thirst. Yu Xing Cao is pungent and cold, and is able to remove stasis of the Blood and Dampness. In clinical practice, these herbs are used to treat lung abscesses, pneumonia, bronchiectasis and pulmonary tuberculosis.

Yi Yi Ren, Bai Jiang Cao, Yu Xing Cao, Ma Chi Xian and Hong Teng enter the Large Intestine meridian. They are effective for treating intestinal abscesses and are used in colitis, appendicitis, dysentery and enteritis. Yi Yi Ren can also be used for tumor in the intestine. Hong Teng and Bai Jiang Cao

expel pus, disperse stasis and reduce pain. Yu Xing Cao is often used for gynecological disorders, such as pelvic inflammation. Ma Chi Xian can reduce toxicity and stop bleeding. It is also applied topically or used in lotions. It is effective for treating cervicitis, endocervicitis and colpomycosis.

23 What are the differences between Qing Hao (*Artemisiae annuae herba*), Yin Chai Hu (*Stellariae radix*) and Chai Hu (*Bupleuri radix*) in regulating the Liver-Qi?

Qing Hao, Yin Chai Hu and Chai Hu enter the Liver meridian. All are cold and gentle herbs. They can disperse and lift the Liver-Qi and so can be used for Liver-Qi stagnation.

Qing Hao has a light fragrant smell, and possesses the ability of penetrating turbidity and dispersing constrained Qi. As it also enters the Gall Bladder meridian, it is able to regulate the function of the Liver and Gall Bladder. It is effective for treating Damp-Heat in the Middle Jiao and constraint of the Liver-Qi and Gall Bladder-Qi. In the latter situation, patients may have symptoms such as tightness in the chest, nausea, dizziness and low-grade fever. In clinical practice, this herb can be used for malaria, hepatitis and jaundice caused by Liver or Gall Bladder disorders.

Yin Chai Hu is sweet, bitter and cold. Bitterness and Cold may reduce Heat; sweetness and Cold may generate the Yin and Body Fluids. This herb is not so strong in dispersing the Liver-Qi as Qing Hao and Chai Hu, but it is very effective for clearing Deficient-Heat, protecting the Yin and Body Fluids of the Liver, and reducing low-grade fever in the initial phase of febrile disease or after infectious diseases.

Chai Hu is a pungent and neutral herb and it is the strongest herb of the three for dispersing the Liver-Qi. It can be used to treat hypochondriac pain and distension, emotional disturbance, irritability and depression. It has no direct function in removing Dampness, unlike the other two herbs. As it has a dispersing property, it can gently disperse Excessive-Heat when the heat is not very strong and is used for cold and influenza infections, and acute infections of the upper respiratory tract.

24 What kind of herbs can be used for reducing Deficient-Heat in febrile disease? What are their characteristics? What are the differences between these herbs and the herbs that tonify the Yin and reduce Empty-Heat?

Qing Hao (*Artemisiae annuae herba*), Yin Chai Hu (*Stellariae radix*), Bai Wei (*Cynanchi atrati radix*), Hu Huang Lian (*Picrorhizae rhizoma*), Mu Dan Pi (*Moutan cortex*), Di Gu Pi (*Lycii cortex*) and Bie Jia (*Trionycis carapax*)** all have the function of reducing Deficient-Heat during acute febrile diseases. Acute febrile disease is a collective term for diseases that are caused by exogenous pathogenic Heat. The pathological changes are characterized by relatively acute onset and predominant Heat signs at the initial stage, and Heat tends to damage the Body Fluids and fluid Essence. In Western medicine, it is regarded as an acute infectious disease caused by bacteria, viruses and other pathogenic microorganisms.

During the process of the disease, when Heat injures the Body Fluids and Yin, the balance of Yin and Yang is disturbed, so the patient may have symptoms like low-grade fever in the evening or during the night. 'Bone steaming' may be present too; this Deficient fever can be seen in the Qi, Nutritive and Blood levels because the Heat has injured the Body Fluids, Yin or Blood. It can also be seen in the early phase of the recovery period of febrile disease. In this situation, the exogenous pathogenic factor is no longer so strong but the Qi and Yin are severely injured. As Heat has consumed the Body Fluids, Yin and Qi, most of the patients complain of dryness of the mouth, tiredness and poor appetite.

Qing Hao is bitter and cold, has a fragrant smell and is light in nature. The fragrant smell and the light nature may disperse constrained Qi and Heat; bitterness and Cold may reduce Heat from the Qi level. The herb enters the Blood so it is able to clear Heat in the Blood. Although this herb cannot nourish the Body Fluids and Yin of the body, its functions of dispersing and reducing Heat as well as cooling the Blood may protect the Yin and Body Fluids. It is often used in the mid and initial phases of febrile disease when the Heat is not high, but is constrained, and there is also stagnation of Qi.

Yin Chai Hu is bitter and cool and enters the Liver and Stomach meridians. It has similar functions to Qing Hao but has a stronger action in descending Deficient-Heat and cooling the Blood. It is more suitable for patients who complain of dryness of the throat and mouth and thirst and have afternoon fever.

Bai Wei is bitter, salty and cold and enters the Lung, Stomach and Kidney meridians. It can reduce Deficient-Heat and cool the Blood. The strong point of this herb is that it can be used not only for acute febrile diseases, but also for chronic disorders, such as in postpartum fever, lingering fever, night sweating and feelings of warmth in the palms and soles of the feet in febrile diseases.

Hu Huang Lian is bitter and cold. Its function is similar to that of Yin Chai Hu in Deficient-Heat, but it cannot cool the Blood. As it enters the Stomach and Large Intestine meridians, this herb is especially effective for treating children's nutritional impairment which is accompanied by abdominal distension and afternoon fever.

Mu Dan Pi is pungent, bitter and cold and enters the Liver, Heart and Kidney meridians. It is the strongest for reducing Heat from the Blood and cooling the Blood. As its pungent taste may disperse Heat and activate the Blood circulation and Qi movement, it is an appropriate herb for treating the syndrome of Heat constraint and Qi and Blood stagnation.

Di Gu Pi is sweet and cold and enters the Lung, Liver and Kidney meridians. Compared with the other herbs mentioned above, it is the strongest apart from Bie Jia in reducing Deficient-Heat, especially when Heat has consumed the Liver-Yin and Kidney-Yin, in which case the patient has fever in the night, 'bone steaming', night sweating and irritability. It can be used for chronic low-grade fever, such as fever in pulmonary tuberculosis, and chronic fatigue syndrome.

Bie Jia is salty and cold and enters the Kidney meridian. It is the strongest of the substances for reducing Deficient-Heat and also has the function of tonifying the Kidney-Yin. It is particularly suitable in conditions where the warm pathogenic factor has invaded the Lower Jiao while the Qi and Yin of the body are severely impaired, which has obvious manifestations of evening or low-grade fever, warmth in the palms and 'bone steaming'.

There are differences between the herbs in this group and those herbs that can reduce Empty-Heat and tonify the Yin of the body. The herbs discussed above treat Heat which is caused by exogenous pathogenic factors; the treatment is given to reduce the Heat and eliminate the exogenous pathogenic factors. These herbs are cold, slightly bitter, pungent and light in property. The herbs that treat deficiency of Yin with Empty-Heat are different. Empty-Heat is caused by long-term Yin deficiency of the internal organs from chronic disease, emotional disturbance,

age and constitution, and there are no exogenous pathogenic factors in the main pathogenic process. The treatment is given to nourish or tonify the Yin and thereby to reduce Heat. These herbs have mainly sweet and cold properties; examples are Sheng Di Huang (*Rehmanniae radix*), Mai Men Dong (*Ophiopogonis radix*) and Bei Sha Shen (*Glehniae radix*).

Comparisons of strength and temperature in herbs that clear Heat

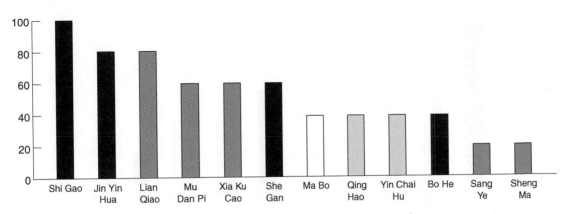

Fig. 3.1 • Comparison of the herbs that disperse Heat and direct it to descend.
Shi Gao (*Gypsum*), Jin Yin Hua (*Lonicerae flos*), Lian Qiao (*Forsythiae fructus*), Mu Dan Pi (*Moutan cortex*), Xia Ku Cao (*Prunellae spica*), She Gan (*Belamcandae rhizoma*), Ma Bo (*Lasiosphaera*), Qing Hao (*Artemisiae annuae herba*), Yin Chai Hu (*Stellariae radix*), Bo He (*Menthae herba*), Sang Ye (*Mori folium*), Sheng Ma (*Cimicifugae rhizoma*).

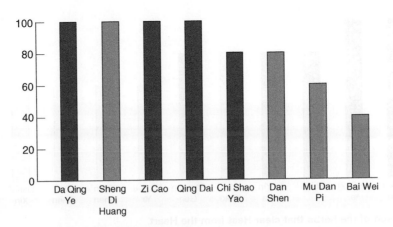

Fig. 3.2 • Comparison of the herbs that cool the Blood.
Da Qing Ye (*Isatidis folium*), Sheng Di Huang (*Rehmanniae radix*), Zi Cao (*Arnebiae/Lithospermi radix*), Qing Dai (*Indigo naturalis*), Chi Shao Yao (*Paeoniae radix rubra*), Dan Shen (*Salviae miltiorrhizae radix*), Mu Dan Pi (*Moutan cortex*), Bai Wei (*Cynanchi atrati radix*).

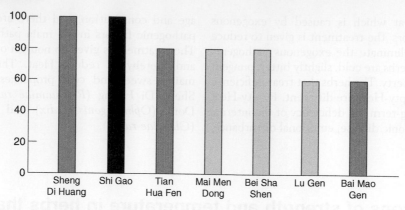

Fig. 3.3 • Comparison of the herbs that clear Heat and generate Body Fluids.
Sheng Di Huang (*Rehmanniae radix*), Shi Gao (*Gypsum*), Tian Hua Fen (*Trichosanthis radix*), Mai Men Dong (*Ophiopogonis radix*), Bei Sha Shen (*Glehniae radix*), Lu Gen (*Phragmitis rhizoma*), Bai Mao Gen (*Imperatae rhizoma*).

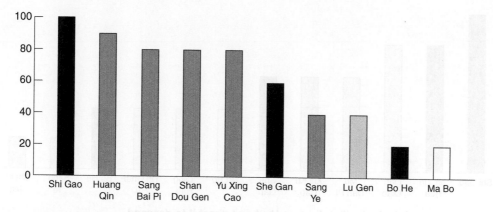

Fig. 3.4 • Comparison of the herbs that clear Heat from the Lung.
Shi Gao (*Gypsum*), Huang Qin (*Scutellariae radix*), Sang Bai Pi (*Mori cortex*), Shan Dou Gen (*Sophorae tonkinensis radix*), Yu Xing Cao (*Houttuyniae herba cum radice*), She Gan (*Belamcandae rhizoma*), Sang Ye (*Mori folium*), Lu Gen (*Phragmitis rhizoma*), Bo He (*Menthae herba*), Ma Bo (*Lasiosphaera*).

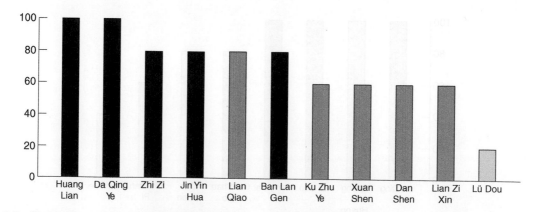

Fig. 3.5 • Comparison of the herbs that clear Heat from the Heart.
Huang Lian (*Coptidis rhizoma*), Da Qing Ye (*Isatidis folium*), Zhi Zi (*Gardeniae fructus*), Jin Yin Hua (*Lonicerae flos*), Lian Qiao (*Forsythiae fructus*), Ban Lan Gen (*Isatidis/Baphicacanthis radix*), Ku Zhu Ye (*Bambusae amarae folium*), Xuan Shen (*Scrophulariae radix*), Dan Shen (*Salviae miltiorrhizae radix*), Lian Zi Xin (*Nelumbinis plumula*), Lü Dou (*Phaseoli radiati semen*).

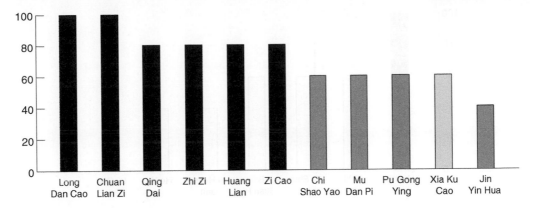

Fig. 3.6 • Comparison of the herbs that clear Heat from the Liver.
Long Dan Cao (*Gentianae radix*), Chuan Lian Zi (*Toosendan fructus*), Qing Dai (*Indigo naturalis*), Zhi Zi (*Gardeniae fructus*), Huang Lian (*Coptidis rhizoma*), Zi Cao (*Arnebiae/Lithospermi radix*), Chi Shao Yao (*Paeoniae radix rubra*), Mu Dan Pi (*Moutan cortex*), Pu Gong Ying (*Taraxaci herba*), Xia Ku Cao (*Prunellae spica*), Jin Yin Hua (*Lonicerae flos*).

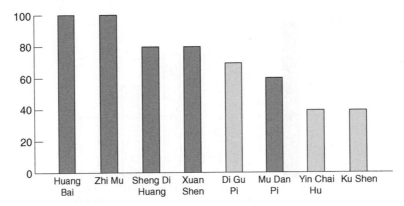

Fig. 3.7 • Comparison of the herbs that clear Heat from the Kidney.
Huang Bai (*Phellodendri cortex*), Zhi Mu (*Anemarrhenae rhizoma*), Sheng Di Huang (*Rehmanniae radix*), Xuan Shen (*Scrophulariae radix*), Di Gu Pi (*Lycii cortex*), Mu Dan Pi (*Moutan cortex*), Yin Chai Hu (*Stellariae radix*), Ku Shen (*Sophorae flavescentis radix*).

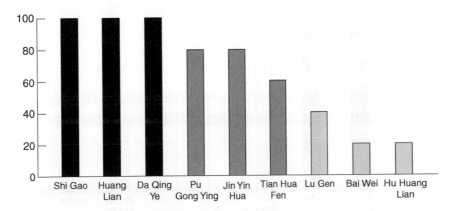

Fig. 3.8 • Comparison of the herbs that clear Heat from the Stomach.
Shi Gao (*Gypsum*), Huang Lian (*Coptidis rhizoma*), Da Qing Ye (*Isatidis folium*), Pu Gong Ying (*Taraxaci herba*), Jin Yin Hua (*Lonicerae flos*), Tian Hua Fen (*Trichosanthis radix*), Lu Gen (*Phragmitis rhizoma*), Bai Wei (*Cynanchi atrati radix*), Hu Huang Lian (*Picrorhizae rhizoma*).

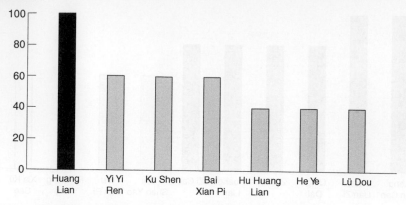

Fig. 3.9 • Comparison of the herbs that eliminate Damp-Heat from the Spleen.
Huang Lian (*Coptidis rhizoma*), Yi Yi Ren (*Coicis semen*), Ku Shen (*Sophorae flavescentis radix*), Bai Xian Pi (*Dictamni cortex*), Hu Huang Lian (*Picrorhizae rhizoma*), He Ye (*Nelumbinis folium*), Lü Dou (*Phaseoli radiati semen*).

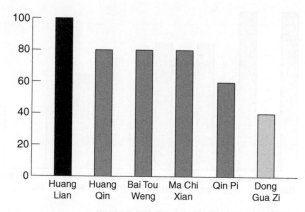

Fig. 3.10 • Comparison of the herbs that clear Damp-Heat from the Large Intestine.
Huang Lian (*Coptidis rhizoma*), Huang Qin (*Scutellariae radix*), Bai Tou Weng (*Pulsatilla radix*), Ma Chi Xian (*Portulacae herba*), Qin Pi (*Fraxini cortex*), Dong Gua Zi (*Benincasae semen*).

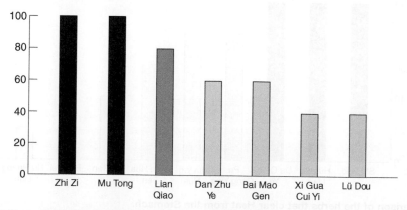

Fig. 3.11 • Comparison of the herbs that clear Heat from the Small Intestine.
Zhi Zi (*Gardeniae fructus*), Mu Tong (*Mutong caulis*)*, Lian Qiao (*Forsythiae fructus*), Dan Zhu Ye (*Lophatheri herba*), Bai Mao Gen (*Imperatae rhizoma*), Xi Gua Cui Yi (*Citrulli exocarpium*), Lü Dou (*Phaseoli radiati semen*).

Chapter **Four**

4

Herbs that drain downwards

泻下药

1 What are the functions of and indications for downward-draining herbs?

Herbs that drain downwards are able to stimulate the intestine, purge accumulation and guide out stagnation, eliminate toxic substances, drain Fire or Cold, and drive out water. These herbs are used in the following conditions.

Constipation

Constipation can be divided into Deficiency and Excess types, which are often caused by insufficient fluid in the intestines or obstruction of the Qi with Heat or Cold. It is often related to bad dietary habits, changes of diet, usage of certain medicines, weakness of the Yin and Blood in elderly people, after giving birth, or it may be habitual constipation. The main symptoms are constipation or difficult bowel movement, abdominal distension, fullness of the stomach and dryness in the mouth. The tongue is slightly purple; the coating is dry, thick, white or yellow in color. The pulse is deep, wiry or deep and thready.

Obstruction in the intestines

The obstruction often has an acute onset. It can be caused by accumulation of feces, Qi, Blood, Heat,

Fire-toxin or Cold in the intestine as well as in the abdomen. The main symptoms are severe abdominal pain, cramp, distension, irregular bowel movement or no bowel movement, fullness of the stomach, nausea, vomiting, reduced appetite, dryness in the mouth, thirst and irritability. The tongue body is red with a dry, yellow or white coating and the pulse is deep, slippery and wiry. This syndrome can be seen in severe constipation, initial stages of simple or partial intestinal obstruction, intestinal adhesion, intussusception and other acute abdominal syndromes.

Fire-toxin accumulation

In the syndrome of Fire-toxin accumulation, when the Fire-toxin has not yet accumulated over a long time and the Blood is not strongly disturbed, the main symptoms are fever, irritability, severe thirst, pain and distension in the abdomen (such as in the initial stage of acute appendicitis), acute pancreatitis, acute cholecystitis, hepatitis and ulcer perforation with mild infection and inflammation. Most of the herbs to treat this disorder are cold in temperature. They can purge the accumulation, drain Excessive-Heat and cool the Blood. They are often used to treat Fire-toxin accumulation in the body. The downward-draining action can move the bowels, and can therefore eliminate Heat and Fire-toxin from the body.

These herbs can also be used to eliminate toxic substances when the Liver and Kidney functions have been impaired and they fail to remove the toxic substances, such as in hepatitis, cirrhosis of the liver and renal failure.

Water accumulation

When the water metabolism is disturbed, water can accumulate in certain places; this is seen in hydrothorax and ascites. This disorder brings about symptoms such as tightness in the chest, shortness of breath and distension of the abdomen. It can also relieve generalized edema. There are herbs which have both cathartic and diuretic effects and can drive out the water and relieve the symptoms.

2 What are the characteristics of downward-draining herbs?

Herbs that drain downwards are able to stimulate the intestines and purge obstructions and Fire-toxins, as well as drive out water. They have the following characteristics in their properties and functions.

Bitter and cold

Most of the herbs that drain downward are bitter and cold because most of the syndromes they treat have substantial accumulation with Excessive-Heat in the intestines. The Heat comes from various sources. First of all, the Stomach and Large Intestine are called the 'family of Bright Yang (Yang Ming)' where Yang and Qi are abundant. Secondly, the Stomach and Large Intestine are the most important organs for transporting food and feces, so the Yang and Qi are active all the time and also produce heat. Thirdly, when there is obstruction in the intestines, as in constipation, the Qi is easily obstructed and Heat will be produced; moreover, most infections produce Heat or Fire-toxin and the accumulation of toxic substances also produces heat when the functions of the liver and kidney are impaired.

Bitterness and Cold both move downwards; Cold, of course, can drain Heat and Fire-toxin. The commonly used bitter and cold herbs are Da Huang (*Rhei rhizoma*), Lu Hui (*Aloe folii extractus*), Qian Niu Zi (*Pharbitidis semen*)*, Gan Sui (*Euphorbiae kansui radix*)*, Da Jǐ (*Knoxiae radix*)*, Shang Lu (*Phytolaccae radix*)* and Ting Li Zi (*Lepidii/Descurainiae semen*).

Salty and cold

Herbs with a salty taste move downwards; they are also able to generate the Body Fluids and soften hardness. A downward-draining substance with a salty and cold property is especially suitable for treating constipation when the feces are very dry and hard. An example is Mang Xiao (*Natrii sulfas*).

Sweet

Herbs with a sweet taste are normally seen among the moist laxatives. Sweetness can harmonize the functions of the intestines and alleviate cramp; examples include Huo Ma Ren (*Cannabis semen*) and Yu Li Ren (*Pruni semen*). Where harsh purgatives or herbs that drive out water possess a sweet taste, this may relatively reduce the speed of the action and reduce the harsh property. Herbs with this characteristic include Fan Xie Ye (*Sennae folium*) and Huo Ma Ren.

Seeds or nuts

Seeds or nuts are gentle laxatives. As they contain lipids, they can lubricate the intestines and ease the expulsion of stools. They are especially suitable for habitual constipation and constipation caused by weakness of Yin and Blood. Commonly used herbs are Huo Ma Ren, Yu Li Ren, Xing Ren (*Armeniacae semen*) and Tao Ren (*Persicae semen*).

Entering the Stomach and Large Intestine meridians, or Spleen, Lung and Kidney meridians

Purgatives mainly enter the Stomach and Large Intestine meridians where their actions are focused; the herbs that drive out water enter the Lung,

Spleen and Kidney meridians, which mainly influence the water metabolism. They are not only able to empty the bowels, but also to drive out water by diuretic action.

Other ways of administration

In order to achieve a good effect of purging the accumulation of or eliminating the toxic substances, herbs that drain downward are used not only orally, but also often in an enema.

3 What are the precautions and contraindications for the use of herbs that drain downwards?

First of all, herbs that drain downwards are harsh herbs; their functions are strong and their speed is high, so they may easily injure the Stomach-Qi and Body Fluids. Moreover, many of them are also poisonous. Compared with other moist laxatives, they should only be taken for a short treatment period and their dosage should be controlled carefully. When the severe symptoms have disappeared, these herbs should be stopped immediately. Long-term usage of the purgatives for constipation may lead to consumption of the Body Fluids in the intestines and make the constipation worse. Since the actions of these herbs are harsh, they are used only for Excessive syndromes and for people with a strong constitution. They are not suitable for people with a weak constitution or chronic diseases. For patients who suffer from Deficiency syndromes but also need these herbs in the treatment of acute or severe accumulation, such as in uremia, these herbs must be used in combination with the tonifying herbs.

Secondly, downward-draining herbs can drain Qi as well as Blood downwards, so they are also not suitable for use during menstruation or in bleeding conditions. They are also contraindicated in pregnancy.

Thirdly, herbs that drain downwards are, in principle, not suitable for patients with Exterior syndromes. It is better to treat the Exterior first and not to drain downwards. Otherwise, the exogenous factors may be led deeper into the body.

When downward-draining herbs are used to treat acute abdominal syndromes, such as acute intestinal obstruction, appendicitis, cholecystitis and pancreatitis, it is also important to remember that these herbs are suitable only for certain periods in the whole pathological process of the disease, or in certain types of disorder. These herbs should only be prescribed by doctors after Western medical examination. If the results of the herbal treatment are not satisfactory, an operation is usually indicated.

4 What are the characteristics of Da Huang (*Rhei rhizoma*), Mang Xiao (*Natrii sulfas*), Fan Xie Ye (*Sennae folium*) and Lu Hui (*Aloe folii extractus*) as purgatives?

These four substances are cold in nature and are commonly used as purgatives. They can be used together or separately according to clinical need.

Da Huang is very bitter and cold and it stimulates the intestines intensively; therefore it can strongly drain Heat and move the stools. It is the most important herb for treating Excessive-Heat accumulation in the intestines and Qi obstruction by the feces. Da Huang can be prescribed when there is high fever, profuse sweating, thirst, constipation, abdominal pain and distension. The patient has a red tongue with a dry, yellow coating and a slippery, wiry and rapid pulse. In clinical practice, it can be used for constipation, irritable bowel syndrome and the primary stage of acute abdominal syndromes.

Mang Xiao has a less strong action in stimulating the intestine, moving stools and draining Heat than Da Huang because it is not as bitter and cold as Da Huang. Mang Xiao characteristically moistens the intestine, softens feces and promotes bowel movement because it is a salty and cold substance. It is particularly suitable for constipation when the feces are very dry and hard.

Da Huang and Mang Xiao are often used together to treat constipation and Excessive-Heat in the intestine. Because Da Huang can purge the bowel and Mang Xiao can soften the feces, they can accentuate each other's therapeutic actions.

Fan Xie Ye is sweet, bitter and cold and enters the Large Intestine meridian. It is moist in nature and is able to moisten Dryness in the Large Intestine, clear Heat and promote bowel movement. The effect of moving the bowels is stronger than that of Da Huang. If a small dosage of Fan Xie Ye is applied, it can also promote the digestion and is used for constipation caused by a bad diet. In clinical practice, it is often used alone as a purgative.

Lu Hui is very bitter and cold and enters the Liver, Heart, Stomach and Large Intestine meridians. It is a very strong herb for purging the bowels and reducing Excessive-Heat. It characteristically drains Liver-Fire and Heart-Fire when Heat has been transported to the Stomach and Large Intestine. Symptoms of this condition include irritability, anxiety, insomnia, a bitter taste in the mouth, thirst and constipation. As its smell is very unpleasant, it is mainly taken in pills instead of in a decoction.

5 What are the characteristics of Da Huang (*Rhei rhizoma*)? What are the differences between the products of this herb?

Da Huang is a commonly used herb in clinical practice. It is a very good purgative agent compared with those in Western medicine. It stimulates the intestines and purges the bowels without severe cramp. Its purgative effect appears 6 hours after taking the herb; Da Huang enema brings a much quicker onset of action.

Da Huang is often used not only as a purgative agent, but also as an agent to relieve toxicity. It can guide out Heat, Damp-Heat or Fire-toxin through the bowels. It can also cool the Blood, invigorate its circulation and eliminate congealed Blood, so it is often used in different kinds of infection, which are considered as a process of Fire-toxin produced in the intestines or in the abdomen. It can also be used for accumulation of toxic substances when the functions of the Liver and Kidney are impaired. Its decoction can also be used as an enema in order to eliminate Fire-toxin in the body.

Da Huang can be used raw or processed. The raw form has a stronger function of purging accumulations in the intestines than the baked form. The raw form should not be cooked for too long, otherwise its purgative action becomes weaker. When Da Huang is fried with alcohol, it is more effective for clearing Excessive-Heat in the Upper Jiao and treating headache, toothache and infection of the eyes. The char-

coal of Da Huang has a better effect in stopping bleeding and eliminating congealed Blood.

6 What are the differences between the products of Mang Xiao (*Natrii sulfas*)?

Mang Xiao is a commonly used purgative substance. Since it is salty and cold and can moisten the intestines and soften the stools, it is often used together with Da Huang (*Rhei rhizoma*) to treat constipation.

The main constituent of Mang Xiao is sodium sulfate. The intestines cannot absorb sulfate, so it stays in the intestines and increases osmotic pressure to return the water in the intestine, stimulate it and soften the feces.

The regularly used product is called Mang Xiao. The impure form of Mang Xiao is called Pu Xiao; it contains salt, calcium sulfate and magnesium sulfate as well as sodium sulfate. Its purgative action is stronger than that of Mang Xiao. *Mirabilitum purum* is called Xuan Ming Fen or Yuan Ming Fen and it is less effective in its purgative action compared with Mang Xiao, but is more effective for topical application to treat stomatitis.

7 What are the differences between Huo Ma Ren (*Cannabis semen*), Yu Li Ren (*Pruni semen*), Xing Ren (*Armeniacae semen*), Tao Ren (*Persicae semen*) and Hei Zhi Ma (*Sesami semen nigricum*) in their laxative effects?

Because all of these seeds or nuts contain lipids, they have the function of moistening the stools and lubricating the intestines and so are able to treat constipation. They also have different characteristics and can be used in different conditions.

Huo Ma Ren is a sweet and neutral herb; it can either promote bowel movement or tonify the Qi and Blood. It is particularly suitable for treating constipation after surgery, giving birth, or in patients who are also suffering from chronic diseases or have a weak constitution. It can also be used to treat hemorrhoids and habitual constipation.

Yu Li Ren is pungent, bitter, sweet and neutral. It enters the Spleen, Small Intestine and Large Intestine meridians. It is moist in nature and has a descending tendency of action. It is able to direct the Qi to descend and promote bowel movement and urination, and is mainly used in Excessive syndromes.

Xing Ren, Tao Ren and Hei Zhi Ma usually are not used as laxatives, but they have the function of moistening the intestines and promoting bowel movement. Xin Ren enters the Lung meridian which is externally–internally related to the Large Intestine meridian, and it is especially used to treat disturbance of the dispersing and descending function of the Lung-Qi that influences the intestines and causes constipation, and vice versa. Tao Ren enters the Lower Jiao, can break up congealed Blood and is more suitable for constipation with signs of Blood stagnation in the intestines, such as in infections, acute abdominal syndromes and hemorrhoids. Hei Zhi Ma is able to nourish the Yin, Essence and Blood and has similar effects to Huo Ma Ren, but the tonifying action is stronger and the action of moving the bowel is weaker than that of Huo Ma Ren.

8 What are the characteristics of Gan Sui (*Euphorbiae kansui radix*)*, Da Jǐ (*Knoxiae radix*)* and Yuan Hua (*Genkwa flos*)*?

These three herbs are all violent cathartic as well as diuretic herbs. They can drain water and drive out congealed fluids by causing diarrhea and promoting urination. They are used only in severe generalized edema or accumulation of fluids in the thoracic or abdominal cavities. According to early studies and experiences, these three herbs are considered incompatible with Gan Cao (*Glycyrrhizae radix*).

The three herbs are often used together, but each has its own characteristics. Gan Sui has the strongest cathartic effect and Yuan Hua has the weakest effect of the three herbs. However, Yuan Hua is the most poisonous herb of the three and Gan Sui is the weakest. Gan Sui particularly drives out the fluid from the meridians, Da Jǐ drives out the fluid from the internal organs and Yuan Hua from the joints and cavities.

Comparisons of strength and temperature in herbs that drain downwards

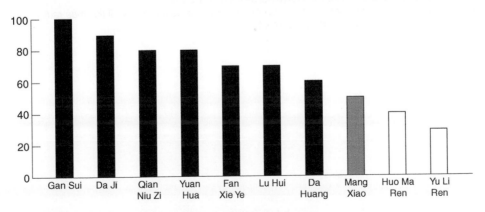

Fig. 4.1 • Comparison of the strength of the downward-draining herbs.
Gan Sui (*Euphorbiae kansui radix*)*, Da Jǐ (*Knoxiae radix*)*, Qian Niu Zi (*Pharbitidis semen*)*, Yuan Hua (*Genkwa flos*)*, Fan Xie Ye (*Sennae folium*), Lu Hui (*Aloe folii extractus*), Da Huang (*Rhei rhizoma*), Mang Xiao (*Natrii sulfas*), Huo Ma Ren (*Cannabis semen*), Yu Li Ren (*Pruni semen*).

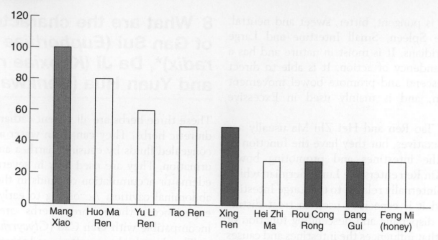

Fig. 4.2 • Comparison of the herbs that moisten the intestines and promote bowel movement.
Mang Xiao (*Natrii sulfas*), Huo Ma Ren (*Cannabis semen*), Yu Li Ren (*Pruni semen*), Tao Ren (*Persicae semen*), Xing Ren (*Armeniacae semen*), Hei Zhi Ma (*Sesami semen nigricum*), Rou Cong Rong (*Cistanchis herba*)**, Dang Gui (*Angelicae sinensis radix*), Feng Mi (*Mel*).

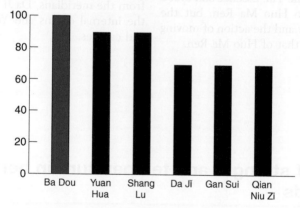

Fig. 4.3 • Comparison of the toxicity of the downward-draining herbs.
Ba Dou (*Crotonis fructus*)*, Yuan Hua (*Genkwa flos*)*, Shang Lu (*Phytolaccae radix*)*, Da Jǐ (*Knoxiae radix*)*, Gan Sui (*Euphorbiae kansui radix*)*, Qian Niu Zi (*Pharbitidis semen*)*.

Chapter **Five**

5

Herbs that expel Wind-Dampness

祛风湿药

1 What are the indications for herbs that expel Wind-Dampness?

Herbs that expel Wind-Dampness are used for treating Bi syndrome. 'Bi' means 'obstruction'. Bi syndrome is also translated as 'Painful Obstruction syndrome'. This syndrome is caused by invasion of Wind, Dampness and Cold, which obstruct the meridians and cause pain in the muscles, tendons, bones and joints. Painful Obstruction syndrome can be divided into four types according to the exogenous pathogenic factors and the characteristics of the symptoms.

Wind Painful Obstruction syndrome

Wind Painful Obstruction syndrome is called 'Xing Bi' in Chinese. 'Xing' means 'moving' or 'walking'. This syndrome is characterized by pain that migrates from joint to joint and from one place to another. The pain worsens during windy weather. Other symptoms and signs include tingling of the limbs, pain with a radiating nature, a normal tongue body with a white, thin coating and a moderate pulse. The pathogenic factors of Wind Painful Obstruction syndrome are Wind, Dampness and Cold, with Wind being the predominant factor. In clinical practice, it is often associated with diseases such as migraine, cervical or lumbar spondylosis, hyperosteogeny and rheumatic fever.

Cold Painful Obstruction syndrome

Cold Painful Obstruction syndrome is called 'Tong Bi'. 'Tong' means 'pain' in Chinese. The syndrome is characterized by severe pain of a fixed, contracting or cramping nature. The pain worsens during winter or cold weather and is relieved by warmth. Other symptoms and signs include cold limbs and a preference for warmth, a purple or blue tongue body with a white, sticky or watery coating and a deep, wiry pulse. The pathogenic factors of this syndrome are Wind, Dampness and Cold, with Cold being the predominant factor. In clinical practice, it is often associated with diseases such as rheumatic fever, rheumatoid arthritis, osteoarthropathy and osteoporosis.

Damp Painful Obstruction syndrome

Damp Painful Obstruction syndrome is called 'Zhuo Bi'. 'Zhuo' means 'to wear' and 'to adhere'. The syndrome is characterized by a fixed, lingering pain and swelling of the joints or muscles associated with a heavy or numb sensation. The pain and swelling worsen during humid and cold weather. The other symptoms and signs are heaviness of the body, edema or difficult micturition, a light purple tongue body with a white, thick coating and a deep, moderate pulse. The pathogenic factors in this syndrome are Wind, Dampness and Cold, with Dampness being the predominant factor. In clinical practice, it can be seen in diseases such as chronic strain of the muscles or other soft tissues and various kinds of arthritis.

Hot Painful Obstruction syndrome

Hot Painful Obstruction syndrome is called 'Re Bi'. 'Re' means 'hotness'. It is characterized by painful and swollen joints with hot or burning sensations. The other symptoms and signs are fever, thirst, scanty urine, a red tongue body with a yellow coating and a rapid, slippery pulse. Hot Painful Obstruction syndrome is a development of the invasion of Wind, Dampness and Cold. First of all, when Wind, Dampness and Cold invade the body, they disturb the Qi movement and the Blood circulation. As the body puts up resistance in order to eliminate these pathogenic factors, Heat is produced in the process. Furthermore, Wind, Dampness and Cold can also turn into Heat if they are not eliminated in time and accumulate in certain meridians and joints. In clinical practice, this syndrome can be seen during the onset and active stage of rheumatic fever or rheumatoid arthritis, as well as frozen shoulder, tenovaginitis, bursal synovitis, pyogenic osteomyelitis and suppurative arthritis.

2 What are the characteristics of herbs that expel Wind-Dampness?

Herbs that expel Wind-Dampness are used for treating Bi syndrome. They are able to expel Wind, transform Dampness and warm the Interior. The characteristics of their properties and functions are as follows.

Pungent taste

Most of the herbs that expel Wind-Dampness are pungent. This gives the herbs the ability to expel Wind from the skin, muscles and bones. As Dampness is associated with Wind, when Wind is expelled by the pungent herbs then Dampness can be partially eliminated too. This function is called 'wind disperses dampness'.

Pungent and warm

Many of the herbs are pungent and warm in nature, and are especially suitable for conditions where Cold or Wind-Cold predominates in the disease. Because the pungent taste can expel Wind and scatter Cold and the warmth can warm the Interior,

warm-pungent herbs can alleviate pain quickly. Warm-pungent herbs are also suitable for usage in the winter, in cold climates and by elderly people. Herbs with a pungent and warm nature include Qiang Huo (*Notopterygii rhizoma*), Du Huo (*Angelicae pubescentis radix*), Wei Ling Xian (*Clematidis radix*), Wu Jia Pi (*Acanthopanacis cortex*) and Qian Nian Jian (*Homalomenae rhizoma*).

Bitter, pungent and warm

Some of the herbs are bitter and pungent, and are especially suitable for treating Damp Painful Obstruction syndrome because bitterness and pungency can dry Dampness and reduce swelling and heavy sensations in the limbs. If the herb is also warm, the ability to expel Wind and Dampness is even stronger. Herbs with these properties are Song Jie (*Pini nodi lignum*), Qian Nian Jian, Hai Feng Teng (*Piperis caulis*), Hai Tong Pi (*Erythrinae cortex*) and Cang Zhu (*Atractylodis rhizoma*).

Salty or sour

Some substances are salty; they are especially suitable for disorders where Wind and Dampness are in the Interior of the body for a considerable time or when the bones are involved. The commonly used salty substances are Wu Shao She (*Zaocys*), Bai Hua She (*Agkistrodon acutus*)* and Wei Ling Xian. Sourness nourishes the Body Fluids and Yin and can therefore moderate cramps and relieve the pain of the tendons and muscles. Mu Gua (*Chaenomelis fructus*) is often used for this purpose.

Entering the Kidney, Bladder and Liver meridians

In Bi syndromes, especially in chronic cases, the bones and tendons are impaired. Herbs that enter the Kidney and Liver meridians are often chosen because the Kidney and Liver govern the bones and tendons. Commonly used substances are Hai Feng Teng, Luo Shi Teng (*Trachelospermi caulis*), Qian Nian Jian, Bai Hua She and Wu Shao She. Herbs that enter the Bladder meridian are often used to activate the Qi and Yang and to expel exogenous pathogenic factors from the skin, subcutaneous region and muscles. This is because the Bladder meridian covers the back of the body, which is considered as the Yang side of the body and is the first to be attacked by pathogenic Wind and Cold. Herbs with such functions include Qiang Huo and Wei Ling Xian.

More forms of administration

Substances that expel Wind-Dampness are not only used orally, but are also applied topically because local use may directly expel the exogenous pathogenic factors, activate the Qi and Blood circulation and ultimately break up the obstruction. The commonly used forms are herbal plasters, lotions and tinctures. In addition, herbal alcohol drink is also frequently used as part of the diet for patients who suffer from chronic Bi syndrome.

3 What are the commonly used methods and herbs for treating Bi syndrome?

Substances that expel Wind-Dampness are mainly pungent, warm and bitter, and enter the Liver, Spleen and Kidney meridians. Pungency has dispersing and moving properties, is able to disperse Wind-Dampness and Cold, and to activate the Qi movement and Blood circulation; bitterness can dry dampness; warmth can scatter Cold, warm the muscles and subcutaneous region and strengthen the function of the Defensive Qi. These substances are able to expel Wind, eliminate Dampness, scatter Cold, invigorate the collaterals, relax the tendons and alleviate pain. Some of the substances also have the function of tonifying the Kidney and Liver and strengthening the bones and tendons.

Substances that expel Wind-Dampness are mainly used for Bi syndromes. Since one or two exogenous pathogenic factors can be predominant in each condition, the symptoms can vary. It is very important to choose the proper herbs according to which of the four types of the Bi syndrome is present, the affected region, the duration of the disease and the constitution of the patient. The commonly used methods and herbs are as follows.

Expelling Wind

This method is mainly used for Wind Painful Obstruction syndrome, which is characterized by migrating pain. Pungent and warm herbs are often used, such as Fang Feng (*Saposhnikoviae radix*),

Qiang Huo (*Notopterygii rhizoma*), Wei Ling Xian (*Clematidis radix*), Hu Zhang (*Polygoni cuspidati rhizoma*) and Wu Shao She (*Zaocys*).

Eliminating Dampness

This method is mainly used for Damp Painful Obstruction syndrome, which is characterized by heaviness and numbness of the limbs. The herbs that are used in this condition are Han Fang Ji (*Stephaniae tetrandrae radix*), Mu Gua (*Chaenomelis fructus*), Bi Xie (*Dioscoreae hypoglaucae rhizoma*), Qin Jiao (*Gentianae macrophyllae radix*), Cang Zhu (*Atractylodis rhizoma*) and Hai Tong Pi (*Erythrinae cortex*).

Scattering Cold and warming the Interior

This method is mainly used for Cold Painful Obstruction syndrome, which is characterized by severe, fixed, cramping pain which worsens in cold weather or in winter. Herbs that can be used in this condition are Fu Zi (*Aconiti radix lateralis preparata*)*, Chuan Wu (*Aconiti carmichaeli radix*)*, Cao Wu (*Aconiti kusnezoffii radix*)*, Gui Zhi (*Cinnamomi cassiae ramulus*) and Xi Xin (*Asari herba*)*.

Clearing Heat and eliminating Wind-Dampness

This method is mainly used for Hot Painful Obstruction syndrome, which is characterized by swelling and red joints with warm or burning sensations. Herbs that can be used are Sang Zhi (*Mori ramulus*), Luo Shi Teng (*Trachelospermi caulis*), Xi Xian Cao (*Sigesbeckiae herba*), Huang Bai (*Phellodendri cortex*) and Yi Yi Ren (*Coicis semen*).

Invigorating the Blood and promoting circulation

This method is mainly used for chronic Bi syndromes or Bi syndromes characterized by stubborn pain. Commonly used herbs are Dang Gui (*Angelicae sinensis radix*), Chuan Xiong (*Chuanxiong rhizoma*), Hong Hua (*Carthami flos*) and Chuan Niu Xi (*Cyathulae radix*).

Dispersing the Lung-Qi, regulating the Qi from the Bladder meridian and expelling exogenous pathogenic factors

This method is mainly used during the onset of Bi syndrome when the exogenous pathogenic factors are in the superficial layer of the body, especially the upper body. The symptoms are sudden onset of pain, swelling of joints, fever, chills and general pain. Commonly used herbs are Qiang Huo, Fang Feng, Gao Ben (*Ligustici sinensis radix*), Ma Huang (*Ephedrae herba*)* and Xing Ren (*Armeniacae semen*).

Invigorating the tendons, opening the collaterals and nourishing the Blood

This method is mainly used for chronic Bi syndrome, where Wind, Dampness and Cold stay in the muscles and tendons for a long period of time, obstructing the Qi and Blood circulation in the collaterals. Patients complain of stiffness of the body, tingling sensations and numbness of the limbs. Herbs that can be used in this condition are Shen Jin Cao (*Lycopodii herba*), Hai Feng Teng (*Piperis caulis*), Sang Zhi, Di Long (*Pheretima*), Dang Gui Wei (*Angelicae sinensis radix extremitas*) and Bai Hua She (*Agkistrodon acutus*)*.

Tonifying the Liver and Kidney, strengthening the tendons and bones

This method is mainly used for chronic Bi syndrome in elderly people and patients with a weak constitution. Patients complain of weakness and stiffness of the joints, especially in the waist and knees, and difficulty with walking. Herbs which can be used for these complaints are Sang Ji Sheng (*Taxilli herba*), Qian Nian Jian (*Homalomenae rhizoma*), Gou Ji (*Cibotii rhizoma*)**, Xu Duan (*Dipsaci radix*), Gu Sui Bu (*Drynariae rhizoma*), Xian Mao (*Curculiginis rhizoma*), Xian Ling Pi (*Epimedii herba*) and Wu Jia Pi (*Acanthopanacis cortex*).

In clinical practice, these methods are often used together. For instance, to treat Wind Painful Obstruction syndrome, methods that expel Wind, invigorate the Blood and nourish the Blood are often used together. To treat Damp Painful Obstruction syndrome, methods that expel Wind, eliminate Dampness, disperse the Lung-Qi and invigorate the sinews are often used together. To treat Cold Painful Obstruction syndrome, methods that scatter Cold, warm the Interior and promote Blood circulation are often used together. To treat chronic Bi syndrome, tonifying methods are often used together with methods for eliminating exogenous pathogenic factors.

4 What are the differences between Qiang Huo (*Notopterygii rhizoma*) and Du Huo (*Angelicae pubescentis radix*)?

Qiang Huo and Du Huo are commonly used herbs to expel Wind, Dampness and Cold from the body and to treat Bi syndrome. In clinical practice, they are often used together to treat rheumatic fever, rheumatoid arthritis and other disorders of the muscles, tendons, nerves and joints which are characterized by pain, heaviness, stiffness, tingling sensations and numbness of the affected area. Qiang Huo and Du Huo were considered to be one in ancient times and were used with little difference in their functions. Later, however, they were recognized to be two different herbs with slight differences in their functions.

Qiang Huo has a pungent, bitter taste and is warm in nature. It enters the Bladder meridian primarily, and the Liver and Kidney meridians secondly. The pungent and warm nature gives Qiang Huo strong dispersing and ascending ability; it is very effective for expelling Wind, Dampness and Cold quickly in the superficial layers of the body such as the skin, subcutaneous region and muscles, especially of the upper body. It is suitable for treating general pain, headache, stiffness of the back (such as in cold and influenza infections), in acute stages of arthritis and in other disorders of the muscles and joints.

Du Huo is also pungent, bitter and warm, but much gentler in nature than Qiang Huo. It enters the Kidney meridian and is especially effective in eliminating Wind, Dampness and Cold from the deeper layers of the body, particularly of the lower body. Because of its nature, Du Huo eliminates pathogenic factors from the body in a more constant and gentler way. It is more suitable for treating chronic cases of arthritis and other disorders of the muscles and joints when the patient complains the pain is in the bones and deep in the joints. Because it enters the Kidney meridian and treats Bi syndrome, Du Huo is more effective for disorders of the knees, back and heels.

Comparing these two herbs in the treatment of Bi syndromes, Qiang Huo is the warmer and has better results in eliminating Cold and relieving pain; Du Huo is more effective for eliminating Damp and has better results in treating heaviness and numbness of the body and joints. In clinical practice, Qiang Huo and Du Huo are often used together because Bi syndromes have chronic, recurrent processes, mostly affecting the whole body, in which pain and heaviness often coexist. Although there are differences between the natures of these two herbs, both are pungent and warm. In patients who suffer from chronic Bi syndrome as well as deficiency of the Yin and Body Fluids, these two herbs, and especially Qiang Huo, should be used with caution. It is wise to add herbs which tonify the Yin and Blood and promote the Blood circulation during the treatment.

5 What are the differences between the two kinds of Wu Jia Pi?

The two kinds of Wu Jia Pi are Nan Wu Jia Pi (*Acanthopanacis cortex*), which means 'Wu Jia Pi from the south', and Bei Wu Jia Pi (*Periploca sepium bunge*), which means 'Wu Jia Pi from the north'. Both are commonly used herbs for treating Bi syndrome. They are pungent, bitter and warm, enter the Liver and Kidney meridians and are able to expel Wind and Dampness, tonify the Liver and Kidney and strengthen the tendons and bones. They are especially suitable for treating Wind and Damp Painful Obstruction syndrome with weakness of the Liver and Kidney. They also have the function of promoting urination, reducing edema and treating swelling of the joints. Comparing these two herbs, Nan Wu Jia Pi is better for expelling Wind-Dampness and strengthening the bones; Bei Wu Jia Pi is more effective for promoting urination and reducing edema.

6 What are the characteristics of Mu Gua (*Chaenomelis fructus*)? What are the differences between Mu Gua and Bai Shao Yao (*Paeoniae radix lactiflora*) for relaxing the tendons?

Mu Gua is sour, warm and aromatic. It primarily enters the Spleen meridian. It can transform Damp-

ness in the Middle Jiao, revive the Spleen and harmonize the Stomach. It can be used for Exterior Damp-Cold in the Middle Jiao, and treat vomiting and diarrhea, cramping pain in the abdomen and even cramp in the legs. It also enters the Liver meridian and transforms Dampness and relaxes the muscles and tendons. It can be used for Damp Painful Obstruction syndrome in which stiffness of the body, cramp in the limbs, swelling of the ankles and difficulty with walking are present. It is an aromatic herb, but its tendency of action is descending; it is commonly used for Dampness in the lower body.

Mu Gua and Bai Shao Yao are both able to relieve cramping pain in the abdomen, cramp of the muscles and tendons of the limbs, and they can be used together. However, there are some differences between their actions.

Mu Gua relaxes the tendons by transforming Dampness and invigorating the collaterals; it treats cramps and stiffness which are caused by dampness. Bai Shao Yao is sour and cold and enters the Liver meridian. As sourness and cold generate Yin, it is able to nourish the Yin and Blood of the tendons, therefore relaxing the muscles, tendons and ultimately alleviating cramp. It treats cramp which is caused by Yin deficiency. If cramp is caused by obstruction of Dampness as well as Yin deficiency, Mu Gua and Bai Shao Yao should be used together.

7 What are the characteristics of Xi Xin (*Asari herba*)*, Wei Ling Xian (*Clematidis radix*), Hai Tong Pi (*Erythrinae cortex*), Xi Xian Cao (*Sigesbeckiae herba*) and Lu Lu Tong (*Liquidambaris fructus*)?

These five herbs have a strong moving ability and are commonly used to treat Painful Obstruction syndrome, but there are some differences between their functions.

Xi Xin is very pungent and warm and enters the Lung, Heart and Kidney meridians. As well as its function of expelling Wind and Cold and releasing the Exterior, its pungent and aromatic smell give it a penetrating ability, allowing it to enter the deeper layers of the body. No matter how deep the pathogenic factors penetrate and how tight the tissues may be, Xi Xin is very effective for eliminating the Wind and Cold, opening up the meridians and collaterals and alleviating pain. In clinical practice, it is often used for Cold Painful Obstruction syndrome, especially chronic cases. It is also used in elderly people and in winter when the pain is severe and deep in the bones, accompanied by other cold signs such as cold limbs and a preference for warmth, a purple or blue tongue body with a white coating and a deep, slow and wiry pulse.

Wei Ling Xian is pungent, salty and warm and enters the Bladder meridian. It has dispersing, moving and opening abilities, moves very quickly and has a fairly strong action in expelling Wind and transforming Dampness, compared with other herbs with similar functions. Compared with Xi Xin, although it is not able to penetrate to the same depth and is less effective in stopping pain, it is very effective for opening up the meridians and collaterals, and treating numbness, paralysis and tingling sensations in the limbs. Because it moves quickly, the therapeutic effect is rapid. Moreover, Wei Ling Xian powder can also be used with alcohol, which strengthens its moving ability.

Hai Tong Pi is bitter, pungent and neutral and enters the Liver and Kidney meridians. It has similar functions to Wei Ling Xian, expelling Wind-Dampness and treating numbness of the limbs. But the speed of Hai Tong Pi is not as great as that of Wei Ling Xian and it is not so strongly and sharply pungent, so its dispersing ability does not spread over as large an area as Wei Ling Xian. It characteristically opens up the meridians and collaterals, directly reaching the affected region. In clinical practice, it is used more for stiffness and numbness of the waist and knees. As it is a neutral herb, it can be used for Bi syndrome with either Cold or Heat symptoms in the pathological changes.

Xi Xian Cao is pungent, bitter and cold and enters the Liver and Kidney meridians. Like Xi Xin, its pungent taste gives it a dispersing ability to enter the deep layers of the body, the tendons and the bones, to search and expel Wind; however, unlike Xi Xin, instead of expelling Cold, it expels Dampness and Heat. In clinical practice, it can be used when the Bi syndrome is in the active stage and the joints are swollen and painful with burning sensations. Like Wei Ling Xian and Hai Tong Pi, it can eliminate Wind-Dampness and treat heaviness and numbness of the limbs. Because it enters the Liver

and Kidney meridians, it is especially effective in treating weakness and stiffness of the knees and back, pain in the bones, numbness and tingling sensations in the limbs—for instance, in hemiplegia and paralysis.

Lu Lu Tong is pungent, bitter and neutral and enters all the meridians. 'Lu' in Chinese means 'road'; 'Tong' means 'open'—hence the name means 'all roads open'. Lu Lu Tong is able to open the meridians and collaterals, expel Wind-Dampness and treat stiffness and numbness of the limbs in Bi syndrome. It can also treat urinary retention, edema and eczema, and can promote lactation of milk after giving birth because it can open up all the meridians and collaterals to promote the movement of water and Qi.

8 What are the characteristics of Fu Zi (*Aconiti radix lateralis preparata*)*, Chuan Wu (*Aconiti carmichaeli radix*)*, Cao Wu (*Aconiti kusnezoffii radix*)*, Xi Xin (*Asari herba*)* and Gui Zhi (*Cinnamomi cassiae ramulus*) for treating Bi syndrome? What are the precautions for using these herbs?

These five herbs are all pungent and hot, are able to scatter internal Cold, dry Dampness, excite the Yang and Qi, and open up the meridians and collaterals. They are also very effective for alleviating pain. In clinical practice, they are often used to treat Bi syndromes which are mainly caused by Cold. In this situation, patients complain of severe pain in the joints, muscles and bones. However, these herbs have different strengths and characteristics, so are used in different conditions.

Fu Zi is very pungent and hot and enters the Heart, Spleen and Kidney meridians. It is swift and violent in its action of spreading warmth, scattering Cold, drying Dampness and warming the meridians. It is often described as the sun; when the sun is rising, the fog disappears immediately. Because of its strength, it is considered to be a herb that enters the 12 meridians. It is used to treat Bi syndromes especially when Cold is predominant with symptoms of cramping, severe pain and stiffness in the muscles, tendons and bones which worsen in cold weather.

Chuan Wu and Cao Wu are similar but stronger in their action compared with Fu Zi. They are also considered stronger for expelling Wind, opening up the meridians and are suitable for treating Bi syndrome where Wind and Cold are predominant, and the main symptoms are numbness of the skin, general pain, severe pain in the joints and bones, stiffness of limbs and cramping in the abdomen.

Xi Xin is pungent and hot and enters the Heart, Lung and Kidney meridians. It is characterized by searching for and expelling Wind and Cold from the deep levels of the body. Xi Xin has good results for alleviating pain in the bones and joints. Apart from treating Bi syndromes, it can also be used for headache, migraine, trigeminal neuralgia, toothache and pain caused by sinusitis.

Gui Zhi is pungent, sweet and warm and enters the Heart, Lung and Bladder meridians. Unlike Fu Zi, which spreads warmth quickly, and unlike Xi Xin, which expels Cold from deep regions, it expels Wind and alleviates pain by warming the meridians, activating and tonifying the Heart-Yang, promoting the Blood circulation and relaxing the tendons. It has a sweet taste, which makes this herb move more slowly than the others; however, as it can tonify the Heart and its action lasts longer, the patient's condition can be improved more steadily. Besides treating Bi syndrome, it can also be used in Raynaud's disease, vasculitis, pulmonary heart disease, rheumatic heart disease, coronary heart disease and dysmenorrhea.

Except for Gui Zhi, the herbs are very poisonous, and especially Cao Wu. They must be used only after processing, and even then the dosage must be controlled carefully. Large dosage or long-term usage may consume the Yin and further injure the Yang, especially when the Yang of the internal organs is weak. Except for Gui Zhi, the herbs are pungent and hot. Moving quickly without staying tendency, they can activate the functions of the internal organs in a short time but the condition of the patient is not improved steadily. Therefore it is advisable to use them combined with sweet and warm herbs, which can tonify the Yang and Qi. Moreover, Chuan Wu and Cao Wu are incompatible with Chuan Bei Mu (*Fritillariae cirrhosae bulbus*), Zhe Bei Mu (*Fritillariae thunbergii bulbus*), Gua Lou (*Trichosanthis fructus*), Ban Xia (*Pinelliae rhizoma*), Bai Lian (*Ampelopsitis radix*) and Bai Ji (*Bletillae tuber*)**.

9 What are the differences in the function of tonifying the Liver and Kidney, strengthening the tendons and bones between Xu Duan (*Dipsaci radix*), Gu Sui Bu (*Drynariae rhizoma*), Sang Ji Sheng (*Taxilli herba*) and Gou Ji (*Cibotii rhizoma*)**?

All of these four herbs are bitter and warm, and enter the Liver and Kidney meridians. They have the function of expelling Wind-Dampness, tonifying the Liver and Kidney and strengthening the tendons and bones. They can treat chronic Bi syndrome which is characterized by stiff joints, sore and painful back and knees, weakness of the legs and difficulty with walking, but there are some differences between their functions.

In Chinese, '*Xu*' means 'successive', 'join' or 'add'; '*Duan*' means 'break'. Therefore the name Xu Duan suggests its function: it can invigorate the Blood, promote healing of the bones and tendons and it is especially suitable for treating trauma and fracture. Xu Duan also has the ability to strengthen the Directing (*Ren*) meridian and treat habitual miscarriage.

In Gu Sui Bu, '*Gu*' means 'bone', '*Sui*' means 'break' and '*Bu*' means 'supplement'. Like Xu Duan, Gu Sui Bu can promote Blood circulation, alleviate pain, and promote healing of the bones and tendons. It is warmer than Xu Duan and enters the Lower Jiao. It warms the Fire of the Gate of Vitality (*Ming Men*) and therefore can also be used for elderly people and patients who suffer from cold sensations in the back and feet, diarrhea, frequent urination, deafness, tinnitus and toothache.

Comparing Xu Duan with Gu Sui Bu, Xu Duan primarily enters the Liver meridian. It promotes healing of the tendons and strengthens them. Gu Sui Bu primarily enters the Kidney meridian and promotes healing of the bones and strengthens them.

Sang Ji Sheng is a gentle herb, neutral and moist; it can nourish the Blood, relax the tendons and is especially suitable for chronic Bi syndrome. It can also calm the fetus and is often used with Xu Duan to treat uterine bleeding in pregnancy and also for prevention of miscarriage.

In Gou Ji, 'Gou' means 'dog' and 'Ji' means 'spine', because the shape of this herb is like the spine of a dog. Gou Ji not only enters the Liver and Kidney meridians, but also enters the Governing (Du) meridian. It is especially effective for strengthening the bones, breaking up obstructions and treating stiffness, weakness and pain in the back or throughout the spinal column.

Because in chronic Bi syndrome both the Liver and Kidney are weak, and the bones, tendons and muscles are all involved in the pathological process, these herbs can be used together to strengthen the therapeutic effects.

10 What are the differences between Bai Hua She (Agkistrodon acutus)* and Wu Shao She (Zaocys)?

Bai Hua She and Wu Shao She are two species of snakes. Both enter the Liver meridian. It is believed that they can reach any part of the body, no matter how deep, because the snake has drilling and moving abilities. They have the ability to expel exogenous Wind from different areas of the body, no matter how deep and for how long the Wind remains. In clinical practice, they are important substances for treating chronic Wind Painful Obstruction syndrome, which is seen in hemiplegia after cerebrovascular accident, facial paralysis and other disorders, which are characterized by stiffness and cramping of the tendons, numbness of the muscles and tingling sensations of the limbs. They can also extinguish internal Wind, control spasms and convulsions, and are also used for epilepsy, convulsions in children and tetanus.

Bai Hua She is sweet, salty, warm and poisonous. Its action in expelling external Wind and extinguishing internal Wind is very strong and quick. Wu Shao She is sweet and neutral; its action is gentler and slower than that of Bai Hua She. In clinical practice, they are often used together to accentuate their effects. They are also often used together with Wu Gong (Scolopendra)* and Quan Xie (Scorpio)* to relieve spasm, and with Di Long (Pheretima) to open up the meridians and collaterals.

11 What are the characteristics of Hai Feng Teng (Piperis caulis), Qing Feng Teng (Sinomenii caulis), Luo Shi Teng (Trachelospermi caulis) and Sang Zhi (Mori ramulus)?

These four herbs are commonly used for expelling Wind-Dampness and unblocking the meridians. When symptoms of stiffness and pain in the joints and muscles are present, they can all be used. In TCM, similes and allegories are used to explain the complicated links between physiology and pathology, as well as the correlation between humans and the natural environment—for instance, the peel of the herb links with the skin; the core, the sprout, links with the Heart; the twig of the plant enters the limbs and meridians; the vine enters the meridians and collaterals. The first three herbs are considered to be the vines and Sang Zhi is the branch. These herbs work particularly on the meridians and collaterals. When Wind-Dampness obstructs the meridians and collaterals and the Qi and Blood fail to nourish and support the meridians and collaterals, the joints and muscles in the affected place become painful, stiff, heavy and numb. These four herbs are particularly suitable for treating such disorders.

Hai Feng Teng is pungent, bitter and slightly warm and enters the Liver and Kidney meridians. Pungency can disperse Dampness and Cold; bitterness can dry Dampness; warmth can scatter Cold and open up the meridians. This herb is usually used for Bi syndromes caused by Wind, Dampness and Cold; here the symptoms are characterized by cramping pain and stiffness in the limbs.

Qing Feng Teng and Sang Zhi are bitter and neutral herbs, and enter the Liver meridian. Both are used for Bi syndrome caused by Wind-Dampness, either with or without Heat or Cold signs. They are able not only to eliminate Dampness, but also to promote urination, which is especially useful when Bi syndrome is accompanied by symptoms such as edema and scanty urine. In addition, these two herbs can be administered in other ways. Qing Feng Teng alcohol drink can be used to reduce numbness, tingling sensations or itchy sensations in the muscles; Sang Zhi can be used in moxibustion to warm the meridian in the locality and expel Wind-Dampness.

Luo Shi Teng is bitter and slightly cold and enters the Heart, Liver and Kidney meridians. Compared with the other herbs in this group, it is more suitable for treating Hot Painful Obstruction syndrome and is especially used for Bi syndrome caused by Heat, Dampness and Wind when the joints and muscles are warm, swollen, contracted and painful.

Also, of these four herbs, Hai Feng Teng and Luo Shi Teng can regulate the Blood circulation. Hai Feng Teng opens up the meridians and can be used with other herbs that promote Blood circulation and treat pains caused by trauma. Luo Shi Teng can also be used to treat trauma, but its action is to cool the Blood, reduce congealed Blood and thereby alleviate pain and swelling.

12 What are the characteristics of Shen Jin Cao (*Lycopodii herba*) and Tou Gu Cao (*Tuberculate speranskia herba*)?

In Chinese, 'Shen' means 'stretching', 'Jin' means 'tendons' and 'Cao' means 'grass'. The name indicates the function of this herb. Although it is a pungent, bitter and warm herb, it is not dry in nature. It enters the Liver meridian and is especially effective for treating disorders of the tendons. It is able to expel Wind, open up the meridians, promote Blood circulation and relax the tendons. It is considered to be an important herb for the tendons. In clinical practice, it is mostly used for chronic Bi syndrome with contracted limbs, difficulty in movement, soreness of the tendons and bones and numbness of the skin. It is often used together with herbs that regulate the blood and tonify the Liver and Kidney.

In Chinese, 'Tou' means 'penetrate', 'Gu' means 'bone' and 'Cao' means 'grass'. As described in the name, Tou Gu Cao is able to reach the bones, expel Wind and eliminate Dampness from the bones. It is a bitter and warm herb and enters the Liver and Kidney meridians. In clinical practice, Tou Gu Cao can be applied when Wind, Dampness and Cold remain in the body for a very long time, and the tendons become very stiff and the joints and the bones are very painful. It is often

used together with herbs that tonify the Kidney and Liver and expel Wind, Cold and Dampness. Tou Gu Cao is also applied topically in lotions. If this herb is cooked with vinegar and the affected limb or joint is placed over the vapor for a considerable amount of time, it can treat spurs, such as spurs on the calcaneus.

13 What precautions should be observed when herbs that expel Wind, Cold and Dampness and treat Bi syndrome are used?

Wind, Cold and Dampness are common exogenous pathogenic factors and Bi syndrome is very commonly seen in clinical practice, so herbs that expel Wind, Cold and Dampness are frequently used. Because they are mostly warm, pungent and bitter, and have a drying nature, they should be used carefully when the patient has a condition of Yin, Blood or Body Fluid deficiency.

Some of these herbs have very good results in alleviating pain and relieving the suffering of the patient, but they are toxic herbs and overdose may lead to poisoning and even death. As toxicity is influenced by the growing habitat of the herbs, the method of processing and the patient's sensitivity, it may vary greatly. Another feature is that the toxic dose is very close to the therapeutic dose, so the dosage and therapeutic duration should be controlled carefully. Some patients think that herbs are natural products and have no side-effects or toxic effects, but this is not completely true. The important thing is to use them properly. There are cases of fatalities; one patient died after taking seven pieces of Ma Qian Zi (*Strychni semen*)* and another died because he doubled the dosage of the herbs himself due to severe pain. Thus it is worth mentioning the toxic herbs that are commonly used to alleviate pain and treat Bi syndrome. These are Fu Zi (*Aconiti radix lateralis preparata*)*, Chuan Wu (*Aconiti carmichaeli radix*)*, Cao Wu (*Aconiti kusnezoffii radix*)*, Ma Qian Zi (*Strychni semen*)*, Lei Gong Teng (*Tripterygii wilfordii caulis*)*, Xi Xin (*Asari herba*)*, Wei Ling Xian (*Clematidis radix*) and Bai Hua She (*Agkistrodon acutus*)*.

Comparisons of strength and temperature in herbs that expel Wind-Dampness

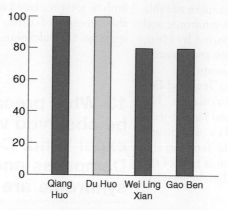

Fig. 5.1 • Comparison of the herbs that expel Wind, Dampness and Cold.
Qiang Huo (*Notopterygii rhizoma*), Du Huo (*Angelicae pubescentis radix*), Wei Ling Xian (*Clematidis radix*), Gao Ben (*Ligustici sinensis radix*).

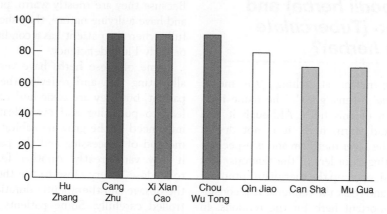

Fig. 5.2 • Comparison of the herbs that expel Wind-Dampness.
Hu Zhang (*Polygoni cuspidati rhizoma*), Cang Zhu (*Atractylodis rhizoma*), Xi Xian Cao (*Sigesbeckiae herba*), Chou Wu Tong (*Clerodendri folium*), Qin Jiao (*Gentianae macrophyllae radix*), Can Sha (*Bombycis mori excrementum*), Mu Gua (*Chaenomelis fructus*).

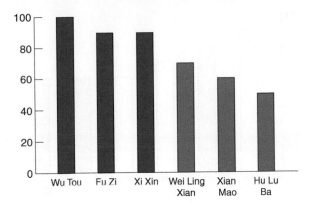

Fig. 5.3 • Comparison of the herbs that expel Cold-Dampness.
Wu Tou (*Aconiti radix*)*, Fu Zi (*Aconiti radix lateralis preparata*)*, Xi Xin (*Asari herba*)*, Wei Ling Xian (*Clematidis radix*), Xian Mao (*Curculinginis rhizoma*), Hu Lu Ba (*Trigonellae semen*).

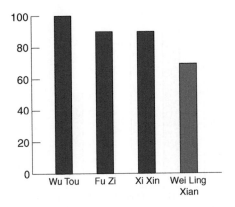

Fig. 5.4 • Comparison of the herbs that expel Cold-Dampness and stop pain.
Wu Tou (*Aconiti radix*)*, Fu Zi (*Aconiti radix lateralis preparata*)*, Xi Xin (*Asari herba*)*, Wei Ling Xian (*Clematidis radix*).

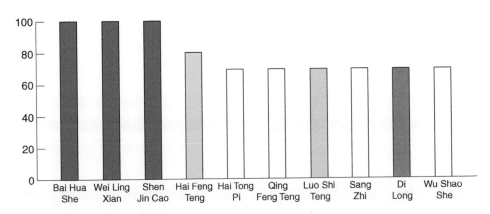

Fig. 5.5 • Comparison of the herbs that expel Wind-Dampness and open the meridians.
Bai Hua She (*Agkistrodon acutus*)*, Wei Ling Xian (*Clematidis radix*), Shen Jin Cao (*Lycopodii herba*), Hai Feng Teng (*Piperis caulis*), Hai Tong Pi (*Erythrinae cortex*), Qing Feng Teng (*Sinomenii caulis*), Luo Shi Teng (*Trachelospermi caulis*), Sang Zhi (*Mori ramulus*), Di Long (*Pheretima*), Wu Shao She (*Zaocys*).

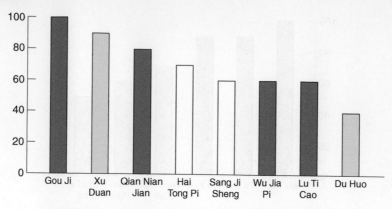

Fig. 5.6 • Comparison of the herbs that tonify the Kidney and Liver and expel Wind-Dampness.
Gou Ji (*Cibotii rhizoma*)**, Xu Duan (*Dipsaci radix*), Qian Nian Jian (*Homalomenae rhizoma*), Hai Tong Pi (*Erythrinae cortex*), Sang Ji Sheng (*Taxilli herba*), Wu Jia Pi (*Acanthopanacis cortex*), Lu Ti Cao (*Pyrola rotundifolia*), Du Huo (*Angelicae pubescentis radix*).

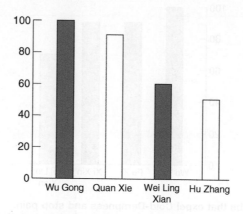

Fig. 5.7 • Comparison of the herbs that expel Wind and relieve pain.
Wu Gong (*Scolopendra*)*, Quan Xie (*Scorpio*)*, Wei Ling Xian (*Clematidis radix*), Hu Zhang (*Polygoni cuspidati rhizoma*).

Chapter **Six**

Herbs that transform Dampness

祛湿药

1 What are the indications for herbs that transform and drain Dampness? What are the characteristics of the syndrome of Dampness accumulation?

Herbs that transform and drain Dampness are used for treating syndromes of accumulation of Dampness in the body. These syndromes are usually due to disturbance of the water metabolism, which is a result of dysfunction of the Lung, Spleen, Kidney, Bladder or San Jiao meridians.

The symptoms of Dampness accumulation are edema, scanty and difficult urination, retention of urine, fullness of the chest, a large amount of phlegm, asthma, distension of the abdomen, diarrhea, pain in the joints and heaviness of the body. If Dampness is complicated with Heat in the Middle or Lower Jiao, then disorders such as jaundice, skin diseases and infections from various pathogenic microorganisms may be present.

Dampness is a Yin pathogenic factor and it has a stagnating tendency. This characteristic is shown not only by the symptoms, such as heaviness, fullness and numbness of the body, but also by a lingering, recurrent or chronic course to the disease.

If Dampness is complicated by other pathogenic factors, especially Heat, it will be very difficult to separate these out because to clear Heat may injure the Spleen-Yang and increase Dampness, and to remove Dampness may injure the Yin and increase Heat, so the course of treatment will be longer than if treating disorders caused by only one exogenous pathogenic factor.

2 What are the characteristics of the herbs that transform and drain out Dampness? What precautions should be observed in the use of these herbs?

Herbs that transform and drain Dampness are able to eliminate it by promoting urination and reducing the accumulation of water; therefore they can treat those syndromes and symptoms caused by the accumulation of Dampness or water. These herbs have the following characteristics.

Bland taste

Since a bland taste has the ability to leach out Dampness by promoting urination, most of the herbs that increase urination and drain out Dampness are bland, including Fu Ling (*Poria*), Zhu Ling (*Polyporus*), Ze Xie (*Alismatis rhizoma*), Hua Shi (*Talcum*), Yi Yi Ren (*Coicis semen*), Tong Cao (*Tetrapanacis medulla*), Che Qian Zi (*Plantaginis semen*) and Deng Xin Cao (*Junci medulla*).

Sweet, bland and cold

Blandness has the ability to leach out water or Dampness and it has a descending tendency in action. Cold can clear Heat, and sweetness and Cold can generate the Yin and Body Fluids, which may have been injured by pathogenic Heat or by the draining action of some herbs. These herbs are suitable for treating water accumulation that is complicated with Heat, especially when the accumulation is in the Lower Jiao. Sweet-bland-cold herbs are also suitable for situations where draining actions are required in this area. The commonly used herbs in this category are Hua Shi, Yi Yi Ren, Tong Cao, Deng Xin Cao, Zhu Ling, Ze Xie and Che Qian Zi.

Sweet, bitter and cold

Some of the herbs are sweet, bitter and cold in nature. They are excellent herbs for treating Damp-Heat accumulation. Because bitterness can dry Dampness and direct Fire downwards, sweetness can tonify the body, and Cold can clear Heat, the bitter-cold nature of these herbs can strongly reduce Heat, and their sweet-cold nature can generate the Yin and Body Fluids, which may have been injured by pathogenic Heat or by the draining action of some herbs. These herbs can be used for a longer period of time than the bitter-cold herbs that dry Dampness and clear Heat. The commonly used herbs are Di Fu Zi (*Kochiae fructus*), Shi Wei (*Pyrrosiae folium*) and Jin Qian Cao (*Lysimachiae herba*).

Entering the Bladder, Kidney and Small Intestine meridians

Because, according to TCM, urination is carried out by the Kidney, the Bladder and the Small Intestine, most of the herbs enter these meridians. They also enter other meridians such as the Lung, Spleen and Large Intestine. They can also regulate the function of these organs and meridians and improve water metabolism.

Moreover, some herbs that drain Dampness can open up meridians and collaterals. They also have the function of increasing the secretion of milk and therefore treat lactation problems.

Herbs that transform and drain out Dampness should be used with caution. Generally speaking, they are suitable only for treating Excess syndromes.

In treatment, herbs that regulate the Liver-Qi or the Qi of the San Jiao meridian should also be used because Qi stagnation may directly obstruct the water passage and cause water accumulation. Furthermore, in treating accumulation of Dampness caused by weakness of the Qi and Yang of the Heart, Lung, Spleen and Kidney, herbs that drain out Dampness can be prescribed only if they are combined with herbs that tonify the Yang and Qi.

Herbs that treat Cold-Dampness have a pungent-warm, bitter-warm or bland nature, and they should be used with caution because they can consume the Yin if they are used in large dosage and for a long period of time. The herbs that treat Damp-Heat have a bitter and cold nature, which can injure the Yang of Spleen and that may increase the dampness accumulation. Therefore, the dosage and treatment period should be carefully considered. Moreover, pregnant women should use these herbs with caution as these aromatic, pungent, bitter and bland herbs can activate Qi and Blood, and the bitter and bland herbs usually move downwards. These actions may bring danger to the pregnancy.

3 What are the commonly used methods for eliminating Dampness?

Dampness is one of the six exogenous pathogenic factors. It is also a pathological product caused by disorder of water metabolism in the body. The associated organs are the Kidney, Bladder, Small Intestine, Spleen, Lung and San Jiao. To eliminate the accumulation of Dampness or water, there are several possibilities. The commonly used strategies are as follows.

Promoting urination and leaching out Dampness

Bland or bland-sweet-cold herbs, which enter the Bladder, Small Intestine and Kidney meridians, can promote urination and reduce accumulation of water or Dampness directly. They are particularly suitable for use where there is water accumulation in the Lower Jiao. The commonly used herbs are Fu Ling (*Poria*) and Ze Xie (*Alismatis rhizoma*).

Drying Dampness

Pungent-bitter-warm herbs can dry Dampness directly. They are particularly suitable when water or Dampness accumulates in the Middle Jiao. The commonly used herbs are Cang Zhu (*Atractylodis rhizoma*), Hou Po (*Magnoliae cortex*), Ban Xia (*Pinelliae rhizoma*) and Du Huo (*Angelicae pubescentis radix*).

Bitter-cold herbs are able to clear Heat and dry Dampness and they are often used for transforming Damp-Heat. Examples are Huang Qin (*Scutellariae radix*), Huang Lian (*Coptidis rhizoma*), Huang Bai (*Phellodendri cortex*) and Zhi Zi (*Gardeniae fructus*).

Expelling Dampness

Pungent herbs have the function of expelling Wind and can also disperse and transform Dampness. These herbs can be used alone if the Dampness accumulates in the Upper Jiao. They can also be used in combination with other methods for treating Dampness in the Middle Jiao and Lower Jiao. The commonly used herbs are Fang Feng (*Saposhnikoviae radix*), Qin Jiao (*Gentianae macrophyllae radix*) and Qiang Huo (*Notopterygii rhizoma*).

Aromatically transforming Dampness

Because aromatic herbs can penetrate turbidity, revive the Spleen and transform Dampness, they are particularly suitable for situations where Dampness obstructs the sense orifices. These herbs are Huo Xiang (*Agastachis herba*), Pei Lan (*Eupatorii herba*), Cao Guo (*Tsaoko fructus*), Sha Ren (*Amomi xanthioidis fructus*) and Qing Hao (*Artemisiae annuae herba*).

Strengthening the function of the Spleen and transforming Dampness

Herbs that tonify the Qi of the Spleen so as to strengthen the function of water transportation and transformation are often used in a Dampness syndrome; examples are Bai Zhu (*Atractylodis macrocephalae rhizoma*) and Huang Qi (*Astragali radix*).

Warming the Kidney-Yang and 'steaming' the Dampness

Pungent-hot herbs that enter the Kidney meridian are able to strengthen the Kidney-Yang, to 'steam' the water, to separate the clean water from the turbid part and accelerate the water metabolism. They are often used for chronic or severe cases of accumulation of water or Dampness in the body. The commonly used herbs are Fu Zi (*Aconiti radix lateralis preparata*)*, Rou Gui (*Cinnamomi cassiae cortex*) and Wu Yao (*Linderae radix*).

Warming the Spleen-Yang and transforming Dampness

Pungent-hot herbs that enter the Spleen meridian are able to strengthen the Spleen-Yang, accelerate the transportation and transformation of the Spleen, and therefore transform Dampness. The commonly used herbs are Sheng Jiang (*Zingiberis rhizoma recens*) and Gan Jiang (*Zingiberis rhizoma*).

Dispersing the Lung-Qi and regulating the water passage

Since water is moved by the Qi in the body, herbs that can disperse the Lung-Qi can also disperse Dampness; examples are Ma Huang (*Ephedrae herba*)* and Jie Geng (*Platycodi radix*).

For the same reason, herbs that direct the Lung-Qi to descend can also be used to regulate the passage of water and eliminate Dampness; examples include Sang Bai Pi (*Mori cortex*), Xing Ren (*Xing Ren*) and Ting Li Zi (*Lepidii/Descurainiae semen*).

Promoting the Qi movement and eliminating Dampness

Since the movement of Qi can accelerate water metabolism, herbs that promote Qi movement can treat accumulation of Dampness. This strategy is often combined with other methods. The commonly used herbs are Xiang Fu (*Cyperi rhizoma*), Chen Pi (*Citri reticulatae pericarpium*), Da Fu Pi (*Arecae pericarpium*) and Hou Po (*Magnoliae cortex*).

4 Fu Ling (*Poria*) can promote urination, tonify the Spleen and calm the Mind. What are its characteristics compared with other herbs which have the same function?

Fu Ling is sweet, bland and neutral, and enters the Heart, Spleen, Stomach, Lung and Kidney meridians. It is able to drain out Dampness by promoting urination. It can also tonify the Spleen and calm the Mind.

Compared with the other herbs that transform Dampness, Fu Ling is characterized by being used for both Damp-Heat and Damp-Cold syndromes to promote urination and drain out Dampness; this is because it is bland and neutral in nature. Because it is sweet and bland, it drains out Dampness without the side-effect of injuring the Yin and Yang of the body. In clinical practice, it is often used for treating accumulation of water and Dampness in the Middle or Upper Jiao, manifesting as edema, heaviness of the body and difficult urination, such as in the diseases of the Kidney, Lung, Liver and Heart.

Comparing Fu Ling with other herbs that tonify the Spleen, its neutral and gentle nature brings this herb its characteristic actions: Fu Ling is white in color and has no taste; it has a gentle action of tonifying the Spleen-Qi but is without a cloying nature. It can therefore be used for treating chronic disorders and for people who have a weak constitution and are very sensitive to the tastes of most herbs. For the same reason, this herb is also recommended in prescriptions for children. It is also an ideal herb for putting in biscuits, cakes, soup or porridge and using in the diet over a longer period of time. Another characteristic of Fu Ling is that it not only tonifies the Spleen, but also transforms Dampness and moves it downwards. Unlike most of the tonifying herbs, which place extra burden on the Stomach and must be used with herbs that regulate the Qi, Fu Ling can be used alone without any side-effects. It is especially useful in patients suffering from edema, difficult urination and diarrhea caused by Spleen deficiency.

Comparing Fu Ling with other herbs that calm the Mind, it is most suitable for treating restlessness, palpitations and insomnia due to deficiency of the Heart-Qi and Spleen-Qi. These patients may also suffer from poor appetite, tiredness, excessive thinking, depression and restless sleep. In most cases, there is a history of chronic disease or long-term mental stress. Fu Ling has no special taste, so it is a good herb for children suffering from restless sleep, crying at night and indigestion.

5 What are the differences between Fu Ling (*Poria*), Fu Ling Pi (*Poriae cocos cortex*), Fu Shen (*Poriae cocos pararadicis*) and Chi Fu Ling (*Poriae cocos rubrae*)?

Fu Ling is sweet, bland and neutral, and enters the Heart, Spleen, Stomach, Lung and Kidney meridi-ans. It is able to drain out Dampness by promoting urination, and tonifies the Spleen. It can also calm the Mind gently.

Fu Ling Pi is the peel of Fu Ling. Unlike Fu Ling, it does not have the function of tonifying the Spleen and calming the Mind, but it is especially effective for transforming Dampness in the skin and subcutaneous regions by promoting urination; therefore it can treat edema and puffiness.

The parts of the fungus around the root are called Fu Shen. Fu Shen has the same function as Fu Ling, but its effect in calming the Mind is stronger, which is why it has 'Shen', meaning 'Mind' or 'Spirit', in its name.

Chi Fu Ling means, in Chinese, 'the red Fu Ling'. In fact, it is completely different from Fu Ling. Although it can promote urination and treat water accumulation in the Lower Jiao, it is cold in nature and is used to treat Damp-Heat syndrome. It cannot tonify the Spleen, nor calm the Mind.

6 Fu Ling (*Poria*), Zhu Ling (*Polyporus*), Ze Xie (*Alismatis rhizoma*) and Yi Yi Ren (*Coicis semen*) are all sweet and bland, and are able to transform and drain out Dampness. What are the differences between the four herbs?

Fu Ling, Zhu Ling, Ze Xie and Yi Yi Ren are all sweet and bland. Sweetness can tonify the body and blandness can drain out Dampness. These four herbs are characterized by being able to drain out Dampness without the side-effects of consuming the Yin and Qi of the body. All four can be used for the situations where Dampness accumulates in the Middle Jiao and Lower Jiao, obstructing the Qi and water passage. Manifestations of this condition are distension of the abdomen, feelings of heaviness in the body, edema in the legs and difficult urination or retention of urine. In clinical practice, the four herbs can be used for ascites, edema and oliguria due to disease of the heart, liver or kidney.

However, there are some differences in their strengths. For promoting urination and draining out

Dampness, Zhu Ling has the strongest action, followed by Ze Xie, then Fu Ling; Yi Yi Ren is the weakest. For tonifying the Spleen and transforming Dampness, Fu Ling is most powerful, followed by Yi Yi Ren, then Ze Xie; Zhu Ling does not have the function of tonifying the Spleen. Moreover, although both Fu Ling and Yi Yi Ren are able to tonify the Spleen, transform Dampness in the Middle Jiao and treat edema and diarrhea, there are still some differences between them. Fu Ling is a neutral herb and it can be applied for either Damp-Heat or Damp-Cold syndromes. It is used more often for syndromes of Dampness accumulation with deficiency of the Spleen-Qi. In clinical practice, it is more suitable for treating chronic gastritis, colitis, malnutrition and chronic hepatitis. Yi Yi Ren is slightly cold and is more suitable for treating syndromes of Damp-Heat accumulation in the Middle Jiao. The symptoms and signs of this include afternoon fever, lower-grade fever, heaviness of the body, diarrhea, a sticky and yellowish tongue coating and a soft, rapid pulse. In clinical practice, it can be used to treat acute enteritis, dysentery, colitis and hepatitis.

Zhu Ling and Ze Xie enter the Kidney and Bladder meridians, and they can treat Dampness accumulation in the Lower Jiao. However, Zhu Ling only has the function of promoting urination and draining out Dampness and is used to treat edema and difficult urination. Ze Xie not only promotes urination but also reduces Empty-Fire from the Kidney and is suitable for treating cystitis and urinary tract infection during menopause.

Of the four herbs, Fu Ling and Yi Yi Ren have a wider range of functions than Zhu Ling and Ze Xie. Fu Ling also enters the Heart, Spleen and Stomach meridians. It has the function of calming the Mind and can be used for treating restlessness, palpitations, restless sleep and pensiveness due to deficiency of the Spleen-Qi and Heart-Qi. Yi Yi Ren can clear Heat and transform pus. It is often used for treating pulmonary abscess and many kinds of infections of the intestine. Nowadays, it is also used in formulas of treating cancers if combined with other herbs. Since Yi Yi Ren enters the Spleen meridian and clears Damp-Heat, it can also be used to treat Hot-Bi syndrome, which is characterized by swollen, warm and painful joints, and heaviness and numbness of the limbs. It is also a commonly used herb to treat skin disorders caused by Damp-Heat; the skin lesions are itchy, weepy and red, such as in eczema.

7 Mu Tong (*Mutong caulis*)* and Tong Cao (*Tetrapanacis medulla*) can both promote urination, drain Damp-Heat and promote lactation. What are the differences between them?

Mu Tong and Tong Cao can both promote urination and drain out Dampness. Both are often used for treating edema and retention of urine as well as scanty, painful, frequent and difficult urination due to Damp-Heat accumulation, such as in acute urinary tract infection, cystitis, pyelitis and prostatitis. Both are also able to promote lactation and are used for insufficient lactation after giving birth.

However, Mu Tong is bitter and cold, and enters the Heart and Small Intestine meridians. It characteristically promotes urination and drains Heat from the Heart via the Small Intestine. Its action in clearing Fire and draining out Dampness is stronger than that of Tong Cao. It is particularly effective for treating Painful Urinary Dysfunction syndrome where the Fire is transmitted from the Heart to the Small Intestine. Since Heart-Fire is often caused by the Liver-Fire, Mu Tong is more suitable for treating urinary disorders which start or worsen under stress and are accompanied by irritability, insomnia, ulceration on the tongue, a bitter taste in the mouth and thirst.

Tong Cao is sweet, bland and cold. It enters the Spleen and Stomach meridians and it is light in nature. Cold can reduce Heat and blandness can promote urination and leach out Dampness. Its action of draining out Dampness and reducing Heat is gentler than that of Mu Tong. It is used only when the Qi and water accumulate in the Lower Jiao. However, compared with Mu Tong, it has less potential to injure the Qi, Yang and Yin as it is not bitter and cold, but sweet and cold, and so it can be used for a longer period of time.

Both Mu Tong and Tong Cao can promote lactation, but Mu Tong achieves this by opening up the meridians and promoting Blood circulation, thereby promoting lactation. Tong Cao enters the Stomach meridian (which passes through the breasts) and then enters the Qi level; it stimulates lactation by promoting the Qi movement. Mu Tong and Tong

Cao are often used together to promote Qi movement and Blood circulation in order to promote lactation.

In addition, since Mu Tong can open up the meridians and promote Blood circulation, it is also used for treating Damp-Heat in the meridians, such as in Hot-Bi syndrome, which manifests as heaviness and numbness of the limbs, and swollen, warm and painful joints. It can also be used for irregular menstruation caused by Damp-Heat in the Lower Jiao and stagnation of the Blood. Tong Cao can clear Heat from the Lung as well as increasing urination.

Mu Tong has, in fact, several names that sound similar. Special attention should be paid to Guan Mu Tong (*Hocquartiae manshurensis caulis*)* which can cause serious kidney damage. It is banned in Western countries and in China. It can be replaced by Chuan Mu Tong (*Clematidis armandii caulis*) or Wu Ye Mu Tong (*Akebiae caulis*) with careful control of both the Chinese names and the Latin equivalents.

8 What are the functions of and differences between Han Fang Ji (*Stephaniae tetrandrae radix*) and Mu Fang Ji (*Aristolochiae fangchi radix*)*?

Han Fang Ji and Mu Fang Ji are very bitter, cold and pungent, and enter the Bladder, Lung and Spleen meridians. Bitterness and Cold can reduce Heat and drain out Dampness. Pungency can expel Wind and alleviate pain. Both herbs are used for eliminating Damp-Heat in the Lower Jiao at the Blood level, promoting urination, and reducing edema and oliguria in pulmonary heart disease, rheumatic heart disease and nephritis. They can also be used for treating painful, swollen and heavy joints and limbs in rheumatic fever. Comparing the functions of these two herbs, Han Fang Ji is stronger in promoting urination and reducing edema; Mu Fang Ji is stronger in expelling Wind and Dampness so as to alleviate pain.

In addition, Mu Fang Ji is considered to be a toxic herb which may lead to serious kidney damage, especially when it is used for a long period of time and with a wrong combination in a formula. It is banned both in Western countries and in China.

9 Yin Chen Hao (*Artemisiae scopariae herba*) and Qing Hao (*Artemisiae annuae herba*) are both able to transform Damp-Heat, reduce low-grade fever and relieve jaundice. What are the differences between them?

Yin Chen Hao and Qing Hao are bitter and cold and have a light, fragrant smell. Both are commonly used for transforming Damp-Heat, eliminating Exterior Damp-Heat and treating symptoms such as heaviness of the head, body and limbs, a sense of constriction in the chest, nausea, loss of appetite, distension in the abdomen and intermittent fever and chills. These symptoms are often seen in sunstroke, summer cold infections, influenza, acute enteritis and dysentery. Both of them can clear Damp-Heat from the Liver and Gall Bladder and relieve jaundice in hepatitis or malaria, in which Damp-Heat accumulates in the Middle Jiao and disturbs the secretion of bile. These two herbs can also reduce low-grade fever and are used for Interior disorders, but the functions and applications are different.

Yin Chen Hao is bitter and slightly cold. Its light and fragrant smell can penetrate the turbid Damp-Heat and separate the Dampness from the Heat. Since Yin Chen Hao enters the Spleen, Stomach, Liver and Gall Bladder meridians, it is particularly effective for treating Damp-Heat accumulation in these organs and meridians. It treats low-grade fever, in which patients complain that their temperature is not high but nevertheless they feel warm inside and the warmth does not radiate to the outside; these symptoms indicate the Heat is constrained by Dampness. Patients may also have symptoms and signs such as tightness in the chest, distension in the abdomen, a white or yellow sticky tongue coating and a soft pulse. Moreover, Yin Chen Hao is also the most important herb for relieving jaundice when Damp-Heat obstructs the bile secretion and the bile is pressed into the Blood. Therefore it is often used for treating acute hepatitis, cholecystolithiasis, angiocholitis, cholecystitis and hemolytic jaundice.

Qing Hao is also a bitter and cold herb, and it is colder than Yin Chen Hao. It also has a light and fragrant smell, but it particularly penetrates into the Blood and Yin levels and disperses Heat there. It also enters the Liver and Gall Bladder meridians and is effective for clearing Heat in these organs and meridians. Compared with Yin Chen Hao, which reduces low-grade fever, it is especially effective for reducing Heat in the Blood and Yin levels when the Blood and Yin have been injured by Heat because its light and fragrant smell can disperse and bring Heat out of the deep layers of the body. It is more often used when patients feel 'bone steaming' and low-grade fever only at night. In this situation, patients have a red tongue body with no coating and a thready, rapid pulse. Compared with Yin Chen Hao, its effect in cooling the Blood and reducing Empty-Heat in treating lower-grade fever is stronger, but it is weaker than Yin Chen Hao in reducing low-grade fever due to Damp-Heat. It can also be used to relieve jaundice in malaria; artemisin, which is extracted from Qing Hao, is able to kill the malaria parasite in vitro so as to reduce jaundice.

Dysfunction syndrome caused by Damp-Heat in which the Heat is more pronounced than the Dampness. The symptoms are very scanty, dark urine, blood in the urine, painful and burning sensations during micturition, irritability, a bitter taste in the mouth, a red tongue without coating, and a wiry and rapid pulse.

Bi Xie is bitter and neutral and enters the Liver, Stomach and Bladder meridians. It does not have the function of clearing Heat, but it is able to separate Dampness from Heat and the clean part of water from the turbid part; it is also good at eliminating Dampness. Bi Xie is particularly used for treating cloudy urine or a large amount of leukorrhea due to Dampness accumulation in the Lower Jiao. In clinical practice, this herb is often used for chronic nephritis. Furthermore, its preparation has an inhibitory effect against some intestinal parasites and many pathogenic fungi.

10 Bian Xu (*Polygoni avicularis herba*), Qu Mai (*Dianthi herba*) and Bi Xie (*Dioscoreae hypoglaucae rhizoma*) can be used in treating Painful Urinary Dysfunction syndrome. What are the differences between them?

Bian Xu, Qu Mai and Bi Xie are all able to promote urination, drain out Dampness and treat Painful Urinary Dysfunction syndrome, which is characterized by frequent, urgent, difficult and painful urination. But there are differences between these three herbs.

Bian Xu is bitter, slightly cold and enters the Stomach and Bladder meridians. Bitterness and Cold can clear Heat and drain out Dampness. It is good at clearing Heat and transforming Dampness when Dampness and Heat are both strong in the Lower Jiao. The manifestations of this condition are difficult and painful urination, scanty urine, a red tongue with a yellow sticky coating and a soft pulse.

Qu Mai is bitter and cold and enters the Blood level of the Heart, Kidney, Small Intestine and Bladder meridians. It is able to clear Heat and cool the Blood in the Small Intestine and drain out Heat. It is especially effective for treating Painful Urinary

11 Qu Mai (*Dianthi herba*), Shi Wei (*Pyrrosiae folium*), Hai Jin Sha (*Lygodii spora*) and Jin Qian Cao (*Lysimachiae herba*) can be used for Blood-Painful Urinary Dysfunction syndrome. What are the differences between them?

These four herbs are able to promote urination and clear Damp-Heat and are used especially for treating Blood-Painful Urinary Dysfunction syndrome when the Damp-Heat in the Lower Jiao has injured the blood vessels. In clinical practice, they are used in the treatment of urinary tract dysfunction, cystitis, cystolithiasis, pyelitis, nephrolithiasis and ureterolithiasis. However, each herb has its own characteristics, thus they are often used together to enhance the therapeutic effects.

Qu Mai is bitter and cold and enters the Blood level. It can strongly reduce Heat from the Heart and Small Intestine and drain out Heat. It is a commonly used herb for treating Painful Urinary Dysfunction syndrome when the Heat is pronounced and has injured the blood vessels.

Shi Wei is sweet, bitter and slightly cold and enters the Lung and Bladder meridians. It can clear Heat from the Lung and regulate the water passage; therefore it can regulate the function of the Bladder. As it can also stop bleeding, it is often chosen to treat Blood-Painful Urinary Dysfunction syndrome.

Hai Jin Sha is sweet, salty and cold and enters the Small Intestine and Bladder meridians. It can clear Heat and transform Dampness by promoting urination. As it is particularly effective for relieving pain in the urinary tract, it can be used for different types of Painful Urinary Dysfunction syndrome. Since pain is pronounced in the Blood- and Stone-Painful Urinary Dysfunction syndromes, Hai Jin Sha is very often used in these two types of disorder.

Jin Qian Cao is bitter, pungent, cool and slightly salty. It enters the Lung, Liver and Gall Bladder meridians. It is able to promote urination and eliminate stones, therefore it can stop bleeding. It is especially suitable for use in Stone-Painful Urinary Dysfunction syndrome when there is blood in the urine.

12 Which herbs can regulate the function of the Bladder and promote urination? What are the applications? How should one use them in clinical practice?

The herbs that regulate the function of the Bladder and promote urination are Fu Ling (*Poria*), Zhu Ling (*Polyporus*), Ze Xie (*Alismatis rhizoma*), Han Fang Ji (*Stephaniae tetrandrae radix*), Hua Shi (*Talcum*), Di Fu Zi (*Kochiae fructus*), Bian Xu (*Polygoni avicularis herba*), Bi Xie (*Dioscoreae hypoglaucae rhizoma*), Shi Wei (*Pyrrosiae folium*), Hai Jin Sha (*Lygodii spora*), Dong Kui Zi (*Malvae semen*) and Che Qian Zi (*Plantaginis semen*).

The indications for using these herbs are edema, retention of urine, oliguria, distension in the abdomen and heaviness of the limbs; the tongue coating is white and the pulse is soft. In clinical practice, these herbs are used for edema, ascites, oliguria and retention of urine in chronic nephritis, diseases of the lung and liver and renal failure or heart failure.

In order to increase the therapeutic effects, these herbs are often used with herbs that regulate the Qi of the Lung and Spleen, regulate the San Jiao water passage, and tonify the Qi and Yang of the Spleen

and Kidney to treat the causes of water accumulation.

13 Which herbs can clear Heat from the Heart and Small Intestine and promote urination? What are the indications for them?

The herbs that clear Heat from the Heart and Small Intestine and drain out Damp-Heat by promoting urination are Mu Tong (*Mutong caulis*)*, Zhi Zi (*Gardeniae fructus*), Qu Mai (*Dianthi herba*), Deng Xin Cao (*Junci medulla*), Dan Zhu Ye (*Lophatheri herba*), Yu Mi Xu (*Maydis stigma*) and Chi Xiao Dou (*Phaseoli semen*).

The indications for using these herbs are irritability, restlessness, thirst, a bitter taste in the mouth, scanty or bloody urine and painful and difficult micturition. The tongue is red with a yellow coating and the pulse is rapid, wiry and slippery. In clinical practice, these herbs are used for treating acute urinary tract infection, cystitis, pyelitis, acute prostatitis and painful and difficult urination in menopausal syndrome.

14 Which herbs can clear Heat from the Lung and promote urination? What are the indications for them?

The herbs that clear Heat from the Lung and promote urination are Shi Wei (*Pyrrosiae folium*), Ban Bian Lian (*Lobelia chinensis herba*), Tong Cao (*Tetrapanacis medulla*), Dong Gua Zi (*Benincasae semen*), Han Fang Ji (*Stephaniae tetrandrae radix*), Sang Bai Pi (*Mori cortex*) and Ting Li Zi (*Lepidii/ Descurainiae semen*).

The indications for using these herbs are coughing with phlegm, wheezing, asthma, edema and difficult urination. The tongue is red with a white coating and the pulse is rapid and superficial, especially in the region of the Lung. The symptoms are caused by obstruction of the Lung-Qi and the Bladder-Qi. In clinical practice, these herbs can be used in asthma, chronic bronchitis, pulmonary emphysema, acute nephritis, pulmonary heart disease, rheumatic heart disease and heart failure.

15 Which herbs can regulate the Spleen, promote urination and drain out Dampness? What are the indications for them?

The herbs that can regulate the function of the Spleen and eliminate Dampness by promoting urination are Fu Ling (*Poria*), Yi Yi Ren (*Coicis semen*), Tong Cao (*Tetrapanacis medulla*), Bi Xie (*Dioscoreae hypoglaucae rhizoma*) and Da Fu Pi (*Arecae pericarpium*).

The indications for using these herbs are scanty urine, retention of urine, difficult urination, edema (especially in the legs), ascites, a large amount of leukorrhea, diarrhea, lack of appetite and heaviness of the body. The tongue is flabby with a thick white coating, and the pulse is soft. In clinical practice, these herbs can be used for chronic prostatitis, chronic pelvic inflammatory disease, chronic hepatitis, nephritis and nephritic syndrome.

16 Which herbs can transform Damp-Heat in the Middle Jiao and Lower Jiao and are used for treating skin diseases and infections? Huang Qin (*Scutellariae radix*), Huang Lian (*Coptidis rhizoma*), Huang Bai (*Phellodendri cortex*) and Long Dan Cao (*Gentianae radix*) are also able to remove Damp-Heat and treat these disorders. What are the differences between these two groups of herbs?

Some herbs that can transform Dampness in the Middle Jiao and Lower Jiao are particularly useful for treating skin diseases and infections. The commonly used herbs are Fu Ling (*Poria*), Yi Yi Ren (*Coicis semen*), Bian Xu (*Polygoni avicularis herba*) and Di Fu Zi (*Kochiae fructus*). These herbs, as well as Huang Qin, Huang Lian, Huang Bai and Long Dan

Cao, are often used in conditions where there is accumulation of Damp-Heat in the Middle Jiao and Lower Jiao, and can treat skin diseases characterized by red, itchy and weepy skin lesions and infections caused by pathogenic microorganisms, including eczema, tinea, pemphigus, herpes zoster, trichomonas vaginitis, monilial vaginitis and vulvitis. However, there are some differences between these two groups of herbs.

First of all, they have different tastes and enter different meridians. The herbs in the first group are mainly bland and cold in nature, and enter the Bladder meridian. In treating Damp-Heat, their action is primarily that of leaching out Damp-Heat by promoting urination because Dampness and Heat are not very easy to separate. The herbs in the second group are very bitter and cold, and enter the Heart, Liver, Stomach and Bladder meridians. Their action is primarily that of strongly reducing Heat and drying Dampness in the Middle or Lower Jiao. They cannot directly leach out Damp-Heat by promoting urination.

Secondly, their strengths and speeds are different. The herbs in the first group, which leach out Dampness, are not harsh or strong in their action of eliminating Damp-Heat and so they can be used for a long period of time. The herbs in the second group, which clear Heat and dry Dampness, are very cold and bitter and can remove Damp-Heat quickly and intensively, but they can injure the Yang and the Qi in the Middle Jiao and Lower Jiao if the dosage is too large or they are used too long.

17 Which herbs can transform Damp-Heat from the Middle Jiao and reduce jaundice? What are the indications for them?

The herbs that transform Damp-Heat in the Middle Jiao and reduce jaundice are Yin Chen Hao (*Artemisiae scopariae herba*), Qing Hao (*Artemisiae annuae herba*), Jin Qian Cao (*Lysimachiae herba*), Yu Jin (*Curcumae radix*), Chi Xiao Dou (*Phaseoli semen*) and Da Huang (*Rhei rhizoma*).

The indications for applying these herbs are jaundice, tightness in the chest, distension of the abdomen, poor appetite, difficult bowel movement, tiredness, heaviness of the body and a low-grade fever. The tongue color is normal or slightly red with a sticky and yellow coating and the pulse is soft. In clinical practice, these herbs can be used for hemolytic jaundice, hepatic jaundice and obstructive jaundice.

18 Which herbs can be used for increasing lactation and what are the indications for them?

The herbs that are used for increasing lactation are Mu Tong (*Mutong caulis*)*, Tong Cao (*Tetrapanacis medulla*), Dong Kui Zi (*Malvae semen*) and Wang Bu Liu Xing (*Vaccariae semen*).

The indications for applying these herbs are problems with milk production caused by Liver-Qi stagnation and obstruction of the Stomach meridians and collaterals. There may be tenderness of the breasts or a primary stage of mastitis. A yellow tongue coating and a wiry pulse are often seen in this condition.

To treat lactation problems due to Qi and Blood deficiency, these herbs can be combined with some

that tonify the Qi and Blood, such as Huang Qi (*Astragali radix*) and Dang Gui (*Angelicae sinensis radix*). In this condition, the indications are milk lactation without tenderness of the breasts, tiredness, dizziness, a pale complexion, a pale tongue and a thready and weak pulse.

19 Which herbs can cool the Blood and treat Blood-Painful Urinary Dysfunction syndrome? What are the indications for them?

The herbs that cool the Blood and stop bleeding, as well as promoting urination, to treat Blood-Painful Urinary Dysfunction syndrome are Shi Wei (*Pyrrosiae folium*), Qu Mai (*Dianthi herba*), Xiao Ji (*Cirsii herba*), Bai Mao Gen (*Imperatae rhizoma*) and Zhi Zi (*Gardeniae fructus*).

The indications for using these herbs are painful and frequent urination, macroscopic or microscopic blood in the urine and pain in the lower abdomen and back. The tongue is red with a thin coating and the pulse is rapid and slippery.

Comparisons of strength and temperature in herbs that transform Dampness

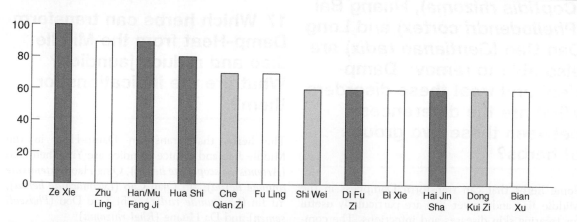

Fig. 6.1 • Comparison of the herbs that regulate the Bladder and promote urination.
Ze Xie (*Alismatis rhizoma*), Zhu Ling (*Polyporus*), Han/Mu Fang Ji (*Stephaniae tetrandrae radix/Aristolochiae fangchi radix*), Hua Shi (*Talcum*), Che Qian Zi (*Plantaginis semen*), Fu Ling (*Poria*), Shi Wei (*Pyrrosiae folium*), Di Fu Zi (*Kochiae fructus*), Bi Xie (*Dioscoreae hypoglaucae rhizoma*), Hai Jin Sha (*Lygodii spora*), Dong Kui Zi (*Malvae semen*), Bian Xu (*Polygoni avicularis herba*).

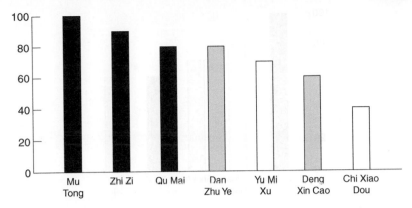

Fig. 6.2 • Comparison of the herbs that regulate the Heart and Small Intestine, promote urination and drain Damp-Heat.
Mu Tong (*Mutong caulis*)*, Zhi Zi (*Gardeniae fructus*), Qu Mai (*Dianthi herba*), Dan Zhu Ye (*Lophatheri herba*), Yu Mi Xu (*Maydis stigma*), Deng Xin Cao (*Junci medulla*), Chi Xiao Dou (*Phaseoli semen*).

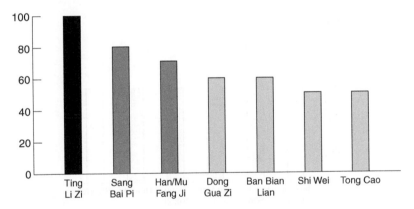

Fig. 6.3 • Comparison of the herbs that regulate the Lung and promote urination.
Ting Li Zi (*Lepidii/Descurainiae semen*), Sang Bai Pi (*Mori cortex*), Han/Mu Fang Ji (*Stephaniae tetrandrae radix/Aristolochiae fangchi radix*), Dong Gua Zi (*Benincasae semen*), Ban Bian Lian (*Lobelia chinensis herba*), Shi Wei (*Pyrrosiae folium*), Tong Cao (*Tetrapanacis medulla*).

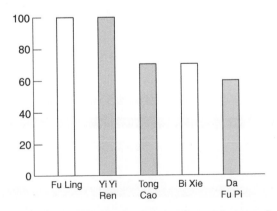

Fig. 6.4 • Comparison of the herbs that regulate the Spleen and Stomach, promote urination and drain Dampness.
Fu Ling (*Poria*), Yi Yi Ren (*Coicis semen*), Tong Cao (*Tetrapanacis medulla*), Bi Xie (*Dioscoreae hypoglaucae rhizoma*), Da Fu Pi (*Arecae pericarpium*).

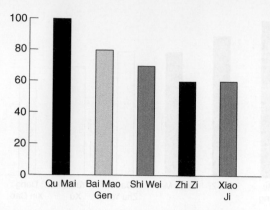

Fig. 6.5 • Comparison of the herbs that promote urination and stop bleeding.
Qu Mai (*Dianthi herba*), Bai Mao Gen (*Imperatae rhizoma*), Shi Wei (*Pyrrosiae folium*), Zhi Zi (*Gardeniae fructus*), Xiao Ji (*Cirsii herba*).

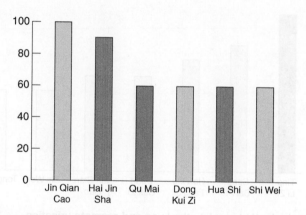

Fig. 6.6 • Comparison of the herbs that promote urination, clear Damp-Heat, stop bleeding and treat Stone-Painful Urinary Dysfunction syndrome.
Jin Qian Cao (*Lysimachiae herba*), Hai Jin Sha (*Lygodii spora*), Qu Mai (*Dianthi herba*), Dong Kui Zi (*Malvae semen*), Hua Shi (*Talcum*), Shi Wei (*Pyrrosiae folium*).

Chapter Seven

7

Aromatic substances for transforming Dampness, for external application, and for opening the orifices

芳香化湿药 外用药 芳香开窍药

1 What are the characteristics of the aromatic herbs and their usage?

Aromatic herbs have a very special function in transforming Dampness and breaking up the blockage of the Qi. They can penetrate into turbid Dampness because their light but sharp smells are able to separate the clean from the turbid. Meanwhile, their light but exceptional smell can wake up (stimulate) the internal organs that have been covered and confused by Dampness. The aromatic and pungent smells of these herbs can, on the one hand, stimulate the Spleen to transform Dampness and treat the causes of Dampness accumulation; on the other hand, they activate Qi movement so as to accelerate the functions of the involved organs.

In clinical practice, the aromatic herbs are often used to remove Dampness from the Middle Jiao, the Spleen and Stomach. They are also used for eliminating Dampness from the Liver and Gall Bladder as well as from the Heart. Some of them can open the orifices and treat 'Lock-up syndrome'. They can also be applied topically to treat open wounds or trauma because they are able to transform the pus, dry Dampness, promote the movement of Qi and Blood, reduce swelling, stop pain and promote healing.

Although the functions of aromatic herbs are similar to those of the herbs that regulate the Qi, herbs that eliminate Dampness and herbs that clear Damp-Heat, they have their own specific characteristics and they do not fit easily into any of the herbal

categories mentioned above. For this reason in many books they are included within the categories of herbs that aromatically transform Dampness, herbs that clear Summer-Heat, herbs that open the orifices and herbs for external usage.

2 What are the indications for and characteristics of the aromatic herbs that transform Dampness in the Middle Jiao?

Herbs that have an aromatic smell are able to transform turbid Dampness in the Middle Jiao and treat the syndrome of Dampness accumulation. This syndrome occurs in certain conditions. First of all, it happens when the Spleen is not able to transform Dampness in situations where there is Excessive-Dampness invasion or deficiency of the Spleen-Qi. Secondly, it can also happen when the Qi movement is disturbed in the Middle Jiao.

In this syndrome, Dampness as well as undigested food, Cold or Heat accumulate in the Middle Jiao and bring about symptoms and signs such as fullness in the chest, distension in the hypochondriac region and abdomen, a poor appetite, a sticky sensation in the mouth, nausea, vomiting, diarrhea or difficult defecation and heaviness of the body. Patients may have a thick, sticky, white or slightly yellow tongue coating and a moderate pulse.

In clinical practice, these herbs are usually used for Excessive syndromes—for example, Dampness invading the Middle Jiao caused by bad eating habits or consumption of unhygienic food, especially during a humid and hot summer. This syndrome can be seen in acute gastroenteritis, dysentery, hepatitis and gastric influenza. These herbs can also be used in Spleen-Qi deficiency syndrome such as in chronic hepatitis, hepatocirrhosis, cholecystitis and uremia, if combined with herbs that tonify the Spleen-Qi and regulate it.

There are many methods and herbs for treating Dampness: some herbs can drain out Dampness by promoting urination, some can dry Dampness directly and some can regulate the Qi to transform Dampness. The aromatic herbs that enter the Spleen and Stomach meridians can penetrate into turbid Dampness, wake up the Spleen which has been covered by Dampness, and stimulate the Spleen-Qi to transform Dampness as well as activating the Qi movement and therefore accelerating the process of transforming Dampness.

3 What are the differences between Huo Xiang (*Agastachis herba*) and Pei Lan (*Eupatorii herba*) in transforming Dampness and reviving the Spleen?

Huo Xiang and Pei Lan both are pungent and aromatic, and enter the Spleen and Stomach meridians. Both are able to transform Dampness in the Middle Jiao, revive the Spleen, improve the appetite and reduce fullness in the Stomach. They are especially often used to treat gastritis, hepatitis, cholecystitis and gastric influenza in the summer when the weather is humid and hot and the functions of Spleen and Stomach become weak.

Huo Xiang is slightly warm, aromatic and pungent. It can penetrate the turbidity and scatter the accumulation of Dampness and Heat. Its action is strong but not harsh and is particularly effective for regulating the Qi in the Middle Jiao, soothing the Stomach-Qi and treating nausea, vomiting and poor appetite.

Pei Lan is a neutral and gentle herb. Its light and fragrant smell can particularly separate the clean from the turbid in the Middle Jiao and revive the Spleen. It is effective for treating a sweet and sticky sensation in the mouth, or foul smell in the mouth,

fullness in the chest, heavy limbs and a heavy sensation in the head. In Chinese, 'Pei' means 'wear' or 'ornament'; 'Lan' means 'orchid'. As Pei Lan has a nice smell, in ancient times it was often put in a small bag and carried by people under their clothes, like people use perfume nowadays.

4 Huo Xiang (*Agastachis herba*), Pei Lan (*Eupatorii herba*), Zi Su Ye (*Perillae folium*) and Xiang Ru (*Moslae herba*) are all able to disperse and transform Dampness and ease the Exterior. What are the differences between them?

These four herbs are aromatic and pungent and are able to expel Wind, Dampness and Summer-Heat, as well as transforming Dampness in the Middle Jiao. They are often used for treating abdominal influenza, acute gastritis and hepatitis accompanied by symptoms and signs such as fever, chills, headache and a heavy sensation in the head, fullness in the chest, gastric and hypochondriac regions, reduced appetite, nausea, vomiting, a thick and white tongue coating and a superficial and moderate pulse.

Of these four herbs, Xiang Ru is the warmest. It is able to induce sweating, disperse Wind and Dampness and release the Exterior. It is especially useful when fever, general pain and heaviness of the body are present but there is no sweating. This herb is also called Summer Ma Huang because it has a similar effect to Ma Huang (*Herba ephedrae*) in inducing sweating, but is gentler. Xiang Ru is more suitable for use in the summer, when the pores are not closed so tightly as in winter. It has also the function of transforming Dampness in the Middle Jiao and treating abdominal pain, vomiting, diarrhea and edema, but its action is not as strong as that of the other three herbs.

Zi Su Ye is a light and aromatic herb. Since it is less warm and pungent than Xiang Ru, it is not able to induce sweating and disperse Dampness. However, it can gently disperse and expel Wind-Cold in the superficial layer of the body and release the Exterior. It can also stop nausea by soothing the Stomach-Qi. It is an ideal herb for alleviating morning sickness and uneasy sensations in the body during early pregnancy because it can harmonize the Qi in the Nutritive and Defensive levels of the body and soothe the Stomach-Qi, and its action is limited to the Upper Jiao and Middle Jiao.

Huo Xiang is an excellent herb for expelling Wind, Cold and Dampness and can also transform Dampness in the Middle Jiao. Compared with Xiang Ru, its action is stronger in transforming Dampness in the Middle Jiao; compared with Zi Su Ye, it not only expels Wind and Cold, but also disperses Dampness in the superficial layers of the body. This is the most commonly used herb for treating cold and influenza infections and acute gastritis, especially in the summer.

Pei Lan is the weakest of the herbs for releasing the Exterior, but it is the strongest in terms of penetrating into the turbidity to separate and transform Dampness. It revives the Spleen and therefore it treats Qi stagnation caused by Dampness. It is especially effective for treating a sticky sensation in the mouth and foul and unpleasant sweet tastes in the mouth, as well as fullness in the chest and gastric region.

5 What are the differences between the functions of Sha Ren (*Amomi xanthioidis fructus*), Bai Dou Kou (*Amomi fructus rotundus*), Cao Dou Kou (*Alpiniae katsumadai semen*) and Cao Guo (*Tsaoko fructus*)?

These four herbs are all aromatic herbs. They are pungent and warm, and enter the Spleen and Stomach meridians. They are able to transform turbid Dampness, regulate the Qi and revive the Spleen. However, the strength of each of the four herbs is different and each also has its own characteristics.

For regulating the Qi in the Middle Jiao and reducing distension and nausea, as well as alleviating pain in the abdomen, Sha Ren is the strongest of the herbs, followed by Bai Dou Kou, then Cao Dou Kou and finally Cao Guo.

For transforming turbid Dampness, warming the Middle Jiao and treating symptoms such as abdomi-

nal pain, preference for warm compresses and drinks, vomiting clear water and diarrhea, Cao Guo is the strongest of the herbs, followed by Cao Dou Kou, then Bai Dou Kou and finally Sha Ren.

As well as these differences, Sha Ren is also able to relieve nausea and calm the fetus and so is used in pregnancy; Bai Dou Kou is particularly good at improving the appetite and reducing distension; Cao Dou Kou can warm and strengthen the Spleen and Cao Guo is used to treat malaria.

6 Which herbs can aromatically transform Dampness from the Liver and Gall Bladder and what are the symptoms in this syndrome?

The herbs that aromatically transform dampness from the Liver and Gall Bladder are Cao Guo (*Tsaoko fructus*), Qing Hao (*Artemisiae annuae herba*), Yu Jin (*Curcumae radix*) and Yin Chen Hao (*Artemisiae scopariae herba*).

These herbs treat the syndrome of Damp-Heat accumulating in the Middle Jiao and obstructing the secretion of bile. Besides the several symptoms of Dampness accumulation in the Middle Jiao, there may also be jaundice, a bitter taste and sticky sensation in the mouth, irritability, tiredness and heaviness of the body. This syndrome can be found in acute hepatitis, cholecystolithiasis, chronic cholecystitis and malaria. Of these four herbs, Cao Guo and Qing Hao are used in the treatment of malaria, whereas Yu Jin and Yi Chen Hao are used to treat hepatitis and cholecystitis.

7 Which herbs can aromatically eliminate Damp-Phlegm from the Heart and what are the symptoms in this syndrome?

The herbs that can aromatically remove Damp-Phlegm from the Heart are Shi Chang Pu (*Acori graminei rhizoma*) and Yu Jin (*Curcumae radix*).

They are used for treating disorders such as poor memory, inability to concentrate, inability to study and mental confusion due to Damp-Phlegm covering the Mind. In this condition, the tongue coating is white and sticky and the pulse is slippery. In order to achieve a better therapeutic effect, these herbs are often combined with other herbs that transform Phlegm and regulate the Qi, such as Yuan Zhi (*Polygalae radix*), Zhu Ru (*Bambusae caulis in taeniam*), Zhi Ke (*Aurantii fructus*) and Chen Pi (*Citri reticulatae pericarpium*).

8 Which aromatic herbs are used externally and what are the indications for use?

The aromatic herbs for external usage are Ru Xiang (*Olibanum*), Yu Jin (*Curcumae radix*), Bing Pian (*Borneol*), Qiang Huo (*Notopterygii rhizoma*), Xi Xin (*Asari herba*)*, Bai Zhi (*Angelicae dahuricae radix*), Rou Gui (*Cinnamomi cassiae cortex*) and She Xiang (*Moschus*)**.

These herbs are usually used in herbal plasters, lotions, pastes or powders. All of them can penetrate the muscles, promote the Qi and Blood circulation, reduce swelling and relieve pain. They are used in the treatment of acute and chronic trauma, strains and open wounds.

Of these herbs, synthetic She Xiang, Bing Pian and Rou Gui can strongly break up the obstructions, reduce swelling and stop pain; Rou Xiang and Yu Jin can effectively promote Blood circulation and relax the muscles; Qiang Huo and Xi Xin can expel Wind-Damp-Cold from the muscles; Bai Zhi can transform Dampness and can be applied to open wounds to promote healing.

In acute infections, these herbs are used together with herbs that reduce Heat-toxin; in conditions of chronic strain, they are used with herbs that open up the collaterals; to treat Bi syndrome, they are used with herbs that expel Wind, Dampness and Cold. These aromatic herbs are also often used externally with herbs that promote Blood circulation. In conditions where there is bleeding or fracture, the herbs should be applied after the bleeding and fractures are corrected.

9 What is Locked-up syndrome?

Locked-up syndrome is an acute, severe and Excess syndrome which may occur alone or develop from

severe disease. The pathological change is sudden disturbance of Qi and Blood, and blockage both of the sensory orifices and of the associations of the internal organs by rebellious Qi, Blood, Phlegm or uprising Yang. Symptoms in this syndrome show obvious signs of blockage of the orifices and a locked-up body, such as loss of consciousness, lockjaw, clenched fists, rigid limbs and lack of urination and bowel movement. In Locked-up syndrome caused by Heat, there are also high fever, irritability, a red face, heavy breath and warm limbs, a yellow, thick tongue coating and a rapid, slippery, forceful pulse. If the Locked-up syndrome is caused by Cold, there are cold limbs, a pale complexion, a white, thick tongue coating and a deep, wiry pulse.

In clinical practice, this syndrome can be found in severe infection, cerebrovascular accident, hepatic coma, uremia, sunstroke, syncope, lightning stroke, drowning and hysteria.

10 Locked-up syndrome and Collapsing syndrome can both occur in coma. What are the differences in the symptoms and the pathological changes between the two syndromes?

In clinical practice, coma may occur in the process of severe diseases such as severe infections, cerebrovascular accident, myocardial infarction, hepatic coma, uremia, loss of a large amount of blood, lightning stroke and drowning. Since these patients have lost consciousness, it is important to make a correct differentiation of the syndrome by observation and palpations before treatment.

Locked-up syndrome is an acute Excess syndrome. The orifices are locked up by disturbance of the Qi and Blood, which are complicated with Phlegm, Heat or Cold, as well as uprising Yang. The symptoms are loss of consciousness, lockjaw, clenched fists, rigid limbs and a wiry, slippery and forceful pulse. The syndrome is seen mainly in cerebrovascular accident, epilepsy, sunstroke, hysteria, severe pain, allergy, syncope, hepatic coma and uremia. Treatment should be given to open the orifices, expel Phlegm, clear Heat or warm the internal Cold and to harmonize the Qi and Blood.

Collapsing syndrome is a Deficiency syndrome. It is caused by disharmony of the Yin, Yang, Qi and

Blood when the Yang and Qi are too weak to hold the Yin and the Blood and to carry on the functions of the internal organs. In this syndrome, patients lose consciousness gradually and they have shallow respiration, shortness of breath, cold limbs, profuse sweating and incontinence of urine. The pulse is very deep and weak. This syndrome occurs in conditions where patients lose a large amount of blood, in severe dehydration, in myocardial infarction and in severe infections. The treatment should be given to strengthen the Qi strongly, and to rescue the Yang. After the patient recovers consciousness, the treatment of tonifying the weakness and harmonizing the functions of the internal organs should start.

11 What are the characteristics of the herbs that open the orifices and what precautions should be observed when they are used?

The substances that open the orifices are used for treating Locked-up syndrome, a severe, acute, Excess syndrome. These substances are very pungent, have strong aromatic smells, move quickly and are able to penetrate the body, break up blockage and revive the Spirit. If combined with other herbs that expel Phlegm, eliminate Heat-toxin or Cold turbidity, they can open the orifices in a very short time. From the viewpoint of Western medicine, these substances are able to stimulate the central nervous system, the peripheral nervous system and the heart, irritate the respiratory mucosa and smooth the muscles.

Since the aromatic components are the main part of substances that open the orifices, and since they are easily destroyed by high temperatures during cooking, substances for opening the orifices are always prepared at low temperature and are often combined with other herbs that eliminate Phlegm, reduce poison and harmonize the Qi and Blood. Some substances such as She Xiang (*Moschus*)** and Niu Huang (*Bovis calculus*)** are substituted by the synthetic versions.

Since Locked-up syndrome is subdivided into Hot Locked-up syndrome and Cold Locked-up syndrome, the substances are also divided into two groups, cold and warm.

The cold substances are used for Hot Locked-up syndrome. They are synthetic Niu Huang (*Bovis calculus*), Bing Pian (*Borneol*), Yu Jin (*Curcumae radix*) and Lian Qiao (*Forsythiae fructus*).

The warm substances are used for Cold Locked-up syndrome. They are synthetic She Xiang (*Moschus*), Su He Xiang (*Styrax*), An Xi Xiang (*Benzoinum*), Shi Chang Pu (*Acori graminei rhizoma*), Huo Xiang (*Agastachis herba*) and Pei Lan (*Eupatorii herba*).

Although these aromatic substances are very necessary for use in acute conditions, even so they should be used with caution. Because these aromatic substances are able to break up the blockage of the orifices and stimulate the Yin, Yang, Qi and Blood, they may scatter and weaken the Qi, so should be used for only a short period of time. After patients are revived from coma, treatment should be given according to the differentiation of the syndrome at that moment. In addition, these substances should not be used in pregnant women, in conditions of heavy bleeding, or during coma in a Collapsing syndrome.

Comparisons of strength and temperature in aromatic substances that transform Dampness, that are for external application and that open the orifices

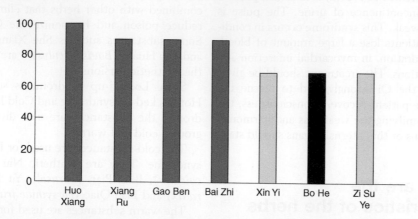

Fig. 7.1 • Comparison of the herbs that aromatically transform turbid Dampness and release the Exterior.
Huo Xiang (*Agastachis herba*), Xiang Ru (*Moslae herba*), Gao Ben (*Ligustici sinensis radix*), Bai Zhi (*Angelicae dahuricae radix*), Xin Yi (*Magnoliae flos*), Bo He (*Menthae herba*), Zi Su Ye (*Perillae folium*).

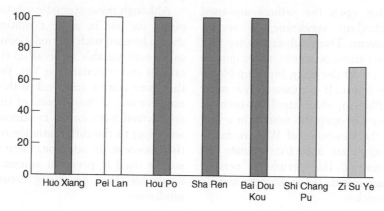

Fig. 7.2 • Comparison of the herbs that aromatically transform Dampness from the Middle Jiao.
Huo Xiang (*Agastachis herba*), Pei Lan (*Eupatorii herba*), Hou Po (*Magnoliae cortex*), Sha Ren (*Amomi xanthioidis fructus*), Bai Dou Kou (*Amomi fructus rotundus*), Shi Chang Pu (*Acori graminei rhizoma*), Zi Su Ye (*Perillae folium*).

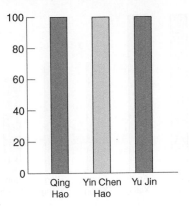

Fig. 7.3 • Comparison of the herbs that aromatically transform Dampness from the Liver and Gall Bladder. Qing Hao (*Artemisiae annuae herba*), Yin Chen Hao (*Artemisiae scopariae herba*), Yu Jin (*Curcumae radix*).

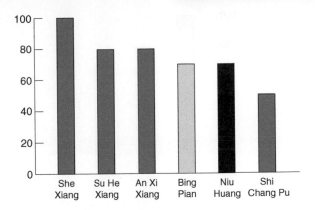

Fig. 7.4 • Comparison of the substances that aromatically open the orifices. She Xiang (*Moschus*)**, Su He Xiang (*Styrax*), An Xi Xiang (*Benzoinum*), Bing Pian (*Borneol*), Niu Huang (*Bovis calculus*)**, Shi Chang Pu (*Acori graminei rhizoma*).

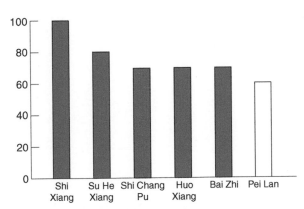

Fig. 7.5 • Comparison of the herbs that aromatically transform turbid Dampness. She Xiang (*Moschus*)**, Su He Xiang (*Styrax*), Shi Chang Pu (*Acori graminei rhizoma*), Huo Xiang (*Agastachis herba*), Bai Zhi (*Angelicae dahuricae radix*), Pei Lan (*Eupatorii herba*).

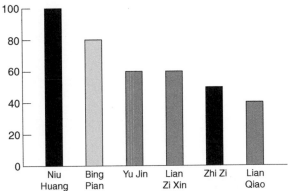

Fig. 7.6 • Comparison of the herbs that clear Heat-toxin and open the orifices. Niu Huang (*Bovis calculus*)**, Bing Pian (*Borneol*), Yu Jin (*Curcumae radix*), Lian Zi Xin (*Nelumbinis plumula*), Zhi Zi (*Gardeniae fructus*), Lian Qiao (*Forsythiae fructus*).

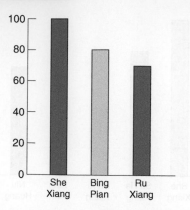

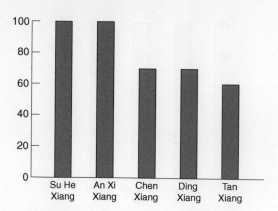

Fig. 7.7 • Comparison of the substances that aromatically reduce swelling and stop pain.
She Xiang (*Moschus*)**, Bing Pian (*Borneol*), Ru Xiang (*Olibanum*).

Fig. 7.8 • Comparison of the substances that aromatically open the orifices, regulate the Qi and relieve pain.
Su He Xiang (*Styrax*), An Xi Xiang (*Benzoinum*), Chen Xiang (*Aquilariae lignum*), Ding Xiang (*Caryophylli flos*), Tan Xiang (*Santali albi lignum*).

Chapter Eight

8

Herbs that transform Phlegm

祛痰药

1 What are the indications for herbs that transform Phlegm? What are visible Phlegm and invisible Phlegm?

Herbs that transform Phlegm are able to treat Phlegm syndrome. Phlegm is a kind of pathological product and it is also a secondary pathogenic factor, which will lead to further pathological changes in the body. Dysfunction of the Lung, Spleen, Kidney and San Jiao can result in accumulation of water. Meanwhile, in pathological conditions, Cold can condense water, Heat can consume water, and stagnation of Qi can obstruct the flow of water. Furthermore, the accumulated water becomes a kind of thick, sticky substance that is called 'Phlegm'. Phlegm interferes with the normal flow of Qi and is also pushed by the Qi to spread through the body, so it may affect all parts of the body, with various manifestations.

Visible phlegm is often seen in clinical practice to accumulate in the Lung, and this can be expectorated. Coughing, wheezing and fullness or stifling feelings in the chest often exist because the Lung-Qi is obstructed.

There is also another kind of Phlegm that is neither visible nor able to be expectorated. This is the so-called 'invisible Phlegm'. It can result in different symptoms when it stays in different parts of the body. When it accumulates in the Stomach, it may cause nausea, vomiting, loss of appetite, and fullness or distension in the upper abdomen. If it is pushed by rebellious rising Qi, then it moves upwards and disturbs the sensory orifices, and the patient experiences dizziness, vertigo, tinnitus and heavy sensations in the head. If the Phlegm obstructs the Heart and disturbs the Mind, it will cause palpitations, restlessness, insomnia, depression, mental confusion, delirium, mania, coma, Wind-stroke and epilepsy. If it obstructs the meridians and collaterals, and blocks the circulation of the Qi and Blood, then corresponding symptoms may occur in the locality. If in the chest, then chest pain and palpitations may be present; if on the face, there may be distortion of the mouth and the eyes; if in the limbs or the trunk, there will be sensations of numbness and heaviness. If Phlegm accumulates for a long period of time and is combined with other pathogenic factors, it can form masses, such as different kinds of tumor.

The most commonly used substances that transform Phlegm may remove visible Phlegm and are also able to disperse the Lung-Qi and direct it downwards; therefore they can stop coughing. Some of the substances are also able to remove invisible Phlegm; however, since the cause of invisible Phlegm is more complicated, in clinical practice they must be used together with other herbs that regulate the Qi, tonify the Spleen-Qi and transform Dampness to increase the therapeutic effects.

2 What are the characteristics of herbs that transform Phlegm? What precautions should be observed when they are used?

Herbs that transform Phlegm are used to treat Phlegm syndromes, which are caused by visible Phlegm and invisible Phlegm. These substances have the following characteristics.

Pungent and bitter

Pungency has dispersing and ascending properties; it has the ability to dissipate thick Phlegm. It is also able to disperse and lift the Qi so as to move the Phlegm. Bitterness has reducing and descending properties; it is able to descend the Qi and eliminate Phlegm. Pungent and bitter herbs have dispersing, ascending and descending capabilities, so they can dissipate thick Phlegm. Almost all the herbs that transform Phlegm have these characteristics.

Salty

Saltiness can soften hardness. Herbs that transform Phlegm with a salty taste are usually used for dissipating invisible Phlegm, which is characterized by a thick even hard nature, such as in chronic lymphadenitis, scrofula and tumors. The substances to treat this kind of Phlegm are Zhe Bei Mu (*Fritillariae thunbergii bulbus*), Hai Zao (*Sargassum*), Kun Bu (*Eckloniae thallus*), Wa Leng Zi (*Arcae concha*), Hai Ge Ke (*Meretricis/Cyclinae concha*) and Meng Shi (*Lapis micae seu chloriti*)*.

Cold or warm in temperature

Herbs that transform Phlegm are cold in temperature and are able to treat Phlegm-Heat syndrome. In this case, the Phlegm is thick, green, turbid and difficult to expectorate. In the syndrome caused by invisible Phlegm, there is mental confusion, a red tongue with a yellow, sticky coating, and a slippery and rapid pulse, which indicates the presence of Phlegm-Heat. The commonly used substances to eliminate Phlegm-Heat are Zhu Li (*Bambusae succus*), Tian Zhu Huang (*Bambusae concretio silicea*), Sang Bai Pi (*Mori cortex*), Chuan Bei Mu (*Fritillariae cirrhosae bulbus*), Gua Lou (*Trichosanthis fructus*), Hai Zao, Kun Bu, Ting Li Zi (*Lepidii/Descurainiae semen*), Hai Fu Shi (*Pumex*) and Hai Ge Ke.

Substances that transform Phlegm that are warm in temperature are able to treat Cold-Phlegm syndrome, which is characterized by copious, white or watery sputum. The commonly used substances are Ban Xia (*Pinelliae rhizoma*), Ju Hong (*Citri erythrocarpae pars rubra epicarpii*), Xing Ren (*Armeniacae semen*), Su Zi (*Perillae fructus*), Tian Nan Xing (*Arisaematis rhizoma*), Bai Fu Zi (*Typhonii rhizoma praeparatum*)* and Bai Jie Zi (*Sinapis albae semen*).

Entering the Lung and Large Intestine meridians

Herbs that enter the Lung and Large Intestine meridians treat mainly visible Phlegm. Besides eliminating Phlegm, most of them are able to stop a cough which is caused by Phlegm accumulation in the Lung and obstruction of the Lung-Qi. The commonly used herbs are Xing Ren, Jie Geng (*Platycodi radix*), Chuan Bei Mu (*Fritillariae cirrhosae bulbus*), Pi Pa Ye (*Eriobotryae folium*), Qian Hu (*Peucedani radix*), Bai Qian (*Cynanchi stauntonii radix*), Zi Wan (*Asteris radix*) and Kuan Dong Hua (*Tussilaginis farfarae*).

Entering the Heart, Stomach, Liver and Gall Bladder meridians

Herbs that enter the Heart, Stomach, Liver and Gall Bladder meridians are able to remove invisible Phlegm. Invisible Phlegm might accumulate in the Stomach, cover the Mind or block the orifices. Invisible Phlegm obstructs the Qi movement and Blood circulation in these meridians and collaterals, causing different symptoms. The commonly used herbs for removing invisible Phlegm are Ban Xia, Zhu Ru (*Bambusae caulis in taeniam*), Zhi Shi (*Aurantii fructus immaturus*), Dan Nan Xing (*Pulvis arisaemae cum felle bovis*), Bai Jie Zi, Bai Fu Zi*, Meng Shi*, Ting Li Zi, Hai Zao, Kun Bu and Hai Ge Ke.

Combining with herbs that transform Dampness and herbs that tonify the Spleen

Phlegm and Dampness are considered in TCM to be substances with the same nature and coming from the same origin. If the pathogen spreads without any form, it is called Dampness; if it accumulates in a particular place and becomes thick and turbid and has a shape, it is called Phlegm. Herbs that transform Phlegm and Dampness can be used together to increase the therapeutic effects of removing Phlegm.

The Spleen is responsible for transforming Dampness. If the Spleen-Qi is deficient, it fails to transport and transform water, and water can accumulate and form Phlegm. There is a saying: 'The Lung is the receptacle of Phlegm and the Spleen is the organ of generating Phlegm.' Herbs that tonify the Spleen-Qi are often used in treating Phlegm syndromes, especially in the chronic disorders.

Herbs that treat Phlegm have a pungent-warm, bitter-warm or pungent-cold nature, and they should be used with caution because pungent, warm and bitter herbs can consume the Yin, and cold herbs can injure the Yang if these herbs are used in large dosage and for a long period of time. Moreover, pregnant women should use these herbs with caution as the pungent and warm herbs can activate Qi and Blood, and the bitter herbs move downwards. These actions may bring danger to the pregnancy.

3 What are the functions and characteristics of Xing Ren (*Armeniacae semen*) and Jie Geng (*Platycodi radix*)?

Xin Ren and Jie Geng both enter the Qi level of the Lung meridian. Both are able to transform Phlegm from the Lung and stop coughing. In clinical practice, they are often used together to treat cold infections and bronchitis. With some other herbs, they can also treat pneumonia, asthma and pulmonary emphysema. However, these two herbs have their own characteristics and they carry out their functions by different methods.

Xing Ren is bitter, warm and slightly poisonous. The bitter taste gives Xing Ren a descending property. Warmth can disperse the accumulation of Phlegm and the stagnation of Qi. It is a kind of seed and it contains oil, which gives this herb a moist nature. The function of Xing Ren is characterized as descending the Lung-Qi and transforming Phlegm in

order to stop coughing. It is particularly useful for treating cough with a large amount of Phlegm, fullness in the chest, shortness of breath and nasal obstruction when exterior pathogenic factors invade the Lung and the Lung-Qi fails to descend.

Jie Geng is pungent, bitter and neutral. It is able to transform Phlegm and stop coughing. The pungent and bitter tastes give Jie Geng dispersing and dissipating capacities. It is light both in weight and in nature; therefore its function is characterized as lifting the Lung-Qi gently but sufficiently. It is suitable for treating cough with Phlegm, stifling in the chest and nasal obstruction due to obstruction of the Lung-Qi.

Comparing Jie Geng and Xin Ren, one moves upwards, the other moves downwards; one disperses the Lung-Qi and the other directs the Lung-Qi to descend. They perfectly match each other to regulate the Lung-Qi, eliminate Phlegm and relieve cough. This is why they are often used together in clinical practice.

4 What are the characteristics of Jie Geng (*Platycodi radix*)?

Jie Geng is bitter, pungent and neutral and enters the Lung meridian. It is light in nature and its function is characterized as ascending and dispersing the Lung-Qi. This feature gives Jie Geng not only the capability of dispersing the Lung-Qi so as to treat cough with Phlegm, but also the possibility of activating the Qi movement in the whole body in order to treat disorders of other organs and meridians. For instance, to treat constipation, or difficult bowel movement due to Qi stagnation in the intestine, besides using purging and descending herbs to stimulate the intestines and promote bowel movement, Jie Geng could also be used to lift the Lung-Qi so as to activate the Qi movement in the Large Intestine because the Lung and Large Intestine are Internally–Externally related. This combination is more effective than if only the descending herbs are used.

Another example is the treatment of difficult urination and edema due to water accumulation in the Lower or Middle Jiao. Besides using herbs that drain water and reduce water accumulation, Jie Geng could be used to disperse the Lung-Qi and open the Upper Jiao so as to accelerate the Qi and water movement in the Middle Jiao and Lower Jiao.

The therapeutic result of this combination is also much better than if draining and reducing herbs are used alone. Since Jie Gen is a special herb for regulating the Qi through opening and lifting the Lung-Qi, it is described in the classics as 'the oar of the boat', which means that Jie Geng may assist the Qi movement in the opposite direction so as to break up various obstructions.

Because Jie Geng is light and ascending in nature and enters the Lung meridian, it is also very often used as a guide to enter the Lung meridian for herbs that do not enter this meridian. For example, in chronic diarrhea due to Spleen-Qi deficiency, patients may also have shortness of breath and weak voice due to Lung-Qi deficiency, and herbs that tonify the Spleen-Qi can easily enter the Lung as well to tonify the Lung-Qi if Jie Geng is used as a guide.

5 What are the differences between Bai Qian (*Cynanchi stauntonii radix*) and Qian Hu (*Peucedani radix*)?

Bai Qian and Qian Hu are often prescribed as 'Er Qian', meaning 'the two Qian', which suggests that these two herbs are often used together. Both are pungent and enter the Lung meridian and are effective for relieving cough. The pungent property gives them the capability of dispersing the Lung-Qi. Meanwhile, the direction of their action is downward; they can effectively descend the Lung-Qi and relieve cough. Both are used for treating fullness in the chest, productive cough and wheezing due to obstruction of the Lung-Qi. They can also be used to treat External syndrome because they are pungent and are able to expel Wind. However, there are some differences between these two herbs, so they can also be used separately in different conditions.

Bai Qian is a warm herb and its action of descending the Lung-Qi is stronger than that of Qian Hu. It is suitable for treating cough, wheezing, asthma and white sputum, which is difficult to expectorate and causes stifling feelings in the chest. Qian Hu is cold in nature and is more suitable for clearing Heat in the Lung and treating cough with green and thick sputum, a sense of constriction in the chest and irritability.

6 What are the differences between Zi Wan (*Asteris radix*), Kuan Dong Hua (*Tussilaginis farfarae*) and Bai Bu (*Stemonae radix*) in relieving cough and transforming Phlegm?

These three herbs all enter the Lung meridian. They have a similar function in moistening the Lung, descending the Lung-Qi, transforming Phlegm and relieving cough. All are warm, pungent and bitter, but they have no drying property and can be used for treating many kinds of cough caused by Exterior or Interior pathogenic factors. They treat cough either in the acute stage or in chronic stages, in Excess or Deficiency syndromes, and in Hot or Cold syndromes. Because of these characteristics, they are widely used in clinical practice. They are often used together to treat bronchitis, pneumonia, upper respiratory tract infection and pertussis.

However, comparing the functions of the three herbs, Zi Wan is the strongest one for transforming Phlegm, Kuan Dong Hua is the most effective one for relieving cough and Bai Bu is the most commonly used to treat chronic cough.

7 What are the differences between Chuan Bei Mu (*Fritillariae cirrhosae bulbus*) and Zhe Bei Mu (*Fritillariae thunbergii bulbus*)?

Chuan Bei Mu and Zhe Bei Mu are bitter and cold, and enter the Lung and Heart meridians. Both can transform Phlegm-Heat, dissipate nodules and treat cough with thick, green sputum that is difficult to expectorate, with dryness in the mouth and nasal cavity. However, they also have their own characteristics.

Chuan Bei Mu is sweet and is less cold than Zhe Bei Mu. Sweetness combined with coldness can generate Yin of the body. This herb is characterized as moistening the Lung, transforming Phlegm and relieving cough. It is effective for treating Phlegm-Heat syndrome with signs of Lung-Yin or Body Fluid deficiency. The symptoms are very sticky and thick sputum, in small amounts, that is difficult to expectorate, or cough without production, dryness in the throat and nasal cavity, chronic cough, paroxysmal cough, cough without Phlegm, stifling in the chest and hypochondriac pain. Together with herbs that nourish the Yin of the body, Chuan Bei Mu is used for treating chronic or acute bronchitis, pneumonia, lung abscess, asthma and tuberculosis. Since it has the function of dissipating thick Phlegm and dispersing constrained Qi in the chest, if combined with herbs that spread the Liver-Qi it can treat depression, 'plum-pit syndrome', pulmonary tuberculosis and nodules.

Zhe Bei Mu is more bitter and colder than Chuan Bei Mu. It has no function in moistening the Lung, but is stronger than Chuan Bei Mu in clearing Heat and reducing Fire. It is also stronger for breaking up congealed Phlegm and is therefore more suitable for treating Phlegm-Heat in the Lung. The manifestations are very sticky sputum, which is difficult to expectorate, a very red tongue with a yellow sticky coating and a slippery and rapid pulse. This herb is also stronger for dissipating nodules than Chuan Bei Mu and it is used to treat red, swollen and painful scrofula or abscesses. Combined with other herbs, it is used to treat tumors.

tion of promoting bowel movement and treating constipation, especially when there is Phlegm-Heat in the Lung.

Comparing the functions of the two herbs, Gua Lou is stronger in the function of clearing Heat and transforming Phlegm; Gua Lou Ren is stronger in moistening the intestine and promoting bowel movement. If combined with herbs that clear Heat, Gua Lou Ren is effective for removing Phlegm-Heat from the intestine and treating colitis and dysentery.

Gua Lou Pi is sweet and cold. It has a similar function to Gua Lou and Gua Lou Ren in transforming Phlegm in the Lung but it is not as strong as the other two in clearing Heat. This herb is characterized as moistening the Lung and throat; therefore it can treat a hoarse, sore throat and thirst due to Dryness in the Lung.

Gua Lou Gen is also called Tian Hua Fen. It has a quite different function from that of the other herbs. It is bitter, sour, cold and slightly sweet, and enters the Lung and Stomach meridians. It has no function of transforming Phlegm, but it can clear Heat from the Lung, generate the Body Fluids and alleviate thirst. In clinical practice, it is used to treat diabetes. It is also able to relieve Heat-toxin and treat sore throat, pneumonia, lung abscess, breast abscess, carbuncles and sores.

8 What are the differences between Gua Lou (*Trichosanthis fructus*), Gua Lou Ren (*Trichosanthis semen*), Gua Lou Pi (*Trichosanthis pericarpium*) and Gua Lou Gen (*Trichosanthis radix*)

These four herbs are from different parts of the same plant, and there are some differences between their functions too.

Gua Lou and Gua Lou Ren are sweet, bitter and cold. They enter the Lung, Stomach and Large Intestine meridians. Both can clear Heat from the Lung, transform Phlegm-Heat and unbind the Qi in the chest. They can treat cough with a large amount of green sputum, distension, constriction and pain in the chest and irritability. In clinical practice, they can be used for treating bronchitis, pneumonia, lung abscess and breast abscess. They also have the func-

9 What are the differences between Tian Zhu Huang (*Bambusae concretio silicea*), Zhu Li (*Bambusae succus*) and Zhu Ru (*Bambusae caulis in taeniam*)?

These three herbs come from bamboo. They are sweet and cold, and have the functions of clearing Heat and transforming Phlegm. However, the three enter different meridians and their strengths are different also, so their clinical applications are different too.

Tian Zhu Huang enters the Heart and Liver meridians, and is effective for dislodging Phlegm, clearing Heat, cooling the Heart and controlling convulsions. It is often used in children when there is high fever, irritability, convulsions and night crying caused by disturbance of the Heart and Liver by Phlegm-Heat. It can also be used to treat fever, shortness of breath and cough with thick sputum in conditions of Phlegm-Heat in the Lung. In clinical practice, it is used for convulsions in infectious diseases, pneumonia, acute bronchitis and influenza.

Zhu Li is the coldest of these three herbs. It enters the Heart, Lung and Stomach meridians. It has a lubricating nature and its function is characterized as strongly eliminating Phlegm-Heat, especially when Phlegm blocks the meridians and collaterals; therefore it is used to treat epilepsy, hemiplegia, facial paralysis, and numbness and tingling or cramp of the limbs. It is also able to open the Heart orifice, and is used when Phlegm-Heat covers the Heart. In this situation, patients lose consciousness and have gurgling sounds in the throat, such as in epilepsy, cerebrovascular accident and myocardial infarction. Zhu Li is also often used for treating mental disorders when Phlegm-Heat covers or disturbs the Mind, such as in schizophrenia.

Zhu Ru is slightly cold, and enters the Lung, Stomach and Gall Bladder meridians. Besides clearing Heat and transforming Phlegm, it is effective for dispersing constrained Qi, eliminating irritability and calming the Mind. It is mainly used for treating restlessness, palpitations, restless sleep, depression and aprosexia, especially after febrile disease or in chronic disease. It is also effective for soothing the Stomach-Qi, clearing Heat and treating nausea and vomiting—for example, in morning sickness of early pregnancy, heatstroke, migraine and Ménière's disease.

10 Ting Li Zi (Lepidii/ Descurainiae semen), Sang Bai Pi (Mori cortex) and Xuan Fu Hua (Inulae flos) are able to direct the Lung-Qi to descend, transform Phlegm and arrest wheezing. What are the differences between their actions?

Ting Li Zi and Sang Bai Pi are cold herbs and enter the Lung meridian. They are able to direct the Lung-Qi downwards, and eliminate Phlegm and water accumulation, thereby reducing obstruction of the Lung-Qi and arresting wheezing. They are used together in clinical practice to treat cough, asthma, fullness in the chest, edema and difficult urination.

Ting Li Zi is very pungent, bitter and cold, and is much stronger than Sang Bai Pi in directing the Lung-Qi downwards and draining water. It is therefore considered to be an agent that drives out water and Phlegm. It also enters the Large Intestine meridian, and can drain Heat, water and Phlegm via bowel movement. It is more suitable for treating the Excess syndromes of Phlegm and water accumulation in the Lung. In these syndromes, the Lung-Qi is obstructed, so the Qi movement is blocked in the San Jiao, Bladder and Large Intestine meridians, such as in asthma, pleuritis, pulmonary heart disease, heart failure, acute nephritis and renal failure. However, since Ting Li Zi is a harsh and cold herb and easily injures the Qi, it is used in Excessive syndromes for only a short time.

Sang Bai Pi is sweet, bland and cold. Coldness can clear Heat, blandness can leach out Dampness, and sweetness can protect the Lung. Sang Bai Pi is gentler than Ting Li Zi in directing the Qi downwards and eliminating the accumulation of water and Phlegm, so it has fewer side-effects and can be used for a longer period of time. In clinical practice, it is often used for treating acute bronchitis, pneumonia, upper respiratory infection and acute nephritis.

Xuan Fu Hua is also able to direct the Qi downwards from the Lung and eliminate Phlegm, relieve cough and arrest wheezing, but it is warm in nature and is more suitable for treating syndromes in which the Lung-Qi is obstructed by accumulation of Cold-Phlegm. Meanwhile, like Ting Li Zi and Sang Bai Pi, Xuan Fu Hua can also leach out water, but its function is a result of directing the Lung-Qi downwards. It is more effective for transforming Phlegm and so is used as an agent especially for dissolving Phlegm. In addition, this herb is also very effective for descending the Stomach-Qi and relieving nausea and vomiting. In clinical practice, Xuan Fu Hua is used for treating bronchitis, pulmonary emphysema, bronchiectasis and acute gastritis.

11 What are the functions of Ban Xia (Pinelliae rhizoma)? What are the characteristics of processed Ban Xia?

Ban Xia is warm, pungent and poisonous, and it enters the Spleen and Stomach meridians. It is able to dry Dampness and transform Phlegm in the

Middle Jiao. When the Dampness is removed, the transportation function of the Spleen is restored, and Phlegm is no longer generated. In clinical practice, Ban Xia is able to treat chronic bronchitis, pulmonary emphysema, and cold and influenza infections with symptoms of coughing up a large amount of white sputum and tightness in the chest. Ban Xia is also very effective for soothing the Stomach-Qi and transforming Damp-Phlegm in the Stomach so as to treat nausea, vomiting, reduced appetite and fullness in the epigastric region; in clinical practice it is used to treat gastritis, anorexia and morning sickness.

However, as raw Ban Xia is poisonous, this herb is often used after processing. There are several processed forms of Ban Xia that are often prescribed, as follows.

Qing Ban Xia, the light Ban Xia

After raw Ban Xia is soaked and rinsed in water until the hot taste is removed, it is cooked with alum. It is then dried and cut in pieces. Qing Ban Xia is warm and pungent, and has a drying nature. It is more suitable for treating Damp-Phlegm accumulation in the Lung, which manifests as coughing with a large amount of sputum, tightness in the chest and nausea.

Jiang Ban Xia, the ginger-processed Ban Xia

After the hot taste is removed by soaking and rinsing in water, Ban Xia is cooked with ginger and alum. It is then dried before being used. Jiang Ban Xia is better at soothing the Stomach-Qi and relieving nausea and vomiting caused by Cold in the Stomach.

Fa Ban Xia, the standard-processed Ban Xia

After the hot taste is removed by soaking and rinsing in water, Ban Xia is soaked with Gan Cao (Radix Glycyrrhizae) and lime. It is dried and crushed before it is used. Fa Ban Xia is particularly effective for drying Dampness in the Middle Jiao and promoting the function of the Spleen and Stomach. It is used to treat fullness in the epigastric region, poor appetite, loose stools, heaviness of the body and tiredness.

Ban Xia Qu, the fermented Ban Xia

After the hot taste is removed by soaking and rinsing in water, Ban Xia is ground and mixed with wheat powder and ginger juice. A dough is made which is then cut into small pieces. After it has fermented, it is dried before being used. Ban Xia Qu is better for strengthening the function of the Stomach and Spleen and promoting digestion. It is used for treating poor appetite, indigestion and a weak constitution.

12 What are the differences between Tian Nan Xing (*Arisaematis rhizoma*) and processed Nan Xing?

Tian Nan Xing is the name of the raw herb. Because the raw herb is poisonous, it is often used after processing. Zhi Nan Xing and Dan Nan Xing are two kinds of commonly used processed products of this herb.

After soaking in alum solution, the herb is rinsed until the hot taste is removed, cooked with fresh ginger, and later dried. The product is called Zhi Nan Xing; this form is pungent, bitter and warm, and enters the Lung, Spleen and Liver meridians. It has a very strong dispersing ability and can intensively dry Dampness, dissolve Damp-Phlegm, treat tightness in the chest and expectorate a large amount of white sputum. It is able to eliminate invisible Phlegm from meridians and collaterals and is used for syndromes of Wind-Phlegm obstruction in the meridians, which manifests as numbness, heaviness and tingling of the limbs, such as in fibrositis, arthritis, facial paralysis and facial spasm.

When the powder of Tian Nan Xing is mixed with bovine bile, it is called Dan Nan Xing (*Pulvis arisaemae cum felle bovis*). Dang Nan Xing is more bitter than Zhi Nan Xing as the pungent and warm nature has been changed to cold and moist. It is characterized as clearing Heat, expelling Phlegm, extinguishing Wind and calming spasm. It can effectively treat cough without production, or scanty green sputum that is difficult to expectorate. It is also able to eliminate invisible Phlegm and treat epilepsy and Wind-stroke, which are caused by Phlegm-Heat covering the Heart.

Although Tian Nan Xing, the raw herb, is poisonous, it is also used in clinical practice. It is very pungent and warm, and is mainly used topically to dissipate congealed blood, reduce swelling and stop pain. It can treat sores, ulcers, carbuncles and trauma.

13 What are the differences between Hai Zao (*Sargassum*) and Kun Bu (*Eckloniae thallus*)?

Hai Zao and Kun Bu are salty and cold, and enter the Liver, Lung and Kidney meridians. Both can clear Heat, transform Phlegm, soften hardness and dissipate nodules. They can also promote urination and reduce edema. In clinical practice, they are often used together to treat nodules such as goiter and scrofula.

There are some differences between the two herbs. Hai Zao is stronger in transforming Phlegm and dissipating nodules; it is more suitable for treating goiter and scrofula. Kun Bu is stronger in softening hardness and reducing the congealed Blood; it is more suitable for treating hepatosplenomegaly, liver cirrhosis and tumors.

14 Which herbs are particularly effective for relieving cough?

The herbs that are particularly effective for relieving cough are able to disperse or descend the Lung-Qi. If they are combined with herbs that transform Phlegm, clear Heat or expel Cold, they can be used for treating an acute or chronic cough in Excess or Deficiency syndromes, or for treating a cough caused by Cold or Heat in the Lung. These herbs can be divided into two groups according to whether they have warm or cold temperatures.

Herbs that relieve cough and are cold in temperature are particularly used when Heat accumulates in the Lung. The commonly used ones are Qian Hu (*Peucedani radix*), Chuan Bei Mu (*Fritillariae cirrhosae bulbus*), Pi Pa Ye (*Eriobotryae folium*), Sang Ye (*Mori folium*) and Sang Bai Pi (*Mori cortex*).

Herbs that relieve cough and are warm in temperature are used when there is no obvious Heat in the Lung, and most are also effective for transforming Phlegm. The commonly used ones are Ju Hong (*Citri erythrocarpae pars rubra epicarpii*), Xing Ren (*Armeniacae semen*), Jie Geng (*Platycodi radix*), Bai Qian (*Cynanchi stauntonii radix*), Zi Wan (*Asteris radix*), Kuan Dong Hua (*Tussilaginis farfarae*) and Bai Bu (*Stemonae radix*).

15 Which herbs are able to clear Heat and transform Phlegm from the Lung?

The herbs that clear Heat and transform Phlegm from the Lung are Zhe Bei Mu (*Fritillariae thunbergii bulbus*), Chuan Bei Mu (*Fritillariae cirrhosae bulbus*), Gua Lou (*Trichosanthis fructus*), Dan Nan Xing (*Pulvis arisaemae cum felle bovis*), Hai Fu Shi (*Pumex*) and Hai Ge Ke (*Meretricis/Cyclinae concha*).

These herbs are particularly effective for treating cough with green, thick sputum that is difficult to expectorate, tightness in the chest, quick breathing, a red tongue with a thick, yellow coating and a rapid and slippery pulse. In clinical practice, these herbs are often used for treating upper respiratory tract infection, acute bronchitis and pneumonia.

These herbs are also often used together with other herbs to treat certain diseases of the Lung. For example, if combined with Shi Gao (*Gypsum*), Huang Qin (*Scutellariae radix*), Jin Yin Hua (*Lonicerae flos*) and Lian Qiao (*Forsythiae fructus*), they can reduce Heat from the Lung and relieve Fire-toxin so as to control infections of the Lung. If combined with Lu Gen (*Phragmitis rhizoma*), Jie Geng (*Platycodi radix*), Yi Yi Ren (*Coicis semen*) and Yu Xing Cao (*Houttuyniae herba cum radice*), they can treat lung abscess and sinusitis.

16 Which herbs are able to moisten the Lung and loosen sputum?

The herbs that moisten the Lung and loosen sputum are Chuan Bei Mu (*Fritillariae cirrhosae bulbus*), Gua Lou (*Trichosanthis fructus*), Pi Pa Ye (*Eriobotryae folium*), Xing Ren (*Armeniacae semen*), Bai He (*Lilii bulbus*), Hai Fu Shi (*Pumex*) and Hai Ge Ke (*Meretricis/Cyclinae concha*).

These herbs are particularly suitable for treating cough without production or with scanty sputum that is difficult to expectorate, and dryness in the nasal cavity, mouth and throat. In some cases, chest pain and difficult breathing are present. The tongue is red with a thin dry, yellow coating, or with no coating, and the pulse is rapid and thready. These suggest that Heat has accumulated in the Lung and the Body Fluids have been consumed.

These herbs are often used for treating upper respiratory infection, acute or chronic bronchitis, pulmonary tuberculosis, pneumonia, influenza, pertussis, pharyngitis, spontaneous pneumothorax, cor pulmonale and silicosis. In order to increase the therapeutic result, these herbs are often used together with herbs that moisten the Lung and nourish the Lung-Yin—for example, Sang Ye (*Mori folium*), Tian Hua Fen (*Trichosanthis radix*), Bei Sha Shen (*Glehniae radix*), Nan Sha Shen (*Adenophorae radix*) and Mai Men Dong (*Ophiopogonis radix*).

17 Which herbs are able to transform Damp-Phlegm?

The herbs that transform Damp-Phlegm are Ban Xia (*Pinelliae rhizoma*), Ju Hong (*Citri erythrocarpae pars rubra epicarpii*), Chen Pi (*Citri reticulatae pericarpium*), Xing Ren (*Armeniacae semen*), Jie Geng (*Platycodi radix*), Zi Wan (*Asteris radix*), Bai Qian (*Cynanchi stauntonii radix*), Xuan Fu Hua (*Inulae flos*) and Bai Jie Zi (*Sinapis albae semen*).

These herbs are particularly effective for treating cough with a large amount of white, thin sputum, fullness in the chest and epigastrium, heavy and cold limbs, tiredness, a white, thick tongue coating and a slippery pulse. They are often used for treating chronic bronchitis, pulmonary emphysema, and cold and influenza infections.

In clinical practice, in order to increase the therapeutic effect to treat the cause of Phlegm, these herbs are often used together with herbs that transform Dampness, such as Fu Ling (*Poria*) and Cang Zhu (*Atractylodis rhizoma*), herbs that strengthen the function of the Spleen, such as Bai Zhu (*Atractylodis macrocephalae rhizoma*), and herbs that warm the Interior, such as Sheng Jiang (*Zingiberis rhizoma recens*).

18 Which herbs are able to disperse the Lung-Qi and direct it to descend, and arrest wheezing?

The herbs that particularly disperse the Lung-Qi and water accumulation and arrest wheezing are Ma Huang (*Ephedrae herba*)*, She Gan (*Belamcandae rhizoma*), Xing Ren (*Armeniacae semen*) and Jie Geng (*Platycodi radix*). They are often used together with herbs that move upwards, such as Xiang Ru (*Moslae herba*), Jing Jie (*Schizonepetae herba*) and Cang Zhu (*Atractylodis rhizoma*).

Herbs that mainly direct the Lung-Qi to descend, reduce the accumulation of Phlegm and water and arrest wheezing are Bai Qian (*Cynanchi stauntonii radix*), Xing Ren (*Armeniacae semen*), Su Zi (*Perillae fructus*), Xuan Fu Hua (*Inulae flos*), Ting Li Zi (*Lepidii/Descurainiae semen*) and Sang Bai Pi (*Mori cortex*). They are often used together with herbs that move downwards, such as Shi Gao (*Gypsum*), Ban Xia (*Pinelliae rhizoma*) and Chen Xiang (*Aquilariae lignum*).

These herbs are particularly suitable for treating wheezing, shallow and quick breathing, coughing with watery sputum, stifling sensations in the chest, edema and difficult urination. In most cases, there is also a purple tongue with a watery coating, and a rapid, restless pulse. In clinical practice, these herbs are often used to treat asthma, pulmonary emphysema, chronic bronchitis, pulmonary heart disease with heart failure, acute nephritis and renal failure.

19 Which herbs are able to soothe the Stomach-Qi, and transform Phlegm and Dampness in the Stomach?

The herbs that soothe the Stomach-Qi and transform Damp-Phlegm are Ban Xia (*Pinelliae rhizoma*), Xuan Fu Hua (*Inulae flos*), Su Zi (*Perillae fructus*), Zi Su Ye (*Perillae folium*) and Pi Pa Ye (*Eriobotryae folium*).

The herbs that soothe the Stomach-Qi and transform Phlegm-Heat and Damp-Heat in the Stomach are Zhu Ru (*Bambusae caulis in taeniam*) and Huang Qin (*Scutellariae radix*).

All of these herbs are able to relieve nausea, vomiting, fullness in the epigastric region, reduced appetite and distension in the abdomen. In most cases, patients have a sticky tongue coating and a rapid, wiry or slippery pulse. In clinical practice, these herbs can be used in the treatment of acute gastritis, hepatitis, morning sickness in early pregnancy, kinetosis, influenza and cold infections, depression, neurosis, anorexia, Ménière's disease and migraine.

20 What are the symptoms and pathogenic changes in the syndrome when Phlegm covers the Mind? What are the commonly used substances to treat this disorder?

Phlegm and Phlegm-Heat may disturb or cover the Heart and cause mental disorders. The syndrome can be subdivided into Yin and Yang types. In the Yin type, the patient is quite dull, has hallucinations, murmurs to him or herself, sometimes cries and sometimes laughs, and has a poor appetite, a white sticky tongue coating and a wiry, slippery pulse. In clinical practice, this syndrome can be seen in depression, phobia, schizophrenia and other mental disorders. The syndrome is often caused by stagnation of the Liver-Qi and Spleen-Qi from disturbance of emotions such as worry, distress and sorrow. When Phlegm combines with the stagnant Liver-Qi, it may cover or disturb the Heart. The treatment principle in this condition is to promote the Qi movement and transform Phlegm. The commonly used herbs are Ban Xia (*Pinelliae rhizoma*), Chen Pi (*Citri reticulatae pericarpium*), Shi Chang Pu (*Acori graminei rhizoma*), Yuan Zhi (*Polygalae radix*) and Fu Ling (*Poria*).

In the Yang type, the manifestations are mental confusion, delirium, mania and excitability, a red tongue with a yellow, sticky coating, and a wiry, slippery and rapid pulse. This syndrome often occurs in patients who have a Yang constitution or are in a condition of Phlegm-Heat; under the influence of violent rage, the Liver-Fire rises up quickly, also pushing Phlegm upwards and covering the Mind. In clinical practice, this syndrome can be found in many kinds of mental disorder such as mania, schizophrenia and in acute cerebrovascular accident. The treatment principle is to transform Phlegm-Heat and to open the Heart orifice. The commonly used herbs are Dan Nan Xing (*Pulvis arisaemae cum felle bovis*), Zhu Ru (*Bambusae caulis in taeniam*), Zhu Li (*Bambusae succus*), Tian Zhu Huang (*Bambusae concretio silicea*), Yu Jin (*Curcumae radix*), Zhi Shi (*Aurantii fructus immaturus*) and Meng Shi (*Lapis micae seu chloriti*)*.

21 Which herbs are able to transform Wind-Phlegm from the meridians and collaterals?

The herbs that transform Wind-Phlegm are Tian Nan Xing (*Arisaematis rhizoma*), Bai Fu Zi (*Typhonii rhizoma praeparatum*)*, Bai Jie Zi (*Sinapis albae semen*), Jiang Can (*Bombyx batrycatus*), Tian Ma (*Gastrodiae rhizoma*)**, Ban Xia (*Pinelliae rhizoma*), Zhu Li (*Bambusae succus*) and Tian Zhu Huang (*Bambusae concretio silicea*).

These herbs are used in clinical practice to treat cramp, numbness, tingling, heaviness and pain in the limbs, facial paralysis, facial spasm, epilepsy, hemiplegia, migraine, neuralgia and arthritis. They are often used together with herbs that regulate the Qi and Blood, expel Wind-Dampness and extinguish internal Wind.

22 Which herbs are able to soften hardness and dissipate nodules?

The herbs that soften hardness and dissipate nodules are Hai Zao (*Sargassum*), Kun Bu (*Eckloniae thallus*), Hai Fu Shi (*Pumex*), Hai Ge Ke (*Meretricis/Cyclinae concha*), Wa Leng Zi (*Arcae concha*) and Zhe Bei Mu (*Fritillariae thunbergii bulbus*). They are used together with some other herbs which also have the function of softening hardness and dissipating nodules, such as Mu Li (*Ostrea concha*), Huang Yao Zi (*Dioscoreae bulbiferae rhizoma*), Xia Ku Cao (*Prunellae spica*) and Xuan Shen (*Scrophulariae radix*).

In clinical practice they are used in the treatment of cervical lymphadenopathy, lymphadenitis, thyroiditis, simple goiter and tumors. In order to increase the therapeutic effects, they are often combined with herbs that regulate the Qi and Blood and reduce Heat-toxin.

Comparisons of strength and temperature in herbs that transform Phlegm

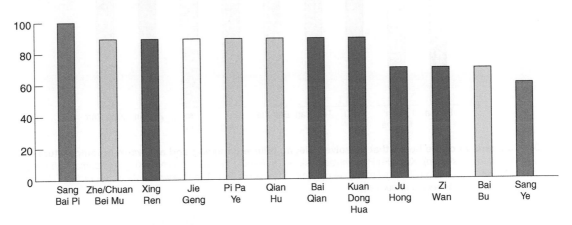

Fig. 8.1 • Comparison of the herbs that relieve coughing.
Sang Bai Pi (*Mori cortex*), Zhe/Chuan Bei Mu (*Fritillariae thunbergii bulbus/Fritillariae cirrhosae bulbus*), Xing Ren (*Armeniacae semen*), Jie Geng (*Platycodi radix*), Pi Pa Ye (*Eriobotryae folium*), Qian Hu (*Peucedani radix*), Bai Qian (*Cynanchi stauntonii radix*), Kuan Dong Hua (*Tussilaginis farfarae*), Ju Hong (*Citri erythrocarpae pars rubra epicarpii*), Zi Wan (*Asteris radix*), Bai Bu (*Stemonae radix*), Sang Ye (*Mori folium*).

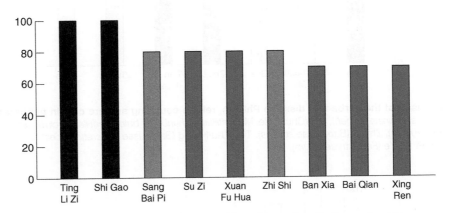

Fig. 8.2 • Comparison of the herbs that direct the Lung-Qi to descend and relieve wheezing.
Ting Li Zi (*Lepidii/Descurainiae semen*), Shi Gao (*Gypsum*), Sang Bai Pi (*Mori cortex*), Su Zi (*Perillae fructus*), Xuan Fu Hua (*Inulae flos*), Zhi Shi (*Aurantii fructus immaturus*), Ban Xia (*Pinelliae rhizoma*), Bai Qian (*Cynanchi stauntonii radix*), Xing Ren (*Armeniacae semen*).

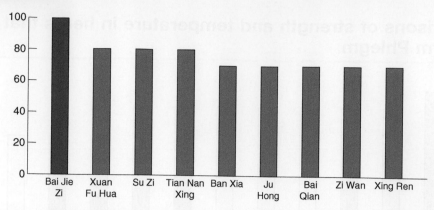

Fig. 8.3 • Comparison of the herbs that dissolve Phlegm, relieve coughing and are warm in temperature.
Bai Jie Zi (*Sinapis albae semen*), Xuan Fu Hua (*Inulae flos*), Su Zi (*Perillae fructus*), Tian Nan Xing (*Arisaematis rhizoma*), Ban Xia (*Pinelliae rhizoma*), Ju Hong (*Citri erythrocarpae pars rubra epicarpii*), Bai Qian (*Cynanchi stauntonii radix*), Zi Wan (*Asteris radix*), Xing Ren (*Armeniacae semen*).

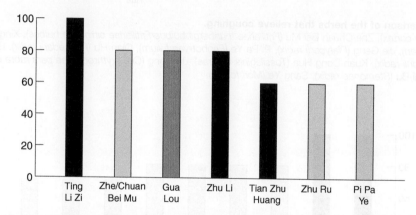

Fig. 8.4 • Comparison of the herbs that dissolve Phlegm, relieve coughing and are cold in temperature.
Ting Li Zi (*Lepidii/Descurainiae semen*), Zhe/Chuan Bei Mu (*Fritillariae thunbergii bulbus/Fritillariae cirrhosae bulbus*), Gua Lou (*Trichosanthis fructus*), Zhu Li (*Bambusae succus*), Tian Zhu Huang (*Bambusae concretio silicea*), Zhu Ru (*Bambusae caulis in taeniam*), Pi Pa Ye (*Eriobotryae folium*).

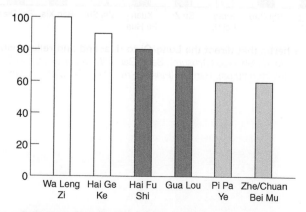

Fig. 8.5 • Comparison of the substances that dissolve thick sputum.
Wa Leng Zi (*Arcae concha*), Hai Ge Ke (*Meretricis/Cyclinae concha*), Hai Fu Shi (*Pumex*), Gua Lou (*Trichosanthis fructus*), Pi Pa Ye (*Eriobotryae folium*), Zhe/Chuan Bei Mu (*Fritillariae thunbergii bulbus/Fritillariae cirrhosae bulbus*).

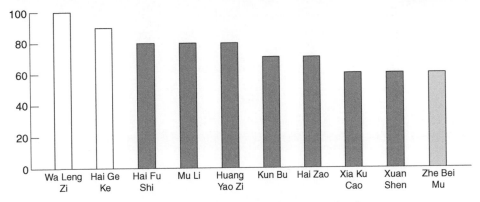

Fig. 8.6 • Comparison of the substances that eliminate Phlegm and soften hardness.
Wa Leng Zi (*Arcae concha*), Hai Ge Ke (*Meretricis/Cyclinae concha*), Hai Fu Shi (*Pumex*), Mu Li (*Ostrea concha*), Huang Yao Zi (*Dioscoreae bulbiferae rhizoma*), Kun Bu (*Eckloniae thallus*), Hai Zao (*Sargassum*), Xia Ku Cao (*Prunellae spica*), Xuan Shen (*Scrophulariae radix*), Zhe Bei Mu (*Fritillariae thunbergii bulbus*).

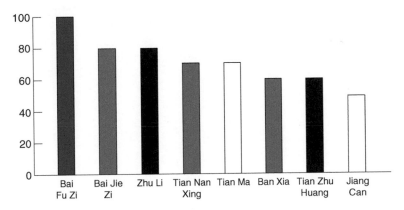

Fig. 8.7 • Comparison of the herbs that eliminate invisible Wind-Phlegm.
Bai Fu Zi (*Typhonii rhizoma praeparatum*)*, Bai Jie Zi (*Sinapis albae semen*), Zhu Li (*Bambusae succus*), Tian Nan Xing (*Arisaematis rhizoma*), Tian Ma (*Gastrodiae rhizoma*)**, Ban Xia (*Pinelliae rhizoma*), Tian Zhu Huang (*Bambusae concretio silicea*), Jiang Can (*Bombyx batrycatus*).

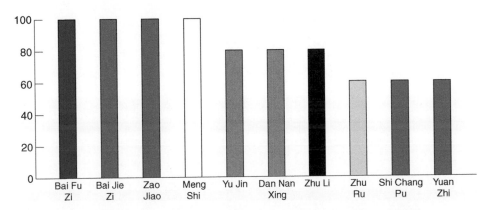

Fig. 8.8 • Comparison of the substances that eliminate invisible Phlegm and open the orifices.
Bai Fu Zi (*Typhonii rhizoma praeparatum*)*, Bai Jie Zi (*Sinapis albae semen*), Zao Jiao (*Gleditsiae fructus*), Meng Shi (*Lapis micae seu chloriti*)*, Yu Jin (*Curcumae radix*), Dan Nan Xing (*Pulvis arisaemae cum felle bovis*), Zhu Li (*Bambusae succus*), Zhu Ru (*Bambusae caulis in taeniam*), Shi Chang Pu (*Acori graminei rhizoma*), Yuan Zhi (*Polygalae radix*).

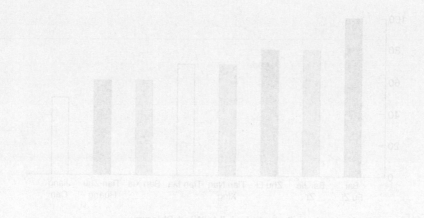

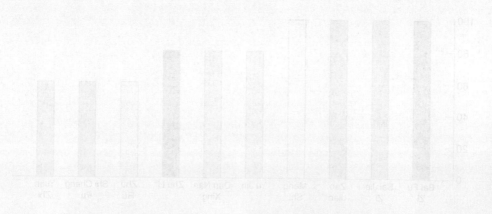

Chapter Nine

9

Herbs that relieve food stagnation; herbs that expel parasites; herbs that induce vomiting

消食药　驱虫药　涌吐药

1 What are the causes of and indications for food stagnation? What precautions should be observed when using herbs that relieve food stagnation?

Herbs that relieve food stagnation are able to promote digestion and dissolve food accumulation. Although food stagnation is not commonly seen nowadays in the developed countries because of the influence of healthy dietary principles, it may still happen in certain situations. First of all, in infants, since the Spleen and Stomach are not fully developed and the parents may lack experience or knowledge of the best diet for children, the child may suffer from indigestion. Secondly, in people with a weak constitution or who suffer from chronic disease, because the functions of the Spleen and Stomach are insufficient, food may tend to stagnate in the Middle Jiao. Thirdly, in elderly people, since the digestion slows with age, indigestion may easily happen. Acute or Excess cases of food stagnation may also occur when on holiday if the diet is changed significantly or the person overindulges.

Food stagnation is caused by the obstruction of the Qi in the Middle Jiao. The main symptoms are fullness in the stomach, belching, nausea, vomiting with a foul smell, distending pain in the abdomen and constipation or diarrhea. The tongue body is normal or slightly red and the coating is thick, white or slightly yellow. The pulse is slippery, forceful and rapid. In chronic cases of food stagnation, especially

in those people with Spleen and Stomach deficiency, symptoms of Qi and Blood deficiency may appear. In children, it may affect their general health and development.

Herbs that relieve food stagnation should be used with caution because they can digest, dissolve and transport food; therefore they may injure the Stomach, Spleen, Qi and Blood too. They are generally used for only a short treatment course. When the accumulated food has been digested, these herbs should be stopped. In people who suffer from indigestion with deficiency of the Spleen and Stomach, these herbs should be used together with herbs that tonify the Spleen and Stomach. In addition, these herbs are normally not used in large dosages, and are often used together with other herbs to enhance the effect, such as herbs that promote the Qi movement, eliminate Dampness or clear Heat in the Middle Jiao. For patients who have a weakness of the Spleen and Stomach, herbs that are slightly warm in temperature are often used to warm the Middle Jiao and accelerate the function of these organs.

2 What are the characteristics of Mai Ya (*Hordei fructus germinatus*), Shen Qu (*Massa medicata fermentata*) and Shan Zha (*Crataegi fructus*)?

These three herbs have the function of promoting digestion. Since they are often used together and are very effective for treating food stagnation, they are given a particular name: Jiao San Xian. In Chinese, 'Jiao' means 'deep-dry-fried', 'San' means 'three' and 'Xian' means 'immortal'. In other words, the name means 'three very effective herbs'. These herbs are often deeply dry-fried until their colors have changed to deep brown. It is believed that they are then more easily digested and work particularly on the Middle Jiao.

These three herbs are often used together because they have different functions and can enhance each other's therapeutic effects. Mai Ya is sweet and neutral, and enters the Spleen and Stomach meridians; it especially aids the digestion of wheat, rice and fruits. Shen Qu is pungent, sweet and warm, and enters the Spleen and Stomach meridians; it particularly aids the digestion of cereals and dispels the effects of alcohol. Shan Zha is sour, sweet and slightly warm, and enters the Spleen, Stomach and Liver meridians; it especially aids the digestion of meat, fat and milk. Because in most cases of food stagnation these foods and drinks are all involved, the three herbs are often used together.

3 Lai Fu Zi (Raphani semen), Mai Ya (Hordei fructus germinatus) and Gu Ya (Oryzae fructus germinatus) are all able to aid the digestion of wheat, rice and fruits. What are the differences between their actions?

These three herbs are all used for stagnation of wheat, rice and fruits, but their strengths are different. Lai Fu Zi is the strongest; it is pungent, sweet and neutral, and enters the Lung and Spleen meridians. It can direct the Lung-Qi to descend, soothe the Stomach-Qi and promote the bowel movement. It can also eliminate Phlegm whether in the Lung or in the Stomach. Lai Fu Zi is especially suitable for use when the food stagnation causes nausea, vomiting and constipation and the tongue has a thick, sticky and white coating.

Mai Ya is gentler than Lai Fu Zi and it can dissolve stagnation of wheat, rice and fruits. But, unlike Lai Fu Zi, it has no function in promoting the Qi movement.

Gu Ya is the weakest herb of the three. It is gentle and slow in action, but its strong point is that it can tonify the Spleen and Stomach, so it can be used for a longer period of time than the others. Gu Ya can also aid the digestion of cereals, so can be used for all starchy foods. It is particularly suitable for people who suffer from indigestion in Deficiency conditions.

4 Shen Qu (Massa medicata fermentata) and Gu Ya (Oryzae fructus germinatus) both can aid the digestion of grains. What are the differences between their actions?

Shen Qu and Gu Ya both can aid the digestion of cereals and reduce the food stagnation, but Shen Qu is stronger than Gu Ya in action. Shen Qu is pungent, sweet and warm and is able to promote the Qi movement, soothe the Stomach-Qi, and aid the digestion of starchy foods which are heavy to the stomach, such as grains and brown bread. It is effective for reducing distension and heavy sensations in the stomach. Gu Ya is much gentler in action than Shen Qu; however, as it has tonifying ability, it can be used for a long time.

Another difference between these two herbs is that Shen Qu is able to dispel the effects of alcohol whereas Gu Ya does not.

5 What are the characteristics of Ji Nei Jin (Gigeriae galli endothelium corneum) and Shan Zha (Crataegi fructus)?

Ji Nei Jin and Shan Zha are two substances that are especially used to aid the digestion of meat and fat. Ji Nei Jin is sweet and slightly cold, and enters the Stomach, Spleen and Bladder meridians. It not only reduces the stagnation of meat, but also aids digestion of all other kinds of food. Its action in relieving food stagnation is quite strong and it is very effective in treating fullness in the Stomach, nausea, vomiting and diarrhea. Since it is cold in temperature, it is also able to reduce Heat and eliminate irritability. It is particularly suitable for use in children with malnutrition when the chronic food stagnation has already produced Heat.

Shan Zha is sweet, sour and slightly warm, and enters the Stomach, Spleen and Liver meridians. Besides its function of dissolving meat, fat and milk accumulations, it is able to break up congealed Blood and promote Blood circulation. It has also recently been found that this herb can lower serum cholesterol level and lower blood pressure, and has been used in the prevention and treatment of arteriosclerosis. Since this fruit has a nice sweet and sour taste, it is often used in the preparation of candy, jam or drinks and has become an ingredient in a healthy diet.

6 What are the characteristics of herbs that expel parasites? What precautions should be observed in their use?

Herbs that expel parasites are able to expel the intestinal parasites, such as roundworm, hookworm, pinworm (threadworm) and tapeworm. Some of them also have the function of eliminating fasciolopsis, schistosome and vaginal trichomonas. Most of these herbs are bitter, pungent, cold or warm, and poisonous. They enter the Stomach, Large Intestine and Spleen meridians. These herbs are not as strong as the modern antiparasitic drugs but they have much less toxicity and can be used repeatedly. They are especially suitable for children and patients suffering from liver and kidney disorders. These herbs are also very often used with other herbs to enhance their therapeutic effect of eliminating parasites and harmonizing the Yin and Yang of the body—for example, herbs that regulate the Qi, purgatives, herbs that promote the digestion, herbs that tonify the Spleen and herbs that clear Heat or warm Cold.

Since these herbs are able to eliminate parasites, most of them, more or less, are poisonous herbs, and therefore the dosage should be carefully controlled. They are usually taken on an empty stomach, are used only once or for 3 days at most as a treatment course. However, some herbs such as Nan Gua Zi (*Curcubitae semen*) and Fei Zi (*Torreyae semen*) are not poisonous, so can be used for a longer period of time.

7 Which herbs can expel *Ascaris* (roundworm)?

The herbs that are very commonly used to expel roundworm are Ku Lian Pi (*Meliae cortex*) and Shi Jun Zi (*Quisqualis fructus*). There are other herbs which have the same function but are not as strong as these two herbs, and they are often used together with these two herbs to accentuate the therapeutic effect. They are He Shi (*Carpesii fructus*), Wu Yi (*Ulmi fructus praeparatus*), Fei Zi (*Torreyae semen*), Bing Lang (*Arecae semen*), Nan Gua Zi (*Curcubitae semen*) and Lei Wan (*Omphalia*).

8 Which herbs can expel *Oxyuroidea* (pinworm or threadworm), *Taenia* (tapeworm) and *Ancylostoma* (hookworm)?

The herbs that can expel pinworm are Ku Lian Pi (*Meliae cortex*), He Shi (*Carpesii fructus*), Fei Zi (*Torreyae semen*), Guan Zhong (*Dryopteridis rhizoma*) and Bing Lang (*Arecae semen*).

The herbs that can expel tapeworm are Bing Lang, Nan Gua Zi (*Curcubitae semen*), Lei Wan (*Omphalia*), Xian He Cao (*Agrimoniae herba*) and Guan Zhong.

The herbs that can expel hookworm are Fei Zi, Bing Lang and Lei Wan.

9 What are the characteristics of Shi Jun Zi (*Quisqualis fructus*) and Ku Lian Pi (*Meliae cortex*)?

Shi Jun Zi and Ku Lian Pi are both effective for expelling roundworm. Shi Jun Zi is sweet and warm, and has a nice smell and taste. As well as expelling roundworm, it can expel pinworm, and it is also able to promote digestion and reduce food and milk stagnation. The fruit contains lipids and has a light laxative action. In clinical practice, it is particularly suitable for use in children. The baked fruit can be eaten directly like a nut, at a dosage of one and a half nuts for each year of age.

Ku Lian Pi is bitter and cold and it is stronger in its action of expelling roundworm than Shi Jun Zi, but it is a toxic herb and can be used only once a day for 2 days. Moreover, fresh Ku Lian Pi is more effective than the dry form. It is often used together with herbs that strengthen the Spleen, as well as with purgative herbs.

10 What are the differences between Shi Jun Zi (*Quisqualis fructus*) and Fei Zi (*Torreyae semen*) in expelling parasites?

Shi Jun Zi and Fei Zi both are fruits and have pleasant smells and tastes after they are dry-fried. They are less toxic than the other herbs and can expel parasites without the side-effect of injuring the Spleen. They can also moisten the intestines and lubricate the stool, so it is not necessary to add extra purgative herbs when these two herbs are used. However, Shi Jun Zi is particularly effective for expelling roundworm and Fei Zi is better for eliminating pinworm, hookworm and tapeworm. Shi Jun Zi is also able to promote digestion and reduce food stagnation, whereas Fei Zi does not have such a function.

11 What are the differences in characteristics between Nan Gua Zi (*Curcubitae semen*) and Bing Lang (*Arecae semen*)?

Nan Gua Zi and Bing Lang are both able to expel many kinds of intestinal parasites, such as tapeworm, roundworm and pinworm. They are more effective for expelling tapeworm if used together; this combination can accentuate their therapeutic action greatly. In addition, Bing Lang is also able to treat schistosome, fasciolopsis and malarial parasite; Nan Gua Zi also treats schistosome. Furthermore, Bing Lang is able to direct the Qi downward, reduce food stagnation, and drain water and Phlegm downwards, as well as promoting bowel movement; these actions may assist the action of expelling the intestinal parasites. Nan Gua Zi can be used with a large dosage and for a longer period of time, as it possesses no characteristic toxic effects.

12 What are the indications for and characteristics of the herbs that induce vomiting? What precautions should be observed in their use?

Herbs that induce vomiting are used when Phlegm, food or toxic substances have accumulated in the stomach. It is possible to expel them through vomiting so as to relieve the accumulation, the toxicity and the obstruction of the Qi. This method is used in intoxication, food stagnation and accumulation of a large amount of Phlegm. The herbs that are able to induce vomiting are Gua Di (*Pedicellus cucumeris*), Li Lu (*Veratri nigri radix et rhizoma*) and Chang Shan (*Dichroae febrifugae radix*).

The method of inducing vomiting to treat diseases was used more often in ancient times than nowadays. There was a famous doctor, Zhang Cong Zheng (1156–1228), who obtained good results by applying the methods of inducing vomiting, sweating and downward draining to expel pathogenic factors, and regulate the Qi and Blood so as to harmonize the Yin and Yang of the body. He wrote a book focusing on the study of these three methods and his clinical experience.

Because the herbs that induce vomiting are very strong and extreme vomiting gives patients an unpleasant sensation, this method is applied only in patients who have Excess syndromes and are in reasonably good health. After vomiting, patients should rest, avoid exposure to wind or start taking food immediately. Moreover, the dosage of the herbs should also be controlled carefully because they are poisonous herbs. If the Phlegm, food or the toxic substances have been expelled through vomiting and the symptoms become less severe, the herbs that induce vomiting should be stopped.

For patients who need to use the vomiting method but have a weak constitution, Ren Shen Lu (*Ginseng cervix*) can be used instead of the other strong herbs to induce vomiting because it is gentler.

If vomiting cannot be stopped after using these herbs, it may injure the Yin, Body Fluids and Qi, so some methods of stopping vomiting should be used. A small amount of She Xiang (*Moschus*)** can stop the vomiting caused by Gua

Di and Chinese onion soup can stop the vomiting caused by Li Lu.

In addition, Li Lu is incompatible with Xi Xin (*Asari herba*)*, Bai Shao Yao (*Paeoniae radix lacti-flora*), Ren Shen (*Ginseng radix*), Bei Sha Shen (*Glehniae radix*), Nan Sha Shen (*Adenophorae radix*), Dan Shen (*Salviae miltiorrhizae radix*) and Ku Shen (*Sophorae flavescentis radix*).

Comparisons of strength and temperature in herbs that relieve food stagnation, that expel parasites and that induce vomiting

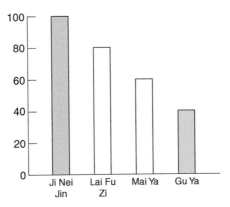

Fig. 9.1 • Comparison of the herbs that promote digestion of wheat, rice and fruits.
Ji Nei Jin (*Gigeriae galli endothelium corneum*), Lai Fu Zi (*Raphani semen*), Mai Ya (*Hordei fructus germinatus*), Gu Ya (*Oryzae fructus germinatus*).

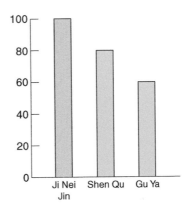

Fig. 9.2 • Comparison of the herbs that promote digestion of cereals and dispel the effects of alcohol.
Ji Nei Jin (*Gigeriae galli endothelium corneum*), Shen Qu (*Massa medicata fermentata*), Gu Ya (*Oryzae fructus germinatus*).

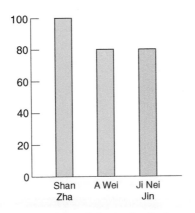

Fig. 9.3 • Comparison of the herbs that promote digestion of meat and remove fat.
Shan Zha (*Crataegi fructus*), A Wei (*Resina ferulae asafoetida*), Ji Nei Jin (*Gigeriae galli endothelium corneum*).

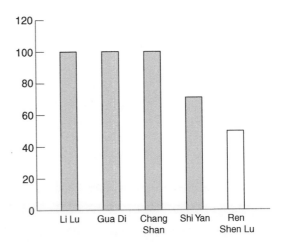

Fig. 9.4 • Comparison of the herbs that induce vomiting.
Li Lu (*Veratri nigri radix et rhizoma*), Gua Di (*Pedicellus cucumeris*), Chang Shan (*Dichroae febrifugae radix*), Shi Yan (*Sal*), Ren Shen Lu (*Ginseng cervix*).

Herbs that regulate the Qi

行气药

1 What are the indications for herbs that regulate the Qi?

Herbs that regulate the Qi are able to regulate, harmonize or spread the Qi so they can treat the syndrome of Qi stagnation. Stagnation of Qi is often caused by emotional disturbance, and accumulation of internal Cold, Heat, Phlegm, water and food. It also occurs in trauma and stagnation of Blood.

The characteristic of the syndrome of Qi stagnation is distension in the affected region. The quality of distension is determined by the degree of the stagnation; generally speaking, *fullness* exists in a mild case, *distension* is seen in an advanced stage, and *pain* occurs in a severe condition.

The syndrome of Qi stagnation varies according to the affected organs and regions. If the Lung-Qi stagnates, the symptoms are breathlessness, stifling in the chest, cough and wheezing. If the Stomach-Qi and Spleen-Qi stagnate, the manifestations are fullness and distension of the entire abdomen, reduced appetite, belching, acid regurgitation, nausea, vomiting, abdominal pain and irregular bowel movement. If the Liver-Qi stagnates, the symptoms are hypochondriac distension and pain, irritability, depression, distension and pain in the breasts, irregular menstruation, and pain in the lower and lateral abdomen. If the Qi stagnates in the meridians, the main symptoms are stiffness, heaviness, numbness or tingling of the limbs and in the affected regions, or migrating pain in the limbs. Most patients with a syndrome of Qi stagnation have a white tongue coating and a wiry pulse when there are no other pathogenic factors.

As well as treating the syndromes mentioned above, in clinical practice these herbs are often used to treat accumulation of water, Phlegm or food and stagnation of Blood, since these pathological factors always cause Qi stagnation and make the original disorder worse. Herbs that regulate the Qi can stimulate the movement of Qi as well as enhancing the effect of other herbs that treat different accumulations. Furthermore, herbs that regulate the movement of the Qi are often used in formulas for tonification because the tonifying herbs are heavy and sticky, so easily disturb the function of transportation and transformation of the Spleen and cause stagnation of Qi.

2 What are the characteristics of herbs that regulate the Qi? What precautions should be observed in their use?

Herbs that regulate the Qi have the following characteristics.

Pungent and warm in nature

Since pungency possesses a moving capability and warmth may activate Qi movement, herbs with warm and pungent properties are able to promote

Qi movement. Almost all the herbs that regulate the Qi have this property, such as Chen Pi (*Citri reticulatae pericarpium*), Wu Yao (*Linderae radix*), Xiang Fu (*Cyperi rhizoma*) and Mu Xiang (*Aucklandiae radix*)**.

Entering the Spleen, Stomach, Liver, Large Intestine and Lung meridians

Since the organs outlined above directly influence the Qi movement of the body, the syndromes of Qi stagnation are also often located in the regions that belong to these organs. Herbs that enter the Stomach and Spleen meridians and treat the stagnation of Qi there are Chen Pi, Zhi Shi (*Aurantii fructus immaturus*), Sha Ren (*Amomi xanthioidis fructus*) and Da Fu Pi (*Arecae pericarpium*). Herbs that enter the Liver meridian and treat the stagnation of Qi there are Xiang Fu, Qing Pi (*Citri reticulatae viride pericarpium*), Chuan Lian Zi (*Toosendan fructus*), Mu Xiang and Wu Yao. Herbs that enter the Large Intestine meridian are Da Fu Pi, Hou Po (*Magnoliae cortex*) and Mu Xiang. (Herbs that enter the Lung meridian and treat the Lung-Qi stagnation are discussed in herbs that stop cough, disperse the Lung-Qi and direct it to descend, and clear Heat from the Lung.)

In addition, since Qi stagnation can be found in most pathological processes, there are a number of herbs that can regulate the Qi movement through other functions, such as herbs that stop cough, dissolve Phlegm, remove food stagnation, drain downward, transform Dampness, warm the Interior, clear Heat and release the Exterior.

Herbs that regulate the Qi should be used with caution in the following conditions.

During pregnancy, heavy menstruation or in bleeding conditions. Since the herbs that regulate Qi are warm and pungent, they can activate the Qi movement, which may cause heavy menstrual bleeding. Herbs that enter the Liver and Kidney meridians should not be used in early pregnancy because they may cause miscarriage.

Conditions of Yin deficiency. Since the herbs that regulate Qi are pungent and warm, they may easily injure the Yin and Body Fluids. Patients with Yin deficiency syndrome or with a Yin-deficient constitution should not use these herbs in large dosages or for a very long period of time.

3 What are the differences in actions between Ju Hong (*Citri erythrocarpae pars rubra epicarpii*), Chen Pi (*Citri reticulatae pericarpium*), Ju Luo (*Citri reticulatae fructus retinervus*), Ju Ye (*Citri reticulatae folium*) and Ju He (*Aurantii semen*)?

All of these herbs come from the tangerine tree and have the function of regulating the Qi. However, each has its own characteristics.

Ju Hong is the reddish layer of fresh tangerine peel. It is pungent, bitter and warm. Pungency has a dispersing property, bitterness causes a descending action, and warmth can dry Dampness and expel Cold. Ju Hong enters the Lung meridian, and is effective for eliminating Damp-Phlegm and stopping cough. It is used for treating a cough with a large amount of sputum that is easy to expectorate caused by Wind and Cold attacking the Lung.

In Chinese, 'Chen' means 'old', and 'Pi' means 'peel'. Chen Pi is the dry tangerine peel, and normally it should be kept for a year before it is used. Compared with the fresh peel, it is more pungent and bitter but less warm. It enters the Stomach and Spleen meridians and is effective for regulating the Qi of these organs. Its aromatic smell can stimulate the Spleen, transform the Dampness and soothe the Stomach-Qi and is often used for distension and pain in the abdomen, reduced appetite, fullness of the stomach, nausea and vomiting.

Ju Luo is sweet, bitter and neutral, and enters the Liver and Lung meridians. According to the concept that the pith of fruit enters the collaterals of the human body, Ju Luo is able to regulate the Qi, open up the collaterals and remove Phlegm there. It is used for treating a chronic cough with Phlegm that is difficult to expectorate, a stifling sensation in the chest and hypochondriac region, such as is seen in chronic bronchitis and emphysema. It can be used together with other herbs such as Si Gua Luo (*Luffae fructus*) and Ju Ye to regulate the Liver-Qi in order to treat pain and distension in the breasts and hypochondrium, such as occurs in premenstrual syndrome and mastopathia.

Ju Ye is pungent, bitter and neutral. Like Ju Luo, it enters the Liver meridian, and it specially regulates the Liver-Qi and breaks down nodules. Its action is stronger than that of Ju Luo. It also enters the Stomach meridian and regulates the Stomach-Qi there. Because the Liver and Stomach meridians pass through the breasts, this herb is able to treat distension and pain of breasts in mastopathia.

Ju He is pungent, bitter and neutral, and enters the Liver and Kidney meridians. It is effective for regulating the Qi, breaking down nodules and stopping pain. According to the concept that seeds move downwards, it is especially used for treating Cold accumulation in the Liver meridian that manifests as cramping pain in the sides of the lower abdomen with a cold sensation, such as occurs in dysmenorrhea, amenorrhea, inguinal hernia and hydrocele of the testis.

4 What are the differences between the functions of Zhi Shi (*Aurantii fructus immaturus*) and Zhi Ke (*Aurantii fructus*)?

Zhi Shi and Zhi Ke come from the same tree. Zhi Shi is the unripe fruit of the bitter orange; Zhi Ke is the big, nearly ripe bitter orange. Both are bitter, slightly cold, and enter the Spleen and Stomach meridians. They can regulate the Spleen-Qi and Stomach-Qi, and treat distension and pain in the abdomen, nausea and vomiting.

Zhi Shi has the stronger bitter taste and it moves downwards strongly. These properties lead to an intensive action of breaking up the obstruction of Qi and the accumulation of Qi, Blood, food or Phlegm, and it can also promote bowel movement. In clinical practice, it can treat severe distension and pain in the chest and abdomen, shortness of breath and constipation, such as is seen in gastroenteritis, intussusception, intestinal obstruction, dysentery, irritable colon, pleurisy and pneumonia.

Zhi Ke also has the function of regulating the Qi, but its action is gentler and slower. It moves horizontally in the Upper Jiao and Middle Jiao. It opens the chest and reduces distension, and is used to treat Qi stagnation in chest, stomach and hypochondrium, which brings about distension in the upper abdomen, stifling in the chest, a reduced appetite, irritability and depression. It also has the function of dissolving Phlegm and treating cough due to Heat in the Lung.

5 What are the differences between Qing Pi (*Citri reticulatae viride pericarpium*), Chen Pi (*Citri reticulatae pericarpium*) and Zhi Ke (*Aurantii fructus*)?

These three herbs all come from tangerine or orange. They can promote Qi movement and reduce distension and pain. Their individual characteristics are as follows.

Qing Pi is the peel of the unripe tangerine. It is warm and bitter, and has the strongest function of regulating Qi of these three herbs. Because it particularly enters the Liver and Gall Bladder meridians, it is effective for promoting the free flow of the Liver-Qi, dissolving Phlegm accumulation and alleviating pain. It is used for treating pain and distension in the chest, breasts and hypochondriac region.

Chen Pi is the dry tangerine peel. It is less warm and bitter than Qing Pi, and it enters particularly the Spleen and Stomach meridians. It regulates the Qi of these organs and is often used for treating distension in the stomach, reduced appetite, nausea and vomiting caused by Qi stagnation in the upper abdomen.

Zhi Ke is the big, nearly ripe bitter orange. Its ability to move the Qi is similar to that of Chen Pi but it focuses on the chest so it is often used to treat tightness in the chest, irritability and depression.

6 What are the characteristics of Xiang Fu (*Cyperi rhizoma*)?

Xiang Fu is a very commonly used herb to regulate the Liver-Qi. It is pungent, sweet, slightly bitter and warm, and enters the Liver and San Jiao meridians. Xiang Fu is an effective and gentle herb for regulating the Qi. It is warm and pungent but without a harsh and drying nature. It promotes Liver-Qi movement but without the possibility of injuring the Yin and Blood of the Liver. It is slightly bitter, so can reduce the slight Liver-Heat that is generated by Liver-Qi stagnation. The sweetness can soften the Liver and moderate the speed of the Qi movement. All these characteristics match the pathological changes in the syndrome of the Liver-Qi stagnation. Because it also enters the San Jiao meridian, which is the passage of the Qi and water, it can effectively spread the Qi throughout the entire body.

In clinical practice, Xiang Fu is used for treating syndromes and symptoms associated with Liver-Qi stagnation, such as distension in the hypochondriac region, feelings of tightness in the chest, irritability, depression, irregular menstruation, dysmenorrhea, distension and pain in the breasts and infertility. Since Xiang Fu is so effective for regulating the Qi, it is regarded in TCM as *the chief of all the herbs that regulate the Qi* and *the first-line choice for treating gynecological disorders*.

7 Which herbs are often used to promote Liver-Qi movement and what are their characteristics?

There are several herbs mainly entering the Liver, Gall Bladder and San Jiao meridians, and they particularly promote Liver-Qi movement. They are Xiang Fu (*Cyperi rhizoma*), Chai Hu (*Bupleuri radix*), Xiang Yuan (*Citri fructus*), Fo Shou (*Citri sarcodactylis fructus*), Mei Gui Hua (*Rosae flos*), Qing Pi (*Citri reticulatae viride pericarpium*), Mu Xiang (*Aucklandiae radix*)**, Wu Yao (*Linderae radix*) and Chuan Lian Zi (*Toosendan fructus*).

Xiang Fu is the most commonly used herb to promote the Liver-Qi movement. Since it is gentle and effective, it can be applied for treating both Excess and Deficiency syndromes that are associated with the Liver-Qi stagnation, such as premenstrual syndrome, menopausal syndrome, irregular menstruation, hypertension, depression, insomnia, hepatitis and peptic ulcer.

Chai Hu is another commonly used herb to regulate the Liver-Qi, and it is also a gentle herb. Unlike Xiang Fu, it is pungent and slightly cold, and has the function of dispersing and lifting the Liver-Qi rather than promoting its circulation. It is particularly suitable for treating constrained Liver-Qi such as in chronic Liver and Gall Bladder diseases, stress and depression with emotions of anger and frustration. Since the tendency of its action is upwards, in syndromes and diseases caused by Liver-Yang rising or Liver-Fire blazing up, such as hypertension and glaucoma, it should be combined with herbs that bring down the Qi.

Xiang Yuan and Fo Shou enter the Liver, Spleen and Stomach meridians. They are bitter, sour and slightly warm. Like Xiang Fu and Chai Hu, both are very effective for promoting Liver-Qi movement and treating hypochondriac pain, distension and depression. Moreover, they are particularly effective when stagnant Liver-Qi has disturbed the Stomach, leading to stifling in the chest and distension in the gastric and hypochondriac regions. They can sooth the Stomach-Qi and treat reduced appetite, vomiting and belching.

Mei Gui Hua has similar functions to Xiang Yuan and Fo Shou and treats the syndrome of Liver-Qi attacking the Spleen and Stomach. However, this herb can promote both Qi and Blood circulation and is a proper herb to treat menstrual disorders due to Qi and Blood stagnation.

Qing Pi is the strongest of these herbs for regulation of the Liver-Qi. Because its action is strong, it may injure the Qi and Yin, especially when there is Yin deficiency, so it is used for only a short period of time and in Excess conditions.

Mu Xiang enters the Gall Bladder, Spleen and Large Intestine meridians. It is able to regulate the Qi in these organs and regions. It is especially effective to treat disorders in which the Liver-Qi overwhelms the Spleen, such as in colitis, peptic ulcer, hepatitis and gastrointestinal neurosis. This herb is quite warm and pungent, and is strong in action, so its dosage should be controlled carefully.

Wu Yao enters the Lower Jiao and can regulate the Liver-Qi in the Liver meridian. It is the warmest of these herbs, and it especially warms the Liver meridian, expels Cold and spreads the Liver-Qi. It is particularly effective for relieving pain in the lateral sides of the lower abdomen and genital area. It treats dysmenorrhea, hernia, frequent urination and urinary incontinence.

Chuan Lian Zi is very bitter and cold. It can very intensively move the Liver-Qi and drain Liver-Fire. As the direction of its action is downwards, it is used for treating syndromes in which Liver-Fire blazes up and the Liver-Qi is constrained. The symptoms are irritability, distension in the hypochondrium, insomnia, quick temper, red eyes, headache, a red tongue with a yellow coating, and a forceful, wiry and rapid pulse. Because Chuan Lian Zi is very bitter and cold, it easily injures the Stomach, and is poisonous, so is not allowed to be used for a long period of time and in large dosages. Overdose may cause nausea, vomiting, diarrhea, dyspnea and arrhythmia.

8 Which herbs are used for regulating the Qi in the abdomen and what are their characteristics?

There are several herbs that have the function of regulating the Qi in the abdomen and treating distension. They are Chen Pi (*Citri reticulatae pericarpium*), Zhi Ke (*Aurantii fructus*), Hou Po (*Magnoliae cortex*), Sha Ren (*Amomi xanthioidis fructus*), Mu Xiang (*Aucklandiae radix*)** , Da Fu Pi (*Arecae pericarpium*) and Zhi Shi (*Aurantii fructus immaturus*).

Chen Pi and Zhi Ke enter the Stomach and Spleen meridians. They especially regulate the Qi in the upper abdomen and treat distension in the epigastric region, with reduced appetite, nausea and vomiting.

Hou Po, Sha Ren and Mu Xiang enter the Middle Jiao, and they regulate the Qi in the whole abdomen and treat distension and pain there. Since they can regulate the Qi in the intestine, they can treat irregular bowel movement and constipation. The action of these three herbs in moving the Qi is stronger than that of Chen Pi and Zhi Ke. Meanwhile, Hou Po and Sha Ren are very effective in transforming Dampness, and treat nausea and vomiting in cases of food stagnation and acute gastroenteritis.

Da Fu Pi and Zhi Shi are able to promote Qi movement in the whole abdomen, especially in the intestines. Both can treat constipation and relieve abdominal pain and distension. Da Fu Pi is also able to promote water metabolism and treat edema and ascites. Zhi Shi is more powerful for removing all kinds of accumulations.

9 Which herbs can influence Qi movement in the body?

In most books of Chinese herbal medicine, herbs that particularly regulate the Qi of the Liver, Stomach and Spleen are discussed as herbs that regulate Qi. However, there is Qi movement in every organ and meridian in a broad sense, and the Qi movement shows itself from the proper functions of the involved organ or meridian, and in the cooperation of the internal organs as well. There are a number of herbs and herbal combinations that can influence Qi movement in the body. They should be considered as herbs that regulate the Qi in a broad sense. Examples are as follows.

Regulating the Lung-Qi, eliminating Phlegm, reducing Fire and regulating Qi in the chest

Ma Huang (*Ephedrae herba*)* disperses and lifts the Lung-Qi and Xing Ren (*Armeniacae semen*) directs the Lung-Qi downwards and transforms Phlegm. They are used together to regulate the Lung-Qi.

Sang Ye (*Mori folium*) disperses Wind-Heat and Sang Bai Pi (*Mori cortex*) clears Heat and directs the Qi of the Lung to descend. They are used together to expel Wind-Heat from the Lung, bring down the Lung-Qi and relieve wheezing.

Jie Geng (*Platycodi radix*) lifts the Lung-Qi and Xing Ren directs the Lung-Qi to descend. Both of them can eliminate Phlegm and stop a cough. They are used together to regulate the function of the Lung and to remove Phlegm.

Xi Xin (*Asari herba*)* disperses the Lung-Qi and Wu Wei Zi (*Schisandrae fructus*) stabilizes the Lung-Qi. They are used together to relieve the Cold type of wheezing.

Ma Huang (*Ephedrae herba*)* disperses the Lung-Qi and disperses Heat from the Lung, and Shi Gao (*Gypsum*) directs the Lung-Qi to descend and clears Heat from the Lung. They are used together to relieve the Heat type of wheezing.

Zhi Zi (*Gardeniae fructus*) directs Heat down from the chest and Dan Dou Chi (*Sojae semen praeparatum*) disperses Heat there. They are used together to treat irritability due to constraint of the Qi and Heat in the chest.

Regulating Qi in the Middle Jiao and promoting digestion

Bai Zhu (*Atractylodis macrocephalae rhizoma*) strengthens the Spleen-Qi and promotes the function of transportation and transformation of the Spleen in the Middle Jiao, and Zhi Shi directs the Qi in the intestines to descend and removes the accumulation of food, Phlegm and Qi. They are used together to promote digestion.

Huang Lian (*Coptidis rhizoma*) directs Stomach-Fire to descend and Sheng Ma (*Cimicifugae rhizoma*) disperses it. They are often used together to reduce constraint of Stomach-Fire and treat toothache.

Ban Xia (*Pinelliae rhizoma*) disperses the stagnation of Stomach-Qi and accumulation of Phlegm, and Huang Qin (*Scutellariae radix*) clears Heat that is generated by the accumulations in the Stomach. They are used together to regulate the Stomach and effectively treat nausea and poor appetite, especially under stress.

Regulating the intestines and promoting bowel movement

Da Huang (*Rhei rhizoma*) reduces Heat and purges accumulation in the intestines and Hou Po (*Magnoliae cortex*) disperses the Qi and directs it to descend. They are used together to promote bowel movement and treat constipation.

Da Huang directs the Qi in the intestines downwards and moves the stool, and Jie Geng (*Platycodi radix*) lifts the Lung-Qi to accelerate the downward movement of the Qi in the Large Intestine. They are used together to treat constipation and distension in the abdomen.

Associating the Heart and Kidney

Huang Lian (*Coptidis rhizoma*) reduces Excessive-Heat in the Heart and Rou Gui (*Cinnamomi cassiae cortex*) strengthens the Kidney-Yang and warms the vital Fire. They are used together to treat insomnia due to disharmony of the Heart and Kidney.

Lifting the Yang and strengthening the Exterior

Huang Qi (*Astragali radix*) strengthens and stabilizes the Defensive Qi, and Fang Feng (*Saposhnikoviae radix*) dispels Wind from the Exterior. They are used together to regulate the opening and closing of the pores, strengthen the body resistance and prevent catching cold.

Regulating the Liver-Qi

Chai Hu (*Bupleuri radix*) lifts and disperses the Liver-Qi, and Bai Shao Yao (*Paeoniae radix lactiflora*) drains Heat downwards and stabilizes the Yin of the Liver. They are used together to treat Liver-Qi stagnation.

Dang Gui (*Angelicae sinensis radix*) tonifies the Blood and promotes the Blood circulation of the Liver, and Bai Shao Yao nourishes the Blood and stabilizes the Yin of the Liver. They are used together

to soften the Liver and treat Liver-Qi stagnation caused by Blood deficiency.

Dispersing and descending constrained Qi and Fire

Chai Hu (*Bupleuri radix*) lifts and disperses the Liver-Qi, and Xiang Fu (*Cyperi rhizoma*) promotes the movement of Liver-Qi. They are used together to treat Liver-Qi stagnation.

Long Dan Cao (*Gentianae radix*) drains Heat forcefully downwards and also drains Fire from the Liver, and Chai Hu lifts and disperses constrained Fire and Qi in the Liver. They are used for treating Excessive Liver-Fire syndrome.

Huang Lian (*Coptidis rhizoma*) descends Fire from the Stomach, and Sheng Ma (*Cimicifugae rhizoma*) lifts and disperses constrained Qi and Fire in the Stomach. They are used together to treat Excessive-Heat in the Stomach.

Shi Gao (*Gypsum*) drains Fire downwards from the Spleen and Stomach, and Fang Feng disperses constrained Heat and Qi in the Spleen and Stomach. They are used to treat Qi constraint in the Middle Jiao and hidden Fire in the Spleen.

Sedating the Liver-Yang

Dai Zhe Shi (*Haematitum*) and Shi Jue Ming (*Haliotidis concha*) descend the Liver-Yang; Qing Hao (*Artemisiae annuae herba*) and Mai Ya (*Hordei fructus germinatus*) lift constrained Qi from the Middle Jiao. They are used together to harmonize the movement of Qi in the process of directing the Liver-Yang to descend.

Calming the Spirit

Long Gu (*Mastodi fossilium ossis*) calms the Heart and Liver, and Chai Hu lifts the Liver-Qi. They are used together to treat restlessness and insomnia.

Ren Shen (*Ginseng radix*) tonifies the Heart-Qi and Wu Wei Zi stabilizes the Heart-Qi. They are used together to calm the Mind and to treat restlessness and palpitations caused by Heart-Qi deficiency.

Harmonizing the Qi and Blood and treating disorders in a certain part of the body

Gui Zhi (*Cinnamomi cassiae ramulus*) disperses the Defensive Qi and Bai Shao Yao (*Paeoniae radix lactiflora*) nourishes the Nutritive Qi. They are used together to harmonize the Ying level and the Wei level.

Tan Xiang (*Santali albi lignum*) and Xie Bai (*Allii macrostemi bulbus*) warm the Heart-Yang and promote Qi movement in the chest; Gui Zhi warms and promotes the Blood circulation. They are used together to strengthen the Heart-Yang, to promote the movement of Heart-Qi and the Blood circulation, and to treat chest pain, shortness of breath and cold limbs.

Comparisons of strength and temperature in herbs that regulate the Qi

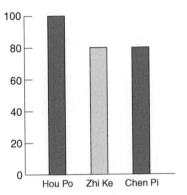

Fig. 10.1 • Comparison of the herbs that regulate the Lung-Qi.
Hou Po (*Magnoliae cortex*), Zhi Ke (*Aurantii fructus*), Chen Pi (*Citri reticulatae pericarpium*).

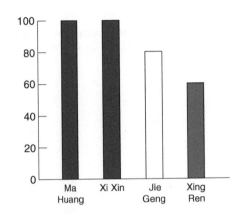

Fig. 10.2 • Comparison of the herbs that disperse the Lung-Qi.
Ma Huang (*Ephedrae herba*)*, Xi Xin (*Asari herba*)*, Jie Geng (*Platycodi radix*), Xing Ren (*Armeniacae semen*).

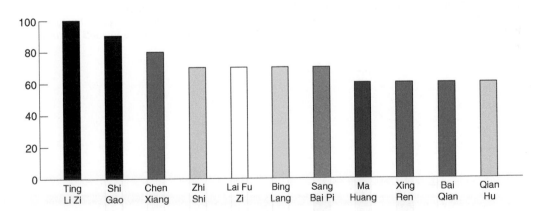

Fig. 10.3 • Comparison of the herbs that direct the Lung-Qi to descend.
Ting Li Zi (*Lepidii/Descurainiae semen*), Shi Gao (*Gypsum*), Chen Xiang (*Aquilariae lignum*), Zhi Shi (*Aurantii fructus immaturus*), Lai Fu Zi (*Raphani semen*), Bing Lang (*Arecae semen*), Sang Bai Pi (*Mori cortex*), Ma Huang (*Ephedrae herba*)*, Xing Ren (*Armeniacae semen*), Bai Qian (*Cynanchi stauntonii radix*), Qian Hu (*Peucedani radix*).

together to harmonize the Ying level and the Wei level of the Blood circulation. They are used together to harmonize the Heart-Yang, to promote the movement and the direction of Heart-Qi and the Blood circulation.

Tan Xiang (santali albi lignum) and Xie Bai (allii macrostemi bulbus) are used to treat chest pain, shortness of breath and to promote Qi movement in the chest. Gui Zhi (cinnamomi cassiae ramulus) is...

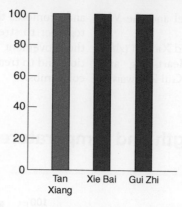

Fig. 10.4 • Comparison of the herbs that regulate the Heart-Qi.
Tan Xiang (*Santali albi lignum*), Xie Bai (*Allii macrostemi bulbus*), Gui Zhi (*Cinnamomi cassiae ramulus*).

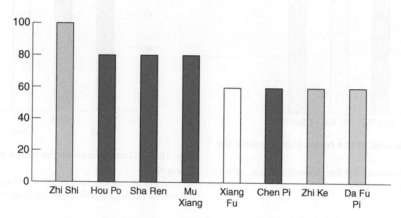

Fig. 10.5 • Comparison of the herbs that regulate the Spleen-Qi and the Stomach-Qi.
Zhi Shi (*Aurantii fructus immaturus*), Hou Po (*Magnoliae cortex*), Sha Ren (*Amomi xanthioidis fructus*), Mu Xiang (*Aucklandiae radix*)**, Xiang Fu (*Cyperi rhizoma*), Chen Pi (*Citri reticulatae pericarpium*), Zhi Ke (*Aurantii fructus*), Da Fu Pi (*Arecae pericarpium*).

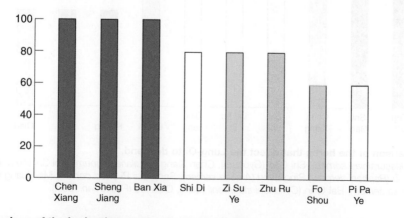

Fig. 10.6 • Comparison of the herbs that soothe the Stomach-Qi.
Chen Xiang (*Aquilariae lignum*), Sheng Jiang (*Zingiberis rhizoma recens*), Ban Xia (*Pinelliae rhizoma*), Shi Di (*Kaki diospyri calyx*), Zi Su Ye (*Perillae folium*), Zhu Ru (*Bambusae caulis in taeniam*), Fo Shou (*Citri sarcodactylis fructus*), Pi Pa Ye (*Eriobotryae folium*).

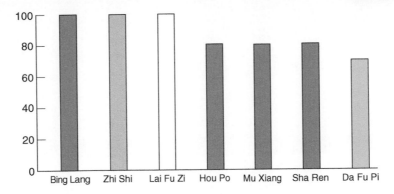

Fig. 10.7 • Comparison of the herbs that regulate the Qi in the Large Intestine.
Bing Lang (*Arecae semen*), Zhi Shi (*Aurantii fructus immaturus*), Lai Fu Zi (*Raphani semen*), Hou Po (*Magnoliae cortex*), Mu Xiang (*Aucklandiae radix*)**, Sha Ren (*Amomi xanthioidis fructus*), Da Fu Pi (*Arecae pericarpium*).

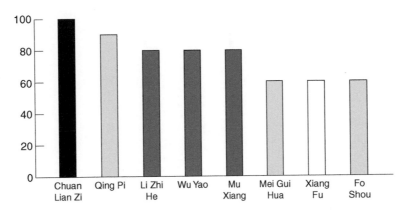

Fig. 10.8 • Comparison of the herbs that regulate the Liver-Qi.
Chuan Lian Zi (*Toosendan fructus*), Qing Pi (*Citri reticulatae viride pericarpium*), Li Zhi He (*Litchi semen*), Wu Yao (*Linderae radix*), Mu Xiang (*Aucklandiae radix*)**, Mei Gui Hua (*Rosae flos*), Xiang Fu (*Cyperi rhizoma*), Fo Shou (*Citri sarcodactylis fructus*).

Chapter Eleven

11

Herbs that regulate the Blood

活血化瘀药

1 What are the causes of Blood stagnation? What are the indications for herbs that promote the Blood circulation?

Herbs that promote the Blood circulation are used for treating syndromes of Blood stagnation. There are different degrees of Blood stagnation. In a mild case, the Blood moves more slowly than it should. If the situation does not change, the Blood stagnates. In a severe case, congealed Blood may be complicated with Phlegm, Heat or Cold, and forms a solid mass that blocks the Blood circulation.

Blood stagnation is caused by several factors. First, both Heat and Cold can lead to Blood stagnation. Heat consumes the Blood and makes it thicker so that the movement of the Blood slows; Cold contracts Blood and lets the Blood circulation slow down. Secondly, Qi stagnation caused by emotional disturbance, stress, anger, excessive pondering or depression over a long period of time can directly result in Blood stagnation. Thirdly, trauma or fracture may directly cause Blood stagnation in the locality. Moreover, Wind, Dampness and Cold that remain for too long in the meridians can also cause Blood stagnation. Accumulation of Phlegm, water, food or parasites in the body for a long period of time may also lead to Blood stagnation. Finally, if the Qi and Blood are deficient, they are not able to promote the Blood circulation so they will also lead to Blood stagnation.

The main symptoms of Blood stagnation are localized pain of a deep, colicky or sharp nature that worsens at night. In severe cases, a solid, immobile mass can be found. Patients who suffer from stagnation of Blood for a long time may have symptoms such as a dark complexion, purple lips and nails, dry skin, amenorrhea, psychiatric disorders, fragile nails and hair. The tongue body is purple with purple spots at the tip or border, and the pulse is wiry and choppy.

In clinical practice, the syndrome of stagnation of Blood can be found in diseases such as myocardial infarction, angina pectoris, acute cholecystitis, biliary ascariasis, acute pancreatitis, acute appendicitis or intestinal obstruction, trauma, strain, sequelae of cerebrovascular accident, rheumatic fever and rheumatoid arthritis, as well as different tumors.

2 What are the characteristics of herbs that promote the Blood circulation?

The Blood circulation needs certain conditions. Blood prefers slight warmth and needs an unobstructed pathway. Too much Cold or Heat may cause pathological changes. Cold can freeze the Blood and results in stagnation. Heat consumes Blood and makes it thicker, so also causes stagnation. Meanwhile, Heat lets the Blood move faster and leave its normal pathway, causing bleeding.

Herbs that promote Blood circulation have the following characteristics according to the physiologic and pathological characteristics of Blood.

131

Pungent, aromatic and slightly warm

Pungency has a moving ability, aromatic smell can penetrate turbidity and reach the deep layers of the body, and warmth may accelerate the actions of the pungent and aromatic properties. Most herbs that promote the Blood circulation are pungent and slightly warm. Such herbs are Chuan Xiong (*Chuanxiong rhizoma*), Ji Xue Teng (*Spatholobi caulis et radix*), Hong Hua (*Carthami flos*), Su Mu (*Sappan lignum*), Yan Hu Suo (*Corydalidis rhizoma*), Wu Ling Zhi (*Trogopterori faeces*), Ru Xiang (*Olibanum*) and E Zhu (*Curcumae rhizoma*).

Pungent, bitter and slightly cold

Since pungency is able to activate the Blood, and bitterness and Cold can clear Heat and prevent Blood consumption from Heat, these herbs are especially suitable for treating Heat in the Blood and Blood stagnation no matter which pathological factor is the initial cause. The commonly used herbs are Dan Shen (*Salviae miltiorrhizae radix*), Yu Jin (*Curcumae radix*), Yi Mu Cao (*Leonuri herba*) and Chi Shao Yao (*Paeoniae radix rubra*).

Pungent, bitter and salty

If congealed Blood exists in the body for a long period of time, it becomes a hard clot or solid mass, and special herbs must be applied to promote Blood circulation as well as to reduce, disperse or dissolve congealed Blood. Since pungency has a dispersing nature, and bitterness and saltiness are able to soften hardness, these properties are often found in herbs that break up or drive out congealed Blood. Such herbs are San Leng (*Sparganii rhizoma*), E Zhu (*Curcumae rhizoma*), Ru Xiang (*Olibanum*), Mo Yao (*Myrrhae*), Wa Leng Zi (*Arcae concha*), Shui Zhi (*Hirudo*), Mang Chong (*Tabanus*)* and Zhe Chong (*Eupolyphaga seu opisthoplatia*)*.

Entering the Heart, Pericardium, Liver and Gall Bladder meridians

The Heart governs the Blood and promotes the Blood circulation. The Liver regulates the amount of Blood in the Blood circulation. As the Pericardium and Gall Bladder are externally–internally related to the Heart and Liver, most of the herbs that promote Blood circulation enter these meridians. Such herbs are Chuan Xiong, Dan Shen, Yue Ji Hua (*Rosae chinensis flos*), Tao Ren (*Persicae semen*) and Hong Hua.

Herbs are divided into different degrees according to the strength of promoting the Blood circulation and removing congealed Blood

Herbs that invigorate the Blood and promote the Blood circulation. These are used for the syndrome of Blood stagnation. The commonly used herbs are Chuan Xiong, Dan Shen, Yue Ji Hua, Yan Hu Suo (*Corydalidis rhizoma*) and Hong Hua.

Herbs that dissolve and dissipate congealed Blood. These are used to treat more severe or chronic syndromes of Blood stagnation, in which the Blood becomes thicker and blood clots are formed. The commonly used herbs are Wu Ling Zhi, Dan Shen, Yu Jin, Ze Lan (*Lycopi herba*), Yi Mu Cao (*Leonuri herba*) and Yue Ji Hua.

Herbs that open the meridians and collaterals and dissolve congealed Blood. These are used to treat chronic Blood stagnation when the meridians and collaterals are blocked for a long period of time. They are particularly used in chronic Bi syndrome. The commonly used herbs are Si Gua Luo (*Luffae fructus*), Wang Bu Liu Xing (*Vaccariae semen*) and Lu Lu Tong (*Liquidambaris fructus*).

Herbs that break up and drive out congealed Blood. These are used to treat severe Blood stagnation, in which a solid and immobile mass is formed. The commonly used herbs are Tao Ren, Ru Xing, Mo Yao, San Leng (*Sparganii rhizoma*) and E Zhu.

Herbs that soften hardness and break up or drive out congealed Blood. These are used to treat a solid mass that is formed by congealed Blood, Phlegm, Dampness, Cold or Heat and toxin. The commonly used herbs are Mu Li (*Ostrea concha*), Wa Leng Zi (*Arcae concha*), Shui Zhi (*Hirudo*), Zhe Chong (*Eupolyphaga seu opisthoplatia*)* and Mang Chong (*Tabanus*)*.

Relieving pain

The pathology of pain in TCM is blockage of the Qi and Blood. Chronic, deep and stubborn pains especially are caused by Blood stagnation; herbs that promote Blood circulation are able to reduce Blood stagnation and open up the meridians, thus relieving pain. The herbs that are particularly effective for relieving pain are Yan Hu Suo, Chuan Xiong, Wu Ling Zhi and Pu Huang (*Typhae pollen*).

Topical usage

Trauma directly causes stagnation of Blood, manifesting as pain, swelling or bleeding in the locality. Herbs that promote Blood circulation are the main part of the treatment when the bleeding has stopped. These herbs can be used not only orally but also topically, such as in lotions, ointments, tinctures and plasters. The commonly used ones are Tao Ren, Hong Hua, Ru Xiang, Chuan Xiong and Dan Shen.

Usage for Bi syndrome

When Wind, Dampness, Cold or Heat invades the meridians, they block the Qi and Blood circulation. Herbs that promote Blood circulation can enhance the actions of the other herbs of expelling Exterior pathogenic factors. In chronic Bi syndrome, there is always Blood stagnation, so the herbs that regulate the Blood are often used in formulas. The commonly used herbs are Chuan Xiong, Su Mu (*Sappan lignum*), Chuan Niu Xi (*Cyathulae radix*) and Jiang Huang (*Curcumae longae rhizoma*).

3 What precautions should be observed when using herbs that promote the Blood circulation?

Herbs that promote the Blood circulation should not be used during pregnancy, in bleeding conditions or during profuse menstruation. Because these herbs are pungent, they let the Blood circulate quickly, and break up congealed Blood or soften hardness. These actions may cause miscarriage and cause heavier bleeding.

Herbs that promote Blood circulation can be used with caution in the following conditions.

Heavy menstruation, miscarriage and bleeding caused by stagnation of Blood

There is a saying: 'If the congealed Blood is not removed, the new Blood is impossible to grow. If the congealed Blood is not removed, the Blood cannot turn back to the normal pathway in the bleeding conditions.' Herbs that promote the Blood circulation can be used for the purpose of stopping bleeding, such as that seen in ectopic pregnancy, pregnancy with metropolypus or uterus myomatosus, adenomyosis or bleeding of a tumor. However, the dosage and course of treatment must be controlled by experienced practitioners.

Patients with weak Spleen and Stomach

As all herbs that promote Blood circulation are quite strong in taste and easily injure the Stomach, the herbs should be taken after meals, especially in patients with chronic Bi syndrome, who have already used Western medicine for a long time, or whose Stomach has been injured too.

Patients with weakness of Qi

Herbs that invigorate the Blood circulation may also activate the Qi movement and these actions can consume the Qi. The herbs should not be used alone when patients suffer from Qi deficiency. The side-effect of herbs that move the Blood is manifested as tiredness after using these herbs. In this situation, herbs that strengthen the Qi and Blood should also be used.

Selecting proper herbs from the strength scale to treat a specific case of Blood stagnation

It is very important to select the correct herbs from the strength scale to treat syndromes of Blood stagnation. If the stagnation is severe, and the applied herbs are too gentle, the congealed Blood will not be eliminated. If the Blood stagnation is mild but the prescribed herbs are very strong, the Qi and Blood can be injured.

The proper herbs should be selected according to the condition and constitution of the patient, the location and nature of the stagnation of Blood, and considering the duration of the disease.

4 What are the characteristics of Chuan Xiong (*Chuanxiong rhizoma*)?

Chuan Xiong is pungent and warm, and enters the Liver, Gall Bladder and Pericardium meridians. Pungency can disperse congealed Blood, and warmth can activate the Blood circulation and dissipate its obstruction. Chuan Xiong is a very effective herb for invigorating the Blood and promoting its circulation. It is characterized by high moving speed and strength. It moves upwards, downwards, inwards and outwards, and can reach every part of the body, so it is regarded as 'the herb that moves the Qi in the Blood'.

In clinical practice, it is often used to remove congealed Blood and stop pain. It is particularly effective in the treatment of headache when the pain is in the sides of the head, such as in headache caused by stress or migraine. It is also used to relieve pain in intercostal neuralgia, coronary heart disease and stenocardia, trauma and arthritis. Since it can reach any part of the body, it can be used to treat cold and cramping pain of the fingers and toes, dysmenorrhea, amenorrhea and irregular menstruation, which are caused by Qi and Blood stagnation complicated by Cold. Combined with other herbs it can be prescribed for Excess, for Deficiency, for Cold or for Heat syndromes.

Although Chuan Xiong is effective for promoting the Blood circulation, it can cause the Qi and Blood to ascend rapidly; therefore it should not be used in patients who suffer from syndromes of Liver-Yang rising, or Liver-Fire or Heart-Fire blazing up—for instance, as seen in hypertension, glaucoma and cerebrovascular accident. Moreover, since this herb is warm and very pungent, a large dosage may consume the Yin and Qi. Patients with Yin deficiency or with a weak constitution should not use this herb in large dosages.

5 What are the characteristics of Dan Shen (*Salviae miltiorrhizae radix*)?

Dan Shen is bitter and slightly cold. It enters the Blood level of the Heart and Liver meridians. It is able to promote the Blood circulation, cool the Blood, calm the Mind and eliminate irritability. It is especially suitable for treating the syndrome of Blood stagnation complicated by Heat. The syndrome is often caused by stress or emotional disturbance, which leads to stagnation of the Liver-Qi or the generation of Heat in the Liver or Heart. In clinical practice, it is used to treat coronary heart disease, stenocardia, hypochondriac pain, heartburn, depression, irritability, insomnia and restlessness. Dan Shen is also used for treating hepatosplenomegaly as it can soften and reduce the size of organs and improve their functions. It is an important herb for treating gynecological disorders, such as dysmenorrhea, irregular menstruation, premenstrual tension syndrome and menopausal syndrome due to Heat and stagnation in the Blood. Dan Shen is also applied topically as lotions or plasters to reduce pain and swelling in conditions of trauma or Hot-Bi syndrome.

According to the relationship of Qi and Blood in TCM, Dan Shen is often used with herbs that spread the Liver-Qi, such as Chai Hu (*Bupleuri radix*), Xiang Fu (*Cyperi rhizoma*) and Qing Pi (*Citri reticulatae viride pericarpium*) in treating Blood stagnation syndrome. It is also used with herbs that reduce Liver-Fire and Heart-Fire such as Long Dan Cao (*Gentianae radix*) and Lian Qiao (*Forsythiae fructus*) in syndromes of Heat in the Liver and Heart meridians.

6 What are the differences between Chuan Xiong (*Chuanxiong rhizoma*) and Dan Shen (*Salviae miltiorrhizae radix*) in promoting the Blood circulation?

Chuan Xiong and Dan Shen are able to promote the Blood circulation and both are commonly used for treating Blood stagnation syndrome. They can effectively relieve pain in the chest and hypochondriac region, pain due to trauma and Bi syndrome.

Chuan Xiong is pungent and warm, and its speed of movement is greater than that of Dan Shen. Its action is also stronger in invigorating the Blood, removing congealed Blood and opening up the meridians.

Dan Shen is bitter and cold; it cools the Blood and moderates the speed of the Blood circulation. Its functions are stronger in dissolving congealed Blood, relieving chest pain, calming the Mind and eliminating irritability than those of Chuan Xiong.

In syndromes complicated by Cold and Heat, stagnation of Qi and Blood, these two herbs can be used together.

7 Dan Shen (*Salviae miltiorrhizae radix*) and Yu Jin (*Curcumae radix*) can both cool the Blood and promote its circulation. What are the differences between their functions?

Dan Shen and Yu Jin are bitter and cold, and enter the Heart and Liver meridians. Both are able to promote the Blood circulation, remove congealed Blood and stop pain. They can also calm the Mind to treat irritability and hypochondriac pain. In clinical practice, they are often used together to treat coronary heart disease, hepatitis, cholecystitis and hepatosplenomegaly.

Dan Shen primarily enters the Heart meridian. Compared with Yu Jin, its function focuses more on the Heart, and it can directly clear Heat in the Heart, cool the Blood and calm the Mind.

Yu Jin primarily enters the Liver meridian. It is not only bitter and cold, but also pungent. Its function focuses more on the Liver meridian and its action in invigorating the Liver-Blood is stronger than that of Dan Shen. Because of the rapidity of its action, it is regarded as 'the herb that moves the Qi in the Blood'. Its action in removing the congealed Blood is also stronger than that of Dan Shen, and it is considered as a herb that is able to break up congealed Blood. It can be used in formulas that treat dysmenorrhea, mastopathia, liver cirrhosis and tumors.

Furthermore, Yu Jin is colder than Dan Shen. It can not only cool the Blood, but also stop bleeding. It is an aromatic herb and is able to penetrate Damp-Heat, clear Damp-Heat and promote bile secretion. In clinical practice, Yu Jin is used for treating Damp-Heat in the Upper Jiao and Middle Jiao. The symptoms are fullness in the chest and epigastric region, jaundice and reduced appetite, such as in malaria and hepatitis. In addition, Yu Jin can spread the Liver-Qi, clear the Liver-Heat and eliminate irritability, as well as treat headache and a tight sensation in the chest caused by Damp-Heat obstruction.

8 What are the differences between Yi Mu Cao (*Leonuri herba*) and Ze Lan (*Lycopi herba*)?

Yi Mu Cao and Ze Lan have similar functions. Both can promote Blood circulation, remove congealed Blood, increase urination and reduce edema. They are the important herbs for treating gynecological disorders and are used for irregular menstruation, amenorrhea, dysmenorrhea, abdominal pain after giving birth and difficult urination. However, there are differences between their properties that influence their applications.

'Yi' means 'benefit', 'Mu' means 'mother' and 'Cao' means 'grass'. The function of this herb is therefore described in its name: 'a plant that benefits mothers'. Yi Mu Cao is pungent, bitter and cold, and enters the Heart and Liver meridians. Pungency has a dispersing ability, and bitterness and Cold can reduce Heat, so this herb can disperse and descend congealed Blood and clear Heat in the Blood. It can be used in many gynecological disorders caused by Blood stagnation and Heat in Blood, such as pelvic inflammation, ovarian cysts, salpingitis, endometritis and endometriosis. It can also be used in bleeding conditions where Blood stagnation is present, such as is seen in menorrhagia and uterus myomatosus.

Ze Lan is pungent and bitter, and enters the Liver and Spleen meridians. Pungency and bitterness can disperse and descend congealed Blood. Unlike Yi Mu Cao, Ze Lan is slightly warm and is able to promote Blood circulation and break up obstructions. It is characterized as removing congealed Blood without the side-effect of injuring the normal Blood, and it is especially suitable for treating stagnation of Blood caused by Cold in the Lower Jiao and in the Blood. It is also an aromatic herb and is able to spread the Liver-Qi and the Spleen-Qi, so it is an excellent herb for treating stagnation of Liver-Qi and Blood and in both Excess and Deficiency cases. In clinical practice, it is often used in menopausal syndrome, irregular menstruation, premenstrual tension, depression, hepatitis and chronic urinary tract infection.

9 What are the characteristics of Hong Hua (*Carthami flos*), Ling Xiao Hua (*Campsitis flos*), Yue Ji Hua (*Rosae chinensis flos*) and Mei Gui Hua (*Rosae flos*)?

These four herbs are all flowers, and all enter the Liver meridian and enter the Blood. They have the function of invigorating the Blood and promoting its circulation. They are often used for treating disorders of menstruation that are due to stagnation of the Liver-Qi and Blood. However, there are differences between their functions.

Hong Hua is pungent and warm, and enters the Heart and Liver meridians. It is the strongest herb of the four for invigorating the Blood and promoting its circulation. If a small dosage is applied, it can regulate the Blood circulation; if a large dosage is applied, it can break up the congealed Blood and stop pain. It can be used for treating syndromes of Blood stagnation, such as seen in uterus myomatosus, endometriosis, amenorrhea, dysmenorrhea, irregular menstruation and infertility. Because it can move the Blood strongly, it may cause bleeding or make it heavier, so the dosage and treatment course should be controlled carefully. During menstruation, this herb should be used in a smaller dosage or stopped for 3 days to avoid heavy menstrual bleeding. As well as treating menstrual disorders, Hong Hua is one of the commonly used herbs to treat trauma. It is effective for reducing swelling and pain. In this case, it can be used both orally and topically.

Ling Xiao Hua is pungent and slightly cold, and enters the Liver and Pericardium meridians. It not only can disperse stagnant Blood and regulate menstruation, but can also cool the Blood, expel Wind and relieve itching. Therefore it is suitable for treating the syndrome of Wind-Heat disturbance in the Blood, in which patients suffer from itching all over the body that worsens with warmth.

Yue Ji Hua is sweet and warm, and enters the Liver meridian. It has a fragrant smell. It can regulate not only the Blood circulation, but also the Liver-Qi. It is a good herb for treating irregular menstruation, premenstrual tension depression, menopausal syndrome and hepatitis due to stagnation of the Liver-Qi and Blood.

Mei Gui Hua is sweet, slightly bitter and warm. Like Yue Ji Hua, it can promote both Qi and Blood circulation of the Liver and is used for treating many gynecological disorders. However, it is characterized as harmonizing the Liver-Qi and Stomach-Qi and is used particularly for the syndrome in which stagnant Liver-Qi attacks the Stomach. The symptoms are fullness in the chest, epigastric and hypochondriac regions, irritability and reduced appetite.

10 Yan Hu Suo (*Corydalidis rhizoma*) and Wu Ling Zhi (*Trogopterori faeces*) are commonly used herbs for alleviating pain. What are the differences between them?

Yan Hu Suo and Wu Ling Zhi enter the Liver and Spleen meridians. Both are able to promote Blood circulation and remove congealed Blood. They are very effective for relieving pain.

Yan Hu Suo is pungent, warm and slightly bitter. It is characterized as entering the Qi and Blood level, and promoting the Qi movement and Blood circulation. It is an excellent herb for relieving pain and its action is steady and strong. In clinical practice, it can be used alone and in TCM is considered to be a painkiller. If it is fried with a little vinegar, this increases its effect in relieving pain.

Wu Ling Zhi is bitter, sweet and warm. It can promote Blood circulation and stop pain but its action is gentler and slower than that of Yan Hu Suo. However, unlike Yan Hu Suo, it has no function in promoting Qi movement. The strong point of this substance is that it dissolves congealed Blood in a gentle but a constant way. It is effective for removing congealed Blood without the side-effect of injuring the normal part of the Blood, so it is used for chronic diseases in which congealed Blood is not easily and quickly removed. In clinical practice, it is often prescribed in formulas for treating gynecological disorders and liver diseases.

11 What are the differences between Chuan Niu Xi (*Cyathulae radix*) and Huai Niu Xi (*Achyranthis bidentatae radix*)?

The growing habitat of Chuan Niu Xi is Si Chuan province; Huai Niu Xi is from the region of the Huai River. Both herbs are bitter, sour and neutral, and enter the Liver and Kidney meridians. Although they have the same name in Chinese, they are actually from two different plants and are different in their functions.

Chuan Niu Xi is characterized as promoting the Blood circulation and directing the Blood downwards. It can treat amenorrhea, abdominal mass, headache and dizziness. It is also effective for directing Heat and Fire downwards, so it is often used for treating hot flushes, headache, dizziness, blurred vision in menopausal syndrome, hypertension and cerebrovascular accident. These disorders are caused by deficiency of the Liver-Yin and Kidney-Yin, and uprising of the Liver-Yang, Liver-Heat, Qi and Blood.

Huai Niu Xi is slightly sweet and sour. It has the function of tonifying the Liver and Kidney, strengthening the tendons and bones, treating weakness in the legs and knees, difficulty in walking and edema in the legs. It has no function in promoting Blood circulation.

12 What are the characteristics of Dang Gui (*Angelicae sinensis radix*) and Ji Xue Teng (*Spatholobi caulis et radix*) in the function of promoting Blood circulation?

Dang Gui and Ji Xue Teng are sweet, slightly bitter and warm, and enter the Liver meridian. Like the other herbs that promote the Blood circulation, they can invigorate the Blood and treat syndromes of Blood stagnation. The differences between these two herbs and the other herbs that promote Blood circulation are that Dang Gui and Ji Xue Teng are able to tonify the Blood and can treat Blood defi-

ciency. Because of this characteristic, these two herbs are particularly suitable for treating syndromes of deficiency of Blood and stagnation of Blood, such as is seen in chronic disease or in patients with a weak constitution.

Unlike Dang Gui, Ji Xue Teng also enters the Kidney meridian. 'Vines enters collaterals', according to the concept of traditional Chinese herbal medicine, so this herb is able to regulate the collaterals and to treat numbness, stiffness and cramping of the limbs and is often used for treating chronic arthritis, the sequelae of cerebrovascular accident and other vascular and neurological diseases.

13 What are the indications for herbs that cool the Blood and regulate its circulation?

There are several herbs that have the ability of promoting the Blood circulation and cooling the Blood, such as Chi Shao Yao (*Paeoniae radix rubra*), Mu Dan Pi (*Moutan cortex*), Yi Mu Cao (*Leonuri herba*), Dan Shen (*Salviae miltiorrhizae radix*) and Yu Jin (*Curcumae radix*). All of them are cold in nature, and enter the Heart or Liver meridians. Since all of them enter the Blood level, they are able to promote the Blood circulation, cool the Blood, and to treat Heat in the Blood and stagnation of the Blood. Meanwhile, these herbs are also used in internal Heat syndromes to prevent the stagnation of Blood in conditions of Heat consuming the Blood. They can be used together or separately. However, there are some differences when they are applied in clinical practice.

Chi Shao Yao is sour, bitter and slightly cold. It is characterized as reducing Excess-Heat in the Blood and regulating the Blood circulation. It can also reduce swelling and pain. In clinical practice, Chi Shao Yao is used to treat abscess, furunculosis, appendicitis, intestinal obstruction and dysmenorrhea. It can also be used topically to treat pain and swelling due to trauma.

Mu Dan Pi is characterized as reducing Empty-Heat in the Blood and regulating the Blood circulation. In clinical practice, it is particularly suitable for treating the syndrome in which Heat disturbs the Blood in conditions of Yin and Blood deficiency. It is used to treat low-grade fever, 'bone-steaming' fever, skin rashes, nose bleeding, blood in the sputum and subcutaneous bleeding.

Yi Mu Cao treats particularly the stagnation of Blood in the Lower Jiao and it is often used for gynecological disorders, such as dysmenorrhea, amenorrhea, irregular menstruation and inflammations.

Dan Shen primarily enters the Heart meridian and is especially effective for clearing Heat in the Heart and promoting the Blood circulation in the chest; it therefore treats irritability, restlessness, palpitations, insomnia and chest pain.

Yu Jin primarily enters the Liver meridian and is especially suitable for clearing Heat and promoting the Blood circulation from the Liver. It is more often used for treating hypochondriac pain due to long-term depression, in premenstrual tension and diseases of the liver and gall bladder.

14 What are the differences between Ru Xiang (Olibanum) and Mo Yao (Myrrhae)?

Ru Xiang and Mo Yao are aromatic herbs. They are very bitter and pungent, and move quickly. They can strongly disperse congealed Blood and direct it to descend, open up the meridians and collaterals, and are very effective for relieving pain. The two herbs are often used together to enhance the therapeutic effect. In clinical practice, they are often applied to reduce pain and swelling in trauma, arthritis and fractures.

Ru Xiang is warm and pungent, and enters the Heart and Liver meridians. Compared with Mo Yao, it promotes not only the Blood circulation, but also the Qi movement. It can also relax tendons. Ru Xiang is especially suitable for conditions where the joints and muscles are very stiff, swollen and painful. It is also more often used topically than Mo Yao.

Mo Yao is neutral and it enters the Liver meridian. Compared with Ru Xiang, it is more bitter and its dispersing action is also stronger. This herb is stronger than Ru Xiang for breaking up congealed Blood and is used not only in trauma and fracture, but also for hard masses, such as tumors.

As both herbs have a strong smell and may easily cause nausea and vomiting, and overdose may injure the Stomach, they are better used in pills or capsules.

15 What are the differences between San Leng (Sparganii rhizoma) and E Zhu (Curcumae rhizoma)?

San Leng and E Zhu are two important herbs that remove congealed Blood and treat tumors. They can strongly promote the Qi movement and Blood circulation, and break up congealed Blood. The two herbs are often used together to enhance their actions because San Leng is stronger in breaking up congealed Blood and E Zhu is stronger in breaking up the restraint of Qi. They are used to treat severe Blood stagnation. In clinical practice, they can be used to treat hepatosplenomegaly, liver cirrhosis, ectopic pregnancy and cancer.

Since San Leng and E Zhu can strongly break up congealed Blood, they can also injure the Qi. When treating patients with Qi deficiency or with a weak constitution, these herbs must be used together with herbs that tonify the Qi.

16 What are the functions of Zhe Chong (Eupolyphaga seu opisthoplatia)*, Shui Zhi (Hirudo) and Mang Chong (Tabanus)*?

These three substances are insects and they are also poisonous. All of them enter the Liver meridian and are able to break up congealed Blood, soften hardness and reduce masses. They are used in the treatment of hepatosplenomegaly, liver cirrhosis and tumors.

In the action of breaking up congealed Blood, Zhe Chong is the weakest of the three and Mang Chong is the strongest. However, all of them can cause the side-effect of injuring of the Qi and Blood. They should be used with caution and, in patients with Deficiency syndromes, combined with herbs that tonify the Qi and Blood.

17 What are the characteristics of Wang Bu Liu Xing (*Vaccariae semen*) and Di Long (*Pheretima*)?

Wang Bu Liu Xing and Di Long are commonly used substances to open up the collaterals. They can eliminate congealed Blood from the collaterals and promote Qi movement and Blood circulation there. They are often used for treating chronic pain, stubborn pain, tingling, stiffness or numbness in the limbs, such as in migraine, sequelae of cerebrovascular accident and other neurological disorders.

However, Wang Bu Liu Xing is also effective for opening up the collaterals of the Liver and Stomach, and promoting secretion of milk, and is used for lack of milk after giving birth owing to stagnation of the Liver-Qi. Di Long is effective in expelling Wind from the meridians and collaterals and is often used in Bi syndrome.

18 Which herbs can be applied topically?

Since herbs that promote the Blood circulation are also good for reducing swelling and relieving pain, many of them can also be used topically in lotions, ointments, tinctures and plasters. Herbs for topical use should be finely ground, easily dissolved or mixed with water, oil or another vehicle, not be irritant to the skin or wounds, and not cause toxic or allergic reactions. The commonly used herbs are Tao Ren (*Persicae semen*), Hong Hua (*Carthami flos*), Ru Xiang (*Olibanum*), Chuan Xiong (*Chuanxiong rhizoma*) and Dan Shen (*Salviae miltiorrhizae radix*).

Comparisons of strength and temperature in herbs that regulate the Blood

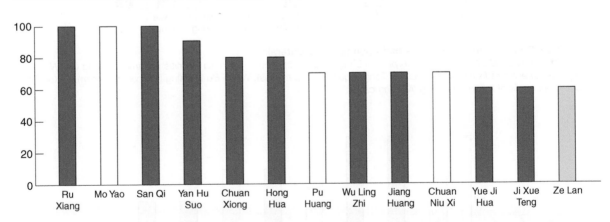

Fig. 11.1 • Comparison of the herbs that promote Blood circulation, stop pain and are warm in temperature.
Ru Xiang (*Olibanum*), Mo Yao (*Myrrhae*), San Qi (*Notoginseng radix*), Yan Hu Suo (*Corydalidis rhizoma*), Chuan Xiong (*Chuanxiong rhizoma*), Hong Hua (*Carthami flos*), Pu Huang (*Typhae pollen*), Wu Ling Zhi (*Trogopterori faeces*), Jiang Huang (*Curcumae longae rhizoma*), Chuan Niu Xi (*Cyathulae radix*), Yue Ji Hua (*Rosae chinensis flos*), Ji Xue Teng (*Spatholobi caulis et radix*), Ze Lan (*Lycopi herba*).

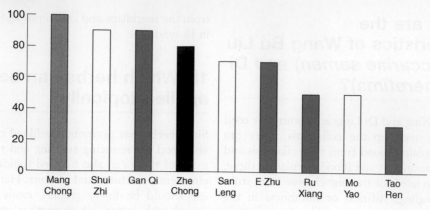

Fig. 11.2 • Comparison of the herbs that break up congealed Blood.
Mang Chong (*Tabanus*)*, Shui Zhi (*Hirudo*), Gan Qi (*Toxicodendri resina*), Zhe Chong (*Eupolyphaga seu opisthoplatia*)*, San Leng (*Sparganii rhizoma*), E Zhu (*Curcumae rhizoma*), Ru Xiang (*Olibanum*), Mo Yao (*Myrrhae*), Tao Ren (*Persicae semen*).

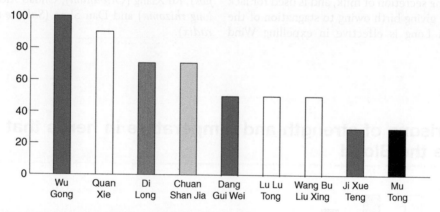

Fig. 11.3 • Comparison of the herbs that open up the collaterals.
Wu Gong (*Scolopendra*)*, Quan Xie (*Scorpio*), Di Long (*Pheretima*), Chuan Shan Jia (*Manitis squama*)**, Dang Gui Wei (*Angelicae sinensis radix extremitas*), Lu Lu Tong (*Liquidambaris fructus*), Wang Bu Liu Xing (*Vaccariae semen*), Ji Xue Teng (*Spatholobi caulis et radix*), Mu Tong (*Mutong caulis*)*

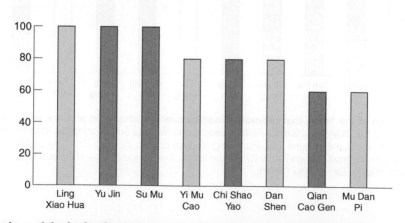

Fig. 11.4 • Comparison of the herbs that invigorate the Blood and are cold in temperature.
Ling Xiao Hua (*Campsitis flos*), Yu Jin (*Curcumae radix*), Su Mu (*Sappan lignum*), Yi Mu Cao (*Leonuri herba*), Chi Shao Yao (*Paeoniae radix rubra*), Dan Shen (*Salviae miltiorrhizae radix*), Qian Cao Gen (*Rubiae radix*), Mu Dan Pi (*Moutan cortex*).

Chapter **Twelve**

12

Herbs that stop bleeding

止血药

1 What are the characteristics of herbs that stop bleeding?

Herbs that stop bleeding are used for acute bleeding conditions and they treat the manifestations rather than the cause of the syndrome. Therefore, when the bleeding is stopped, the patient should be treated according to the differentiation of the syndromes.

Herbs that stop bleeding have the following characteristics.

Sour or astringent

Sour and astringent substances possess an astringent property—that is, they reverse abnormal leakage of blood and their tendency of action is inwards. They treat the symptom of bleeding rather than its cause and are often used in different bleeding conditions as a first aid procedure. The commonly used substances are Bai Ji (*Bletillae tuber*)**, Ou Jie (*Nelumbinis nodus rhizomatis*), Zong Lü (*Stipulae trachycarpi fibra*), Hua Rui Shi (*Ophicalcitum*) and Zao Xin Tu (*Terra flava usta*).

Cold and bitter

Coldness can clear Heat and bitterness can reduce Fire. Since bleeding is often caused by Heat, especially in acute cases, there exist herbs that not only can stop bleeding, but also can clear Heat. They are

used as herbs that treat both the cause and the symptoms of the disorder. They are Da Jì (*Cirsii japonici herba seu radix*), Xiao Ji (*Cirsii herba*), Ce Bai Ye (*Platycladi cacumen*), Huai Hua (*Sophorae flos*), Di Yu (*Sanguisorbae radix*) and Bai Mao Gen (*Imperatae rhizoma*).

Promoting the Blood circulation and stopping bleeding

It does not sound logical that the functions of moving the Blood and stopping bleeding should coexist in one herb. Nevertheless, these herbs do exist and they are particularly used when bleeding is caused by obstruction due to congealed Blood, such as in menorrhagia caused by trauma, hysteromyoma or heavy bleeding due to retained placenta. The herbs that can remove congealed Blood and stop bleeding are San Qi (*Notoginseng radix*), Qian Cao Gen (*Rubiae radix*), Pu Huang (*Typhae pollen*), Xue Yu Tan (*Crinis carbonisatus*) and Hua Rui Shi.

Usage of charred herbs

In TCM, it is considered that bleeding will be stopped by the use of black, charred herbs. In clinical practice, as good results with this method have substantiated the concept, many herbs are charred particularly for the purpose of stopping bleeding. The commonly used herbs are Da Jì, Xiao Ji, Pu Huang, Ou Jie, Zong Lu and Xue Yu Tan.

2 What precautions should be observed when using herbs that stop bleeding?

Herbs that stop bleeding are particularly used in acute conditions so as to control the bleeding in time. However, after the bleeding has stopped, or even when there is still some bleeding present, herbs that treat the cause should also be used. For example, if the bleeding is caused by Heat, such as in colitis, dysentery and enteritis, herbs that clear Heat and cool the Blood should be used. If the bleeding is caused by Qi deficiency, herbs that tonify the Qi should be prescribed to hold the Blood, such as in thrombocytopenia. If the bleeding is caused by Yin deficiency with Yang rising, such as in cerebrovascular accident, herbs that direct the Yang downwards must be added.

Herbs that stop bleeding are effective for treating many kinds of bleeding conditions. However, when the bleeding is very heavy and presents a danger to the patient, the person should be sent to hospital immediately. If it is impossible to reach a hospital, a large dose of Ren Shen (*Ginseng radix*) should be applied, together with the herbs that stop bleeding, to hold the Qi in order to control the Blood and stop bleeding.

Since most of these herbs have a sour, astringent or cold nature that may cause stagnation of Blood, these herbs should be used for a short period of time only or combined with herbs that can gently disperse the stagnation.

3 What are the differences between Da Jì (*Cirsii japonici herba seu radix*) and Xiao Ji (*Cirsii herba*)?

Da Jì and Xiao Ji are sweet and cold, and both enter the Liver and Heart meridians. The fresh or raw herbs are able to cool the Blood and stop bleeding. If they are charred, they acquire an astringent property, and then they can also stabilize the Blood and stop bleeding. In clinical practice, they are often used in combination to enhance the effect of stopping the bleeding. These two herbs are also effective for treating jaundice and other disorders of bile secretion, and hypertension.

Da Jì is colder than Xiao Ji and has a stronger action in reducing Heat, cooling the Blood and stopping bleeding. It is used for bleeding caused by Heat, such as seen in pulmonary tuberculosis, gastric ulcer, menorrhagia or diseases of the liver.

Xiao Ji is not so cold, and its function of cooling the Blood and stopping bleeding is gentler than that of Da Jì. It is especially effective for reducing Heat in the Lower Jiao and in treating bleeding caused by Damp-Heat in the Lower Jiao, such as seen in acute urinary tract infection, cystitis and pyelonephritis.

4 Xiao Ji (*Cirsii herba*) and Bai Mao Gen (*Imperatae rhizoma*) can both treat blood in the urine. What are the differences between them when they are used in clinical practice?

Xiao Ji and Bai Mao Gen are sweet and cold. Both can cool the Blood and stop bleeding. They can also promote urination and eliminate Damp-Heat from the Lower Jiao. They are especially effective for treating bloody urine caused by Damp-Heat in the Lower Jiao, which injures the local blood vessels and disturbs the local Blood circulation. However, there are some differences between these two herbs in clinical practice.

Xiao Ji enters the Heart and Liver meridians. Besides cooling the Blood and stopping the bleeding, it can also promote urination and reduce edema, so it is often used for treating nephritis. It can also be used to treat hypertension, hepatitis and hyperlipemia.

Bai Mao Gen enters the Lung and Stomach meridians. Compared with Xiao Ji, its effect in cooling the Blood and stopping the bleeding in the Lower Jiao is weaker. However, it stops bleeding not only in the Lower Jiao, but also in the Upper Jiao, so can be used in conditions such as nose bleeding and hemoptysis. It also generates the Body Fluids and relieves thirst. It is more suitable for use in patients suffering from thirst, a dry mouth and nose, who at the same time have symptoms in the Lower Jiao, such as acute urinary tract infection, nephritis and other febrile diseases.

5 Huai Hua (*Sophorae flos*), Huai Jiao (*Sophorae fructus*) and Di Yu (*Sanguisorbae radix*) are often used for treating intestinal hemorrhage. What are the differences between these three herbs?

These three herbs are all bitter and cold, and their tendency of movement in the body is downward. They enter the Liver and Large Intestine meridians, are effective for clearing Heat in the Lower Jiao, cooling the Blood and stopping bleeding, and are used for the treatment of colitis, dysentery and hemorrhoids. In clinical practice, they are often combined to increase the therapeutic effects. However, there are differences between them.

Huai Hua is slightly cold, and its ability to clear Heat and cool the Blood is not as strong as that of the other two herbs, but it has a stronger function in stopping bleeding than Huai Jiao. It is an important herb for treating dysentery and hemorrhoids. Since it enters the Liver meridian, and as a flower it has a tendency to ascend and disperse constrained Heat, it can cool the Liver, clear Heat in the head and benefit the eyes. It is used for the treatment of hypertension and dry, burning sensations in the eyes.

Huai Jiao is colder than Huai Hua, and its functions of clearing Heat and reducing Fire are also stronger. Since it moves downwards, it is very effective for treating hemorrhoids and it is often put in creams for topical use. Like Huai Hua, it also has the function of clearing Heat in the Liver and is used to treat hypertension, headache and dizziness.

Di Yu is bitter, sour and cold. It not only cools the Blood and stops bleeding, but also contracts and holds the Blood. It treats bleeding in the Lower Jiao and is used for colitis and menorrhagia. As it is also able to reduce swelling and stop pain, it is suitable for treating external hemorrhoids.

6 What are the differences between raw Pu Huang (*Typhae pollen*) and charred Pu Huang?

Pu Huang is a gentle herb; it is sweet and neutral, and enters the Pericardium and Liver meridians. As the raw form can promote the Blood circulation and dissolve congealed Blood, it is used to treat irregular menstruation, dysmenorrhea and abdominal pain after giving birth. Furthermore, it is also effective for stopping bleeding and so it is used for bleeding conditions. It is a good choice for bleeding caused by Blood stagnation.

If Pu Huang is charred, it acquires warm and astringent properties, and is stronger than raw Pu Huang for stopping bleeding in any part of the body. However, unlike the raw herb, it does not promote Blood circulation.

7 What are the characteristics of San Qi (*Notoginseng radix*)?

San Qi is a very effective herb for stopping bleeding. It is sweet, slightly bitter and warm, and enters the Liver and Stomach meridians. Sweetness can slow down the development of a critical situation, warmth can unblock the meridians and bitterness can purge congealed Blood. San Qi is effective in breaking up congealed Blood and harmonizing it. As soon as the congealed Blood has disappeared, the Blood turns back to its normal pathway, and the bleeding will stop. If the Blood circulates properly, the swelling is reduced and the pain stops.

Since San Qi can treat bleeding due to Blood stagnation, it can stop bleeding without the side-effect of causing new Blood stagnation, so it is widely used in the treatment of trauma, wounds, skin ulcers, carbuncles, epistaxis, hematemesis, uterine bleeding, blood in the urine and intestinal hemorrhage. It can be applied both internally and topically.

8 Ai Ye (*Artemisiae argyi folium*), Pao Jiang (quick-fried *Zingiberis rhizoma preparatum*) and Zao Xin Tu (*Terra flava usta*) are substances for warming the Interior and stopping bleeding. What are the differences between them?

Ai Ye is warm and aromatic, and enters the Liver, Spleen and Kidney meridians. It is able to warm the

143

Interior, expel Cold, stop bleeding and alleviate pain. Its function focuses on the Blood level of the Lower Jiao. It is effective for treating menorrhagia, and uterine bleeding during pregnancy or due to hysteromyoma when there is Cold in the Lower Jiao and the Blood. This herb can also be used topically. Also, Ai Ye is the substance from which moxa sticks are made and, used in moxibustion, it can penetrate the skin and meridians, warm the Qi and Blood and expel internal Cold.

Pao Jiang is bitter and warm, enters the Spleen and Liver meridians and also enters the Blood level. Although, like Ai Ye, it can warm the Interior, stop bleeding and alleviate pain, its function focuses on the Middle Jiao. It is especially effective for treating

bleeding due to Spleen-Yang and Qi deficiency, which then fail to control the Blood. Such bleeding may be located in the Stomach, intestines or Uterus.

Zao Xi Tu is warm and astringent, and enters the Spleen and Stomach meridians. It warms the Interior and stops bleeding in both the Middle Jiao and Lower Jiao, such as is seen in bleeding from the Stomach, intestines or Uterus. Moreover, it binds up the intestines and stops diarrhea. It is more suitable for conditions of Spleen-Yang deficiency, such as seen in chronic colitis, which manifests as abdominal pain and cramping, diarrhea, intestinal hemorrhage, cold hands and feet, and a pale complexion.

Comparisons of strength and temperature in herbs that stop bleeding

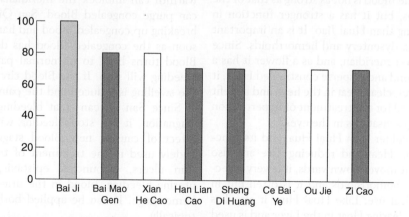

Fig. 12.1 • Comparison of the herbs that stop bleeding from the Lung.
Bai Ji (*Bletillae tuber*)**, Bai Mao Gen (*Imperatae rhizoma*), Xian He Cao (*Agrimoniae herba*), Han Lian Cao (*Ecliptae herba*), Sheng Di Huang (*Rehmanniae radix*), Ce Bai Ye (*Platycladi cacumen*), Ou Jie (*Nelumbinis nodus rhizomatis*), Zi Cao (*Arnebiae/Lithospermi radix*).

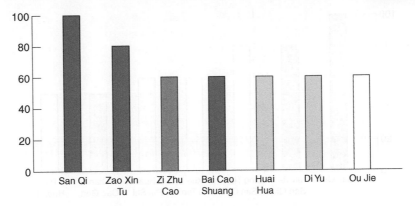

Fig. 12.2 • Comparison of the herbs that stop bleeding from the Stomach and intestines.
San Qi (*Notoginseng radix*), Zao Xin Tu (*Terra flava usta*), Zi Zhu Cao (*Callicarpae folium*), Bai Cao Shuang (*Fuligo plantae*), Huai Hua (*Sophorae flos*), Di Yu (*Sanguisorbae radix*), Ou Jie (*Nelumbinis nodus rhizomatis*).

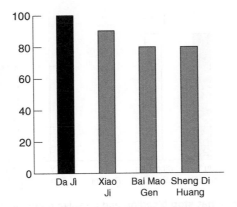

Fig. 12.3 • Comparison of the herbs that stop bleeding from the urinary tract.
Da Jì (*Cirsii japonici herba seu radix*), Xiao Ji (*Cirsii herba*), Bai Mao Gen (*Imperatae rhizoma*), Sheng Di Huang (*Rehmanniae radix*).

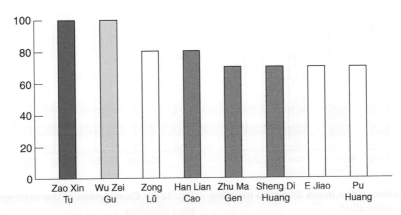

Fig. 12.4 • Comparison of the herbs that stop bleeding from the Uterus.
Zao Xin Tu (*Terra flava usta*), Wu Zei Gu (*Sepiae seu sepiellae os*), Zong Lü (*Stipulae trachycarpi fibra*), Han Lian Cao (*Ecliptae herba*), Zhu Ma Gen (*Boehmeriae radix*), Sheng Di Huang (*Rehmanniae radix*), E Jiao (*Asini corii colla*), Pu Huang (*Typhae pollen*).

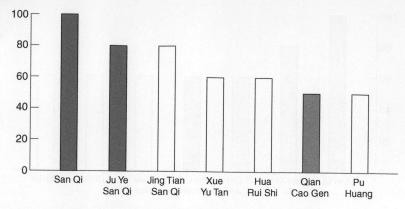

Fig. 12.5 • Comparison of the substances that stop bleeding from trauma.
San Qi (*Notoginseng radix*), Ju Ye San Qi (*Gynura segetum*), Jing Tian San Qi (*Sedi aizoon herba*), Xue Yu Tan (*Crinis carbonisatus*) Hua Rui Shi (*Ophicalcitum*), Qian Cao Gen (*Rubiae radix*), Pu Huang (*Typhae pollen*).

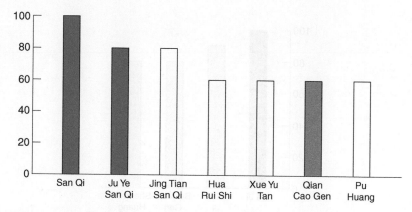

Fig. 12.6 • Comparison of the herbs that stop bleeding and dissolve congealed Blood.
San Qi (*Notoginseng radix*), Ju Ye San Qi (*Gynura segetum*), Jing Tian San Qi (*Sedi aizoon herba*), Hua Rui Shi (*Ophicalcitum*), Xue Yu Tan (*Crinis carbonisatus*), Qian Cao Gen (*Rubiae radix*), Pu Huang (*Typhae pollen*).

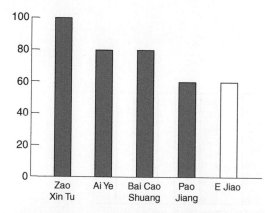

Fig. 12.7 • Comparison of the herbs that stop bleeding and are warm in temperature.
Zao Xin Tu (*Terra flava usta*), Ai Ye (*Artemisiae argyi folium*), Bai Cao Shuang (*Fuligo plantae*), Pao Jiang (quick-fried *Zingiberis rhizoma preparatum*), E Jiao (*Asini corii colla*).

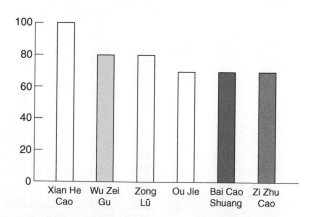

Fig. 12.8 • Comparison of the astringent herbs that stop bleeding.
Xian He Cao (*Agrimoniae herba*), Wu Zei Gu (*Sepiae seu sepiellae os*), Zong Lü (*Stipulae trachycarpi fibra*), Ou Jie (*Nelumbinis nodus rhizomatis*), Bai Cao Shuang (*Fuligo plantae*), Zi Zhu Cao (*Callicarpae folium*).

Chapter Thirteen

Herbs that warm the Interior

温里药

1 What are the functions of and indications for the herbs that warm the Interior?

Herbs that warm the Interior are able to expel Cold, rescue the Yang from collapse, warm the meridians and internal organs, and alleviate pain. They are used for internal Cold syndrome.

Internal Cold syndrome develops under two conditions. First, it is caused directly by invasion of exogenous pathogenic Cold. This invades the body through the skin and subcutaneous tissues, and then enters the meridians and internal organs. It obstructs the spreading of Yang, the movement of the Qi and the circulation of the Blood, such as is seen in Bi syndrome. In addition, if there is inappropriate consumption of cold food and drink, exogenous pathogenic Cold can directly enter the Stomach and accumulate in the Middle Jiao, such as is seen in acute gastritis, enteritis and gastric influenza. Secondly, internal Cold can develop from deficiency of the Yang of the internal organs, and especially from deficiency of the Kidney-Yang, Spleen-Yang and Heart-Yang. In most cases, the two causes coexist.

Internal Cold syndromes can be seen in the following patterns.

Accumulation of exogenous pathogenic Cold in the meridians and internal organs

Here an acute onset of the disorder appears after exposure to cold, rain or snow, or consumption of a large amount of cold drink and food. Patients may suffer from cramping pain in the limbs, abdominal pain, diarrhea, cold extremities or dysmenorrhea. There is a pallid complexion, a white tongue coating and a wiry and deep pulse.

Kidney-Yang deficiency

This syndrome can be found in elderly people and in people with a poor constitution or with chronic disease. They may suffer from cold extremities, cold in the back and cold knees, frequent urination, impotence, infertility, dysmenorrhea, aqueous-grainy diarrhea and edema. A light purple tongue body with a white and moist coating and a deep, slow and weak pulse are found in most cases. These symptoms can be seen in chronic nephritis, pyelitis and hypofunction of the pituitary gland, the adrenal cortex or the thyroid gland.

Spleen-Yang deficiency

This syndrome is often seen in people with chronic digestive disorders. They suffer from abdominal pain of a cramping nature, diarrhea or soft stools without a strong smell, edema, distension of the abdomen and a poor appetite, and have a preference for warm drinks rather than cold. A pale tongue body with a thick white coating and a weak and slow pulse are often seen. This pattern can be found in chronic colitis, peptic ulcer, chronic enteritis, liver disease, hypothyroidism and chronic nephritis.

Heart-Yang deficiency

This syndrome exists in people who are under stress or emotional distress for a long period of time. The symptoms and signs are palpitations, shortness of breath, chest pain and an oppressive sensation, cold limbs, depression, a bluish tongue body with purple spots, and a deep, wiry and irregular pulse.

Collapse of Yang

Collapse of Yang is caused by serious disturbance of the balance between Yin, Yang, Qi and Blood under the influence of pathogenic factors. When the Blood and Yin are suddenly weakened, or the Qi and Blood are suddenly obstructed, they fail to support the Yang, so the Yang collapses. This syndrome can be seen in critical conditions, especially after the collapse of Qi, such as seen in shock caused by myocardial infarction, myocarditis, severe blood loss, trauma, severe dehydration or allergy. The main symptoms are extremely cold extremities, a cold sensation that cannot be alleviated by warmth, a pallid complexion, an apathetic expression, slow reactions, shallow breathing and profuse sweating. The tongue body is pale and the pulse is thready, weak and deep.

Cold in the meridians

Both exogenous pathogenic Cold and internal Cold from Yang deficiency of the internal organs can exist in this pattern. The main symptoms are cold and severe pain in the limbs, cramp in the muscles, stiffness of the body, dysmenorrhea and cramping pain in the sides of the lower abdomen. These symptoms worsen with cold. The tongue body is bluish, its coating is white and the pulse is wiry, deep and slow.

Pain

When Cold obstructs the movement of the Qi and circulation of the Blood, it can directly cause pain which is characterized by sudden onset, cramp and a preference for warmth, such as seen in Cold Painful Obstruction syndrome, dysmenorrhea and muscle strain.

2 What are the characteristics of herbs that warm the Interior and expel Cold? What precautions should be observed in their usage?

Herbs that warm the Interior and expel Cold are able to stimulate and warm the Yang, scatter Cold, rescue the Yang from collapse, open up the meridians, promote Qi movement, invigorate the Blood circulation and alleviate pain. They have the following characteristics.

Very pungent and hot

Most of the herbs that warm the Interior are very pungent and hot. Pungency can disperse Cold, open up the meridians, and promote Qi movement and the Blood circulation. Heat can directly reduce Cold, warm the Interior and relieve cramp caused by Cold.

Entering the Heart, Spleen and Kidney meridians

The Heart-Yang, Spleen-Yang and Kidney-Yang are very important for maintaining the function of other internal organs. They stimulate Qi movement and the Blood circulation, and can promote digestion and water metabolism. Some herbs mainly warm the Yang of one of these three organs. The herbs that are used to warm the Heart-Yang are Gui Zhi (*Cinnamomi cassiae ramulus*) and Rou Gui (*Cinnamomi cassiae cortex*). The herbs that are often used to warm the Spleen-Yang are Gan Jiang (*Zingiberis rhizoma*), Gao Liang Jiang (*Alpiniae officinari rhizoma*), Wu Zhu Yu (*Evodiae fructus*), Hua Jiao (*Zanthoxyli fructus*) and Xiao Hui Xiang (*Foeniculi fructus*). The herbs that are used for warming the Kidney-Yang are Fu Zi (*Aconiti radix lateralis preparata*)* and Rou Gui.

Some herbs are very pungent and hot, their speed of scattering Cold and spreading warmth is very high, and they are considered to enter the 12 regular meridians; an example is Fu Zi.

The herbs that can expel exogenous pathogenic Cold from the superficial region of the body were detailed in the chapters on herbs that release the

Exterior (Ch. 2) and herbs that expel Wind-Dampness (Ch. 5). Some of these can also be used for treating Interior Cold syndromes.

In clinical practice, herbs that warm the Interior and expel Cold should be used with caution. First, these herbs are very pungent and hot, and they can consume the Yin and Body Fluids. If used for too long or in too large a dosage, they may bring about side-effects such as dryness in the mouth, throat and nasal cavity, thirst, sore throat, constipation, itching and dry skin, a burning sensation in the Stomach and palpitations. Patients with Yin and Blood deficiency should not use them. Secondly, many patients with Blood deficiency often show symptoms of internal Cold. In this condition, herbs that warm the Interior should not be used in large amounts. Thirdly, these herbs are pungent and harsh, and are able to stimulate the Blood circulation, so should not be used in bleeding conditions or in pregnancy. However, if the bleeding causes the collapse of Yin, and further collapse of the Yang, herbs that tonify the Qi and herbs that rescue the Yang can be used together. Fourthly, in the condition of Yang collapse, herbs that rescue the Yang should be applied in time. If the Yang is extremely weak and the internal Cold exceeds its maximum, and there is a fierce conflict between the Cold pathogenic factor and the hot herbs, a small amount of cold herbs, which serves as an 'opposing assistant', should be added in with the larger amount of hot herbs in order to achieve the proper therapeutic result.

3 What are the differences between herbs that stimulate the Yang and those that tonify the Yang?

Herbs that stimulate the Yang and those that tonify the Yang are two different kinds of herbs, and are used in different conditions.

Herbs that stimulate the Yang

Herbs that stimulate the Yang are also called 'herbs that warm the Interior' or 'herbs that expel internal Cold'. They are pungent and hot, and can directly scatter internal Cold. They are used for treating Excessive internal Cold syndromes. They can also stimulate the Yang of the internal organs, and accel-

erate their functions so as to disperse the internal Cold in both Excess and Deficiency conditions. The commonly used herbs are Fu Zi (*Aconiti radix lateralis preparata*)*, Gan Jiang (*Zingiberis rhizoma*) and Wu Zhu Yu (*Evodiae fructus*). In clinical practice, the therapeutic effect of these herbs is rapid, and results in raising of the blood pressure, body temperature and heart rate, and a reduction in the reaction time of the patient. These herbs are particularly used in critical conditions, such as shock or heart or renal failure.

As these herbs are very pungent and hot, however, they can easily consume Yin and Body Fluids, so should not be used for a long period of time. In the treatment of chronic internal Cold syndromes caused by Yang deficiency, the effect of these herbs in warming the Yang and expelling Cold is neither reliable nor stable. If these herbs are used for a longer period of time, they may also consume the Yin, further damage the Yang and complicate the patient's condition.

Herbs that tonify the Yang

Herbs that tonify the Yang are sweet and slightly warm. They can tonify the weakness of the Yang of the internal organs by replenishing the shortage of Essence. They can warm the Yang and promote its function gently. They are particularly used for treating Deficiency of the Yang in chronic diseases, especially deficiency of the Kidney-Yang. They improve the condition of patients slowly but steadily. The commonly used herbs are Du Zhong (*Eucomniae cortex*), Gou Ji (*Cibotii rhizoma*)**, Yi Zhi Ren (*Alpiniae oxyphyllae fructus*) and Tu Si Zi (*Cuscutae semen*).

In many books, herbs that stimulate the Yang and those that tonify the Yang are often called 'herbs that warm the Yang' or 'herbs that strengthen the Yang'. This leads to confusion. However, there are some herbs that are pungent, hot and sweet, and have functions both of stimulating the Yang and of tonifying the Yang. These include Rou Gui (*Cinnamomi cassiae cortex*), Ba Ji Tian (*Morindae radix*), Yin Yang Huo (*Epimedii herba*) and Gui Zhi (*Cinnamomi cassiae ramulus*). They can be used in both Excess and Deficiency conditions.

In clinical practice, herbs that stimulate the Yang and herbs that tonify the Yang can be used together to treat the syndrome of Yang deficiency with internal Cold.

4 What are the commonly used strategies for warming the Interior and expelling Cold?

Herbs that warm the Interior and expel Cold are pungent and hot. They treat Excessive internal Cold syndrome. They are also often used together with tonifying herbs to treat the internal Cold syndrome caused by Yang deficiency. However, there are several different methods and strategies for warming the internal organs and meridians and expelling Cold. They are often used together in clinical practice to increase the therapeutic results of warming the Interior.

Stimulating the Yang, warming the internal organs and the meridians, and expelling Cold directly

This method is carried out by pungent and hot herbs, which are able to warm the Interior and expel Cold directly. It is used to treat Excessive internal Cold syndrome characterized by cold extremities, cramping of the muscles, stiffness of the body and severe pain. The tongue body is often bluish with a white coating, and the pulse is deep and wiry. The commonly used herbs are Fu Zi (*Aconiti radix lateralis preparata*)*, Gan Jiang (*Zingiberis rhizoma*), Wu Yao (*Linderae radix*), Ai Ye (*Artemisiae argyi folium*), Gui Zhi (*Cinnamomi cassiae ramulus*) and Rou Gui (*Cinnamomi cassiae cortex*).

Stimulating the Yang and tonifying the Yang

This method is particularly used for treating internal Cold syndrome caused by Yang deficiency, which is characterized by cold sensations and weakness in the back and knees, frequent urination, loose stools, edema, impotence and tinnitus. The tongue body is pale and the coating is white and moist. The pulse is deep, weak and slow. The commonly used herbs are Ba Ji Tian (*Morindae radix*), Yin Yang Huo (*Epimedii herba*), Rou Gui and Tu Si Zi (*Cuscutae semen*).

Tonifying the Qi in order to strengthen the Yang

Since the Qi is a part of the Yang, and it can strengthen the function of internal organs, long-term

deficiency of Qi may lead to deficiency of Yang. Herbs that tonify the Qi are often used when the Yang is weak and internal Cold exists. The commonly used herbs are Huang Qi (*Astragali radix*) and Ren Shen (*Ginseng radix*).

Promoting the movement of Qi

When internal Cold accumulates in the body, from whatever the cause, it may contract the meridians, collaterals and muscles. The Qi becomes obstructed and pain may appear in the affected area. Herbs that promote Qi movement and are warm in nature are used in these conditions to assist the herbs that expel Cold to open up the meridians and to alleviate pain. Examples are Wu Yao, Mu Xiang (*Aucklandiae radix*)**, Qing Pi (*Citri reticulatae viride pericarpium*) and Xiao Hui Xiang (*Foeniculi fructus*).

Eliminating Cold-Dampness

When Cold accumulates in the body, no matter whether in conditions of Excess or Deficiency, it obstructs the meridians. It also obstructs the movement of Qi and the circulation of water, so that Cold-Dampness develops. Moreover, when the Yang is weak or the Cold exceeds its maximum, the Yang is not able to 'steam' the Yin; in consequence, the water metabolism becomes very slow and water may accumulate in certain parts of the body. In this condition, herbs that are warm in nature and that have the function of transforming Dampness should be used—for example, Cang Zhu (*Atractylodis rhizoma*), Bai Zhu (*Atractylodis macrocephalae rhizoma*), Sheng Jiang (*Zingiberis rhizoma recens*) and Cao Dou Kou (*Alpiniae katsumadai semen*).

Assisting in an opposite way to treat the syndrome of Yang collapse

When the Yang collapses, internal Cold is in excess inside the body, and it counteracts the attempts of pungent and hot herbs to enter the body because they have completely different natures. Patients may react to the conflict that ensues by vomiting up the herbal drink and they may have symptoms such as irritability, an irregular pulse and other uneasy sensations. The method of solving this problem is to add a small amount of a cold herb, such as Zhu Dan Zhi (*Pulvis bovis*) or Huang Bai (*Phellodendri cortex*), into a larger amount of hot herbs to moderate the conflict between the pathological cold and the hot herbs. Another method of moderating the conflict is to ask the patients to leave taking the herbal drink until it is cooler. This strategy is called 'assisting in an opposite way'.

Applying sweet herbs to reduce the speed of the harsh herbs

To consolidate the result of warming the Interior, a good method is to use pungent and hot herbs to spread the warmth in the body, and to use sweet herbs as well to keep the pungent herb from moving too quickly. This gives a better therapeutic result. An example is the combination of Fu Zi with Zhi Gan Cao (*Glycyrrhizae radix preparata*).

5 What are the differences between the functions of Fu Zi (*Aconiti radix lateralis preparata*)* and Rou Gui (*Cinnamomi cassiae cortex*)?

Fu Zi and Rou Gui are both pungent and hot, and both can warm the Kidney-Yang, strengthen the Kidney-Fire, scatter internal Cold and alleviate pain, but there are some differences between their functions.

Fu Zi is very pungent and hot, and it has a drying and harsh nature. Because it moves very quickly in the body, it is considered to be a herb that enters the 12 meridians. It has the quickest action in warming the Interior and expelling Cold out of all the herbs that warm the Interior. Rou Gui is less pungent and hot than Fu Zi, but it has a sweet taste and it enters only the Kidney meridian. These properties make Rou Gui especially effective for warming the Lower Jiao in order to warm the Kidney and scatter Cold there. As it is sweet, it does not move as quickly as Fu Zi. The strong point of this herb is that it spreads the warmth in a steady and strong way. It is used for severe internal Cold accumulation in the Lower Jiao, which cannot be scattered in a very short time.

Fu Zi is vigorous in warming and stimulates the Kidney-Yang, promoting the functions of the internal organs so that it can rescue the Yang from collapse; Fu Zi is considered the most important herb for treating Yang collapse. Rou Gui is not used to treat the syndrome of Yang collapse because it is not as hot and does not work as quickly as Fu Zi. However, it is able to warm and tonify the Fire of the Gate of

Vitality (*Ming Men*), and it is used for treating floating Yang syndrome, a syndrome that appears when the Kidney-Yang is extremely weak and internal Cold in the Lower Jiao is at its maximum. In this situation, the Cold pushes the Yang to go upwards, and the manifestations are a flushed face, a floating red color that appears only on the cheeks, heavy sweating, weak and cold limbs, a pale or light purple tongue body with a moist coating, and a weak and rootless pulse. This floating Yang syndrome is a dangerous situation like collapse of Yang. Rou Gui can warm and strengthen the Fire of the Gate of Vitality and it can disperse Cold; therefore it is able to lead the floating Fire back to its source.

Fu Zi can spread warmth quickly through the whole body through the 12 regular meridians, and scatter Cold and Dampness in the body like the sun disperses fog. This is the reason that it is a very commonly used herb to treat Bi syndrome which is caused by Cold, Dampness and Wind. Rou Gui stays in the Lower Jiao and spreads warmth there. It especially warms the Kidney meridian and treats impotence, infertility, amenorrhea and urination disorders.

Both of these two herbs can alleviate pain. Fu Zi can spread warmth, scatter Cold, dry Dampness and open up the meridians. It has very good results in alleviating pain no matter where it is. Rou Gui warms the Kidney and the Blood, scatters Cold and stimulates the Blood circulation to alleviate pain, especially when the pain is in the abdomen, back and knees.

Because of these characteristics, Fu Zi and Rou Gui are often used together in clinical practice to enhance the actions of warming and strengthening the Kidney-Yang, warming the meridians and alleviating pain.

6 What are the differences between Fu Zi (*Aconiti radix lateralis preparata*)* and Gan Jiang (*Zingiberis rhizoma*)?

Fu Zi and Gan Jiang are both very pungent and hot. Both of them move quickly and can scatter internal Cold, spread warmth and alleviate pain. They are often used together in acute or chronic disorders, such as in Yang Collapsing syndrome and chronic Bi syndrome. There are some differences between these two herbs, however.

151

Fu Zi is a very pungent and hot herb. It enters the 12 meridians and moves without any staying tendency. It spreads the Yang in the body very quickly, and treats internal Cold syndrome by this method. Gan Jiang is also very pungent and hot, but it enters the Spleen, Stomach, Heart and Lung meridians, and it moves a little bit slower than Fu Zi. Its tendency of action remains in the Middle Jiao. It is particularly effective for warming the Spleen and Stomach, and treating cramping and cold in the abdomen and vomiting and diarrhea due to internal Cold in the Middle Jiao.

Fu Zi enters the 12 meridians, but especially the Kidney meridian. It can strongly warm and strengthen the Kidney-Yang, and rescue the Yang from collapse. Gan Jiang enters primarily the Spleen meridian and it cannot directly warm the Kidney-Yang. However, it can warm the Middle Jiao and disperse Cold and dry Dampness there. It may accentuate the function of Fu Zi in warming the Kidney and rescuing the Yang. Because of this, these two herbs have become the most commonly used combination for treating Yang Collapsing syndrome.

7 What are the differences between Sheng Jiang (*Zingiberis rhizoma recens*), Gan Jiang (*Zingiberis rhizoma*) and Pao Jiang (quick-fried *Zingiberis rhizoma preparatum*)?

Sheng Jiang, Gan Jiang and Pao Jiang come from the same part of the plant. All are warm in nature and work on disorders in the Middle Jiao, but they have different characteristics.

Sheng Jiang, the fresh ginger root, is pungent and slightly warm. It primarily enters the Stomach meridian, moves without any tendency to stay, and is able to disperse Damp-Cold and to direct the Stomach-Qi downwards. It treats mainly acute stomach-ache, vomiting and nausea. Since it can also expel exterior Wind and Cold, it is especially suitable for treating acute gastritis, gastric influenza and cold infections.

Gan Jiang, the dried ginger root, is more pungent and hotter than the fresh one, and it primarily enters the Spleen meridian. It can either move or stay in the organ and meridian. It disperses Cold, dries

Dampness and treats abdominal pain with a cold and cramping nature, diarrhea and poor appetite, such as seen in chronic colitis, dysentery and nephritis.

Unlike Sheng Jiang and Gan Jiang, Pao Jiang (quick-fried ginger) is not pungent and hot, but bitter and warm. It enters the Spleen meridian. Since it is not pungent, it has more of a staying tendency in its action. It particularly warms the Middle Jiao, and stops bleeding and diarrhea caused by internal Cold, such as seen in chronic colitis, dysentery, dysmenorrhea and polymenorrhea.

These three herbs are often introduced by comparisons such as: '*Sheng Jiang is rather moving than staying, Gan Jiang is either moving or staying, and Pao Jiang is rather staying than moving.*'

8 What are the differences between Fu Zi (*Aconiti radix lateralis preparata*)* and Wu Tou (*Aconiti radix*)*?

Fu Zi and Wu Tou are the roots of the same plant. They are very pungent, hot and poisonous. Both can warm the Interior and expel Cold. The main difference between their functions is that Fu Zi, the lateral root of the plant, is able to warm and strengthen the Kidney-Yang and rescue the Yang from collapse. The thin and long root is considered to have a stronger and quicker action and is used in critical situations. Wu Tou, the main root of the plant, does not have the function of strengthening the Kidney-Yang and is not able to rescue the Yang from collapse; however, it has a stronger ability than Fu Zi to expel Wind and Cold, and can strongly warm the meridians and alleviate pain.

Fu Zi and Wu Tou are both used for Bi syndrome, and their slight difference is described as: '*Fu Zi particularly expels Cold, and Wu Tou particularly expels Wind.*'

9 What are the differences between Rou Gui (*Cinnamomi cassiae cortex*) and Gui Zhi (*Cinnamomi cassiae ramulus*)?

Rou Gui and Gui Zhi are different parts of the same tree. They are pungent, sweet and hot. They enter the Blood and warm it. They can also warm the meridians and alleviate pain, but there are some differences between their functions.

Rou Gui is the bark; it enters the Kidney meridian only, and its action focuses on the Lower Jiao. It is able to expel Cold and warm the Kidney and Liver meridians. It is used to treat Kidney-Yang deficiency, manifesting as cold and weakness in the back and knees, impotence, infertility, amenorrhea, dysmenorrhea, diarrhea and frequent urination.

Gui Zhi is the twig of the tree; it enters the Heart meridian primarily. Compared with Rou Gui, it is less hot and pungent, but the young twig has an aromatic smell that gives this herb a thin pungent property, which makes it move quickly and lightly. It can particularly warm the Blood, stimulate the Heart and promote the Blood circulation; therefore it can treat cold hands and feet, cramping of the muscles and pain due to Cold obstruction in the Blood circulation.

In comparing the ability of these two herbs to expel Cold and warm the Interior, Gui Zhi is more active and mainly works on the periphery, whereas Rou Gui stays in the Lower Jiao and warms the base of the body. Both can alleviate pain and are used in Bi syndrome: Rou Gui is mainly used for chronic and severe pain due to Kidney-Yang deficiency; Gui Zhi is mainly used for pain due to obstruction of the Blood circulation by Cold in the meridians. In addition, Gui Zhi also enters the Lung and Bladder meridians. As it is able to expel Wind and Cold in the superficial layer, it can treat Exterior syndrome. On the other hand, as Rou Gui can strengthen the Fire of the Gate of Vitality and lead the Fire back to its source, it is used for floating Yang syndrome.

10 What are the differences between Wu Zhu Yu (*Evodiae fructus*), Gan Jiang (*Zingiberis rhizoma*) and Fu Zi (*Aconiti radix lateralis preparata*)* in the function of expelling interior Cold?

These three herbs are all very pungent and hot. All move quickly and have no tendency to stay. They can scatter Cold quickly and warm the Interior, but their functions have different characteristics.

Fu Zi enters the Kidney meridian primarily. It warms the Interior and can disperse Cold caused by the Kidney-Yang deficiency. Gan Jiang enters the Spleen meridian and warms the Middle Jiao; it is used in Excessive-Cold and Deficient-Cold syndromes of the Middle Jiao. Wu Zhu Yu enters and warms the Liver meridian. It directs the Liver-Qi to descend and treats its uprising caused by Excessive-Cold in the Liver meridian. As it can also spread the Liver-Qi, it can be used when the Liver-Qi attacks the Stomach. The indications for using Wu Zhu Yu are: headache, particularly on the top of the head, cramping pain with cold sensations in the Stomach or in the sides of the lower abdomen, vomiting of clear fluid, and a wiry and slow pulse. This pattern can be found in disorders such as migraine, hypertension, peptic ulcer, chronic gastritis and dysmenorrhea.

11 What are the differences between Rou Gui (*Cinnamomi cassiae cortex*) and Ai Ye (*Artemisiae argyi folium*) in the function of warming the Qi and Blood in the Lower Jiao?

Rou Gui and Ai Ye are warm in nature and both enter the Lower Jiao. They can warm the Qi and Blood and expel Cold, and treat dysmenorrhea, infertility and abdominal pain. However, there are some differences between their functions.

Rou Gui is very pungent and hot. It is able to warm the Blood and activate its circulation. However, it is not suitable for bleeding conditions, or for pregnant women, even when there is cold in the Lower Jiao. Ai Ye is gentler in both taste and temperature. It can warm the Liver, Kidney and Spleen meridians, and is especially suitable for regulating the menstruation and stopping bleeding caused by Cold in the Lower Jiao. It can be used for miscarriage, polymenorrhea and dysmenorrhea. It is considered an important herb for gynecological and obstetric disorders.

12 What are the differences between Ai Ye (*Artemisiae argyi folium*) and Pao Jiang (quick-fried *Zingiberis rhizoma preparatum*) in the function of warming the meridians and stopping bleeding?

Ai Ye and Pao Jiang are pungent and warm. Both can warm the Qi and Blood, expel Cold from the meridians and stop bleeding. However, Ai Ye enters the Lower Jiao and the Liver and Kidney meridians. It warms the Blood and stops bleeding caused by Yang deficiency in the Lower Jiao. It is often used for profuse menstrual bleeding, functional uterine bleeding and bleeding during pregnancy.

Pao Jiang is bitter and warm. It enters the Middle Jiao and the Spleen meridian. It particularly warms the Middle Jiao and stops bleeding caused by Yang deficiency of the Spleen, such as seen in peptic ulcer, chronic colitis and dysentery.

13 What are the differences between Sheng Jiang (*Zingiberis rhizoma recens*) and Gao Liang Jiang (*Alpiniae officinari rhizoma*) in the function of warming the Stomach?

Sheng Jiang and Gao Liang Jiang are pungent and warm. Both enter the Stomach meridian and are able to expel Cold and warm the Stomach. However, Sheng Jiang is more pungent than warm; it regulates the Qi, disperses Dampness and soothes the Stomach-Qi. It treats cold sensations in the Stomach, nausea and vomiting, such as seen in cold or influenza infections.

Gao Liang Jiang is hotter and more pungent than Shen Jiang. As its heat is greater than its pungency, its action is stronger in warming the Stomach and alleviating pain. It can be used for cramping pain in the upper abdomen, vomiting of clear fluid and preference for warm drinks. These disorders can be seen in chronic gastritis and gastroduodenal ulcer.

14 Xiao Hui Xiang (*Foeniculi fructus*), Cao Dou Kou (*Alpiniae katsumadai semen*), Hua Jiao (*Zanthoxyli fructus*) and Ding Xiang (*Caryophylli flos*) all can warm the Middle Jiao and expel Damp-Cold. What are the differences between their functions?

These four herbs are pungent and warm, and enter the Spleen and Stomach meridians. They can warm the Middle Jiao and expel Cold and Dampness. They are used to treat abdominal pain, distension, poor appetite, vomiting and diarrhea. However, they have different characteristics.

Xiao Hui Xiang is an aromatic herb that can disperse Cold and promote Qi movement; therefore it is able to alleviate pain and improve the appetite. Cao Dou Kou is also an aromatic herb; unlike Xiao Hui Xiang, which promotes Qi movement, its strong point is drying Dampness and warming the Spleen. Because of this, it can treat nausea, vomiting, diarrhea and poor appetite. Hua Jiao has similar functions to Cao Dou Kou, but it is much warmer, so its action in drying Dampness and dispersing Cold is stronger than that of Cao Dou Kou. Since it is a poisonous herb and it moves quickly in the Middle Jiao, it is used only for acute Excessive Damp-Cold syndrome for a short therapeutic duration, such as for severe pain and cramping in the abdomen, frequent and urgent bowel movement and watery stools. Ding Xiang, like Xiao Hui Xiang, can regulate the Qi, but it is especially able to descend the Stomach-Qi and treat belching and hiccups.

Besides warming the Middle Jiao, Xiao Hui Xiao can also promote the Qi movement in the Lower Jiao. It enters the Kidney and Liver meridians, and treats abdominal pain, distension and cramping in the sides of the lower abdomen and hernia. Hua Jiao and Ding Xiang are able to warm the Kidney-Yang and treat Cold in the lower back and abdomen, diarrhea, impotence and cold extremities.

15 Which herbs can soothe the Stomach-Qi and treat vomiting? What are their characteristics?

The commonly used herbs to soothe the Stomach-Qi and stop vomiting are Ban Xia (*Pinelliae rhizoma*), Zi Su Ye (*Perillae folium*), Sheng Jiang (*Zingiberis rhizoma recens*), Gao Liang Jiang (*Alpiniae officinari rhizoma*), Wu Zhu Yu (*Evodiae fructus*), Hua Jiao (*Zanthoxyli fructus*), Cao Dou Kou (*Alpiniae katsumadai semen*), Xiao Hui Xiang (*Foeniculi fructus*), Ding Xiang (*Caryophylli flos*), Huang Qin (*Scutellariae radix*), Huang Lian (*Coptidis rhizoma*) and Zhu Ru (*Bambusae caulis in taeniam*).

The characteristics of these herbs can be summarized briefly as follows:

- Ban Xia especially treats nausea when there is Phlegm in the Stomach and Lung
- Zi Su Ye and Sheng Jiang treat vomiting in Exterior syndrome
- Gao Liang Jiang can warm the Stomach strongly, stop vomiting and relieve pain
- Wu Zhu Yu treats vomiting of clear fluid when there is severe headache in the top of the head
- Hua Jiao, Cao Dou Kou and Xiao Hui Xiang are able to warm the Spleen, and to regulate the Qi in the Middle Jiao in order to regulate the Stomach-Qi and stop vomiting
- Ding Xiang can descend the Stomach-Qi and treat belching and hiccup
- Huang Qin, Huang Lian and Zhu Ru are cold in nature and are used for vomiting caused by Heat or Phlegm-Heat in the Stomach.

Comparisons of strength and temperature in herbs that warm the Interior

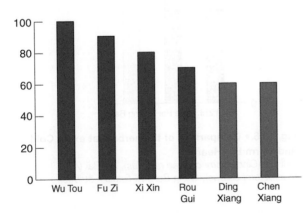

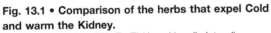

Fig. 13.1 • Comparison of the herbs that expel Cold and warm the Kidney.
Wu Tou (*Aconiti radix*)*, Fu Zi (*Aconiti radix lateralis preparata*)*, Xi Xin (*Asari herba*)*, Rou Gui (*Cinnamomi cassiae cortex*), Ding Xiang (*Caryophylli flos*), Chen Xiang (*Aquilariae lignum*).

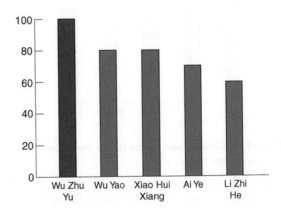

Fig. 13.2 • Comparison of the herbs that expel Cold and warm the Liver.
Wu Zhu Yu (*Evodiae fructus*), Wu Yao (*Linderae radix*), Xiao Hui Xiang (*Foeniculi fructus*), Ai Ye (*Artemisiae argyi folium*), Li Zhi He (*Litchi semen*).

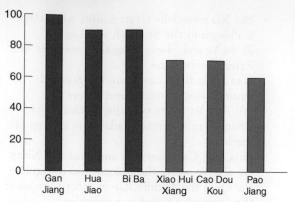

Fig. 13.3 • Comparison of the herbs that expel Cold and warm the Spleen.
Gan Jiang (*Zingiberis rhizoma*), Hua Jiao (*Zanthoxyli fructus*), Bi Ba (*Piperis longi fructus*), Xiao Hui Xiang (*Foeniculi fructus*), Cao Dou Kou (*Alpiniae katsumadai semen*), Pao Jiang (quick-fried *Zingiberis rhizoma preparatum*).

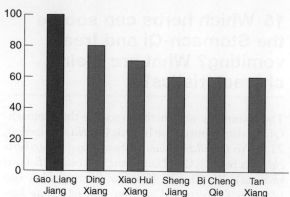

Fig. 13.4 • Comparison of the herbs that expel Cold and warm the Stomach.
Gao Liang Jiang (*Alpiniae officinari rhizoma*), Ding Xiang (*Caryophylli flos*), Xiao Hui Xiang (*Foeniculi fructus*), Sheng Jiang (*Zingiberis rhizoma recens*), Bi Cheng Qie (*Litseae fructus*), Tan Xiang (*Santali albi lignum*).

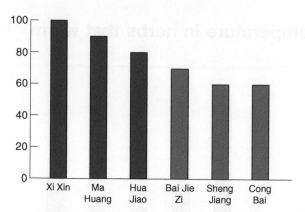

Fig. 13.5 • Comparison of the herbs that expel Cold and warm the Lung.
Xi Xin (*Asari herba*)*, Ma Huang (*Ephedrae herba*)*, Hua Jiao (*Zanthoxyli fructus*), Bai Jie Zi (*Sinapis albae semen*), Sheng Jiang (*Zingiberis rhizoma recens*), Cong Bai (*Allii fistulosi bulbus*).

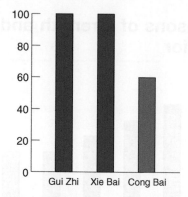

Fig. 13.6 • Comparison of the herbs that expel Cold and warm the Heart.
Gui Zhi (*Cinnamomi cassiae ramulus*), Xie Bai (*Allii macrostemi bulbus*), Cong Bai (*Allii fistulosi bulbus*).

Chapter Fourteen

Herbs that tonify

补益药

1 What are the functions of tonifying herbs and their indications? What precautions should be observed in their usage?

Tonifying herbs possess tonifying, nourishing, supplementing and strengthening abilities. They are used to treat Deficiency syndromes. As the main substances of the body are the Qi and Essence, which further generate the Blood, Body Fluids, Yin and Yang, the Deficiency syndromes can be generally divided into four types: deficiency of the Qi, deficiency of the Blood, deficiency of the Yin and deficiency of the Yang. They can be further subdivided into the deficiency of specific organs, such as Kidney-Yin deficiency, Spleen-Qi deficiency or Heart-Blood deficiency. Deficiency syndromes may also exist in patients with a weak constitution, in those in the recovery period of diseases, as well as in elderly people and children; in these patients, it is hard to determine which organ is weak and which part should be tonified, as the condition of the patient is generally weak.

The tonifying herbs can be divided into four categories: tonifying the Qi, tonifying the Blood, tonifying the Yin and tonifying the Yang. As the Essence is the basic material of the Qi, Blood, Yin and Yang, tonifying the Essence is included within these four categories. In order for the practitioner to master the functions and applications of tonifying herbs, it

is important to compare the characteristics of herbs in different categories as well as those within a single category. Although they all possess tonifying ability, the strength, speed, temperature and nature of each is quite different. For instance, Ren Shen (*Ginseng radix*) can tonify the Qi, and its action is quick and strong, therefore it is suitable for treating severe Qi deficiency and is used in the critical condition of Qi collapse. Dang Shen (*Codonopsis radix*) and Fu Ling (*Poria*) can also tonify the Qi but their action is much gentler and slower than that of Ren Shen. They are especially useful for treating chronic deficiency of the Qi, or conditions in which the patient is unable to bear the strong tonifying herbs. Some herbs such as Shu Di Huang (*Rehmanniae radix praeparata*) and Huang Qi (*Astragali radix*) are very effective for tonifying Qi deficiency, but their rich and cloying nature places a burden on the Stomach and Spleen; therefore herbs that regulate the Qi to promote digestion should be used in the meantime. In patients who suffer from chronic disease, elderly people or patients with a generally weak constitution, herbs that are neutral and light without a cloying nature should be used—for example, Bai Bian Dou (*Dolichoris lablab semen*), Yu Zhu (*Polygonati odorati rhizoma*) and Bai He (*Lilii bulbus*); they can be used for a longer period of time. There are herbs that tonify certain organs and are particularly suitable for weakness of that organ—for instance, Huang Qi tonifies the Spleen-Qi and Lung-Qi, whereas Bai Zhu (*Atractylodis macrocephalae rhizoma*) tonifies only the Spleen-Qi.

Before herbs are used to treat Deficiency syndromes, clear differentiation of the syndromes is required—for instance, whether the Qi is involved in the Deficiency syndrome, or whether the Blood, or even the Yin and Yang, are also involved. One thing that should be mentioned is that the mental state could powerfully influence the person's vitality. Depression, fear, worry or pondering leads to tiredness, as does stress or physical exertion. This is a common complaint that resembles that seen in a Deficiency syndrome, but, in these cases, the symptom of tiredness alters according to the mental and physical condition, and the tongue and pulse do not show obvious weakness of the internal organs.

The tonifying herbs are used for treating Deficiency syndrome; they are not suitable for use in conditions where substantial excessive pathological products are present, such as Phlegm, food and water accumulation, or stagnation of Qi and Blood. Because of their rich and cloying nature, the tonifying herbs may retain these pathological products in the body. For the same reason, they are not suitable for use in conditions where there are exogenous pathogenic factors. However, in many cases, Deficiency syndromes are complicated with Excess pathological factors, or internal disorders are complicated with external factors, and the factor of Deficiency often plays a causative role in the pathological process, so in these circumstances tonifying herbs can be used in combination with herbs that eliminate Excess pathological factors and exogenous pathogenic factors.

Many tonifying herbs have a sweet and cloying nature, and are therefore not easily digested. As they may cause distension of the abdomen and reduced appetite, they should be combined with herbs that promote Qi movement in the Stomach, Spleen and Large Intestine, especially in patients with deficiency of the Middle Jiao, elderly people and children.

In addition, for treating chronic Deficiency syndromes, the treatment should take place in courses. Generally speaking, winter is a better season to start tonifying treatment than summer because winter is the time of storing and the digestive capability is stronger than in summer. Another way of starting the treatment is following the changes of Yin and Yang in nature: to treat Yin deficiency the treatment should be given in spring and summer; to treat Yang deficiency the treatment should be given in autumn and winter.

2 What are the methods of 'direct tonifying' and 'indirect tonifying'?

Direct tonifying and indirect tonifying are commonly used strategies in Chinese herbal medicine. Both are used for treating Deficiency syndromes. 'Direct tonifying' means to tonify the weak part of the body directly. For example, Shu Di Huang (*Rehmanniae radix praeparata*) can tonify the Kidney-Essence if there is Kidney-Essence deficiency; Huang Qi (*Astragali radix*) can tonify the Spleen-Qi and Dang Gui (*Angelicae sinensis radix*) can tonify the Liver-Blood directly if there is Spleen-Qi and Liver-Blood deficiency.

'Indirect tonifying' means to tonify the body according to the relationship of the Zang Fu organs as well as the relationship of the Qi and Blood. According to the Five Elements theory, the five Zang organs are related by physiology and pathology. By following the cycle of generation, a basic treatment principle for Deficiency syndrome is developed. This principle is: 'if there is deficiency in one organ, tonify the mother organ'. That is one strategy of indirect tonifying.

Although the five organs can be tonified according to this principle, in clinical practice, some methods are more often used and are more effective than others. For instance, suppose that a patient complains that he often catches cold, his nose is blocked and he also sweats easily. Meanwhile, he has a pale face, his tongue body is pale and flabby with a white coating and his pulse is soft and weak. According to the symptoms and the examinations, the diagnosis is weakness of the Lung-Qi. Therefore, according to this principle, the treatment starts with tonifying the Spleen-Qi, the mother organ of the Lung. When the Spleen-Qi is sufficient, it lifts the Qi to the Lung, thereby strengthening the Exterior. Huang Qi and Bai Zhu (*Atractylodis macrocephalae rhizoma*) are often used in this condition. This is called '*fertilizing the Earth in order to generate the Metal*'. There is another reason why this method is frequently used in clinical practice. It is believed that the Spleen is the source of the Qi and the Lung is the container of the Qi; therefore, to tonify the Lung-Qi, one should start with tonifying the Spleen-Qi. This is why all the herbs that tonify the Lung-Qi and strengthen the Exterior enter both the Lung and Spleen meridians; examples include Huang Qi and

Ren Shen (*Ginseng radix*). Another commonly used indirect tonifying pattern is called '*nourishing the Water to receive the Wood*'. It is used in conditions where the Liver-Yin and Blood are so weak that the Liver-Yang escapes the control of the Yin and so it rises up. The treatment method here is to tonify strongly the Kidney-Yin, the mother organ of the Liver, in order to tonify the Liver-Yin and control the Liver-Yang. Because the Kidney and Liver are both located in the Lower Jiao, the Kidney contains the Essence and the Liver contains the Blood; the Kidney-Essence can turn into Blood so as to supplement the Liver-Yin and Blood, and to control the Liver-Yang. This method is very often used for hypertension, glaucoma, menopausal syndrome and diabetes, with symptoms such as headache, dizziness, tinnitus, dry and painful eyes, blurred vision, hot flushes, tingling or numbness of the extremities, a deep red or purple tongue body with or without a thin coating and a thready and wiry pulse. Indirect tonifying can also be used in other conditions—for example, tonifying the Liver-Blood so as to treat Heart-Blood deficiency in the treatment of mental disorders. For instance, one can use Dang Gui, Shu Di Huang, Bai Shao Yao (*Paeoniae radix lactiflora*) and Suan Zao Ren (*Ziziphi spinosae semen*), which tonify the Blood and enter the Liver meridian, to treat palpitations, restlessness and insomnia.

The indirect tonifying strategy also follows the relationship between Qi and Blood, Yin and Yang of the body or in one organ. According to the concepts that 'the Qi is the commander of the Blood, the Blood is the mother of the Qi' and 'the Yin exists on the Yang and the Yang exists on the Yin', methods are used to tonify the Qi in order to generate the Blood in the condition of Blood deficiency, and to tonify the Yin in order to generate the Yang in the condition of Yang deficiency. The former is often used in critical situations where the patient has lost a large amount of blood in a short time and it is impossible to supply the blood in a very short period of time. Here Ren Shen and Huang Qi should be used first to strengthen the Qi in order to control and generate the Blood. The latter is often used in situations where the Kidney-Yang is weak—for instance, in elderly people, patients suffering from cold in the back, knees and extremities, clear urine and loose stools. Treatment can be given to tonify the Kidney-Yin strongly, whilst simultaneously using smaller amounts of gentle, sweet and warm herbs to warm the Kidney-Yang, instead of just using hot and pungent herbs to activate the Kidney-Yang, which

may consume the Kidney-Yin and, furthermore, also injure the Kidney-Yang.

Comparing the strategy of direct tonifying with that of indirect tonifying, the direct tonifying method can be used alone, whereas the indirect tonifying method is often used with the first method, especially in chronic cases. In the herbal literature, there can be found herbs which have the functions of tonifying both the mother organ and the child organ, the Yin and the Yang, although they have a particular emphasis—for example, Huang Qi primarily tonifies the Spleen-Qi and secondly the Lung-Qi; Dang Gui primarily tonifies the Liver-Blood and secondly the Heart-Blood; Shu Di Huang mainly tonifies the Kidney-Essence and the Kidney-Yin, but gently tonifies Kidney-Yang as well.

3 What is the opinion of the 'school of tonifying the Spleen' in the herbal literature?

The concept of the earth being the center can be found in Chinese classics of philosophy and agriculture. In TCM, the idea that the Spleen and Stomach are the principal organs in tonification has a very long history too. In the Jin dynasty, a famous physician Li Dong Yuan wrote a book named *Discussion on the Spleen and Stomach* (AD 1249), which completed the theory and treatment based on this concept, and tonifying the Spleen has become a real school of thought since that time.

The 'school of tonifying the Spleen' is also called 'the school of fertilizing the Earth'. People in this school hold the opinion that the Spleen (together with the Stomach) is the foundation of life. After a person is born, the growth and development depend on the condition of the Spleen and Stomach. The Spleen and Stomach are in the Middle Jiao and are responsible for receiving, digesting and transforming food and drink into Essence, Qi, Blood and Body Fluids. Afterwards, the Spleen transports them into the Lung and spreads them throughout the whole body. The unused part of the food and drink is eliminated from the Large Intestine. Although this transportation is partially carried out by the dispersing function of the Lung and the transporting function of the intestines, the Qi of the Lung and intestines also comes from the Spleen.

Furthermore, as the Spleen and Stomach are in the Middle Jiao, which connects the Upper Jiao and

Lower Jiao though lifting and descending the water and the Qi, it is a key control system of the body in both physiology and pathology.

Moreover, in practice, tonifying the body through the Spleen is easier and quicker than doing this through other organs. The therapeutic effects show strong support for this school. The Post-Heaven Essence and Qi generated from the Spleen are relatively easier to restore and strengthen compared with the Pre-Heaven Essence and Qi, which are stored in the Kidney. As the Kidney-Essence does not increase much after a person is born, the whole development of the person requires the supplementation of the Spleen-Essence and the Blood. This is a very positive viewpoint in terms of life and health because it implies that one can improve one's well-being by strengthening the Spleen, no matter how weak a constitution one is born with and how weak the Kidney-Essence and the Kidney-Qi are. Therefore, although the constitution is determined by the Kidney-Essence and Qi, the condition of health can be changed and improved by developing and strengthening the function of the Spleen and Stomach. For instance, one person may be born with a very good constitution, and so has the capability to have a healthy and a long life, but that certainly will not happen if the Kidney-Essence has been consumed quickly and the Spleen is impaired badly by not taking good care of them—for instance, living in a very busy, stressful or unrestrained way for many years, or suffering from fear, anxiety, stress or starvation, such as lived in war or natural disasters. Conversely, a premature baby, although originally having a weaker Pre-Heaven Qi and Essence, may be taken good care of so that the function of the Spleen is supported and developed, and live in a healthy way both physically and mentally, so that overall the person's health is better, and the life is longer, than in the former case.

For these reasons, the concept and the treatment of protecting and strengthening the Spleen are very widely used in clinical practice. This idea also influences the nursing and dietary ideas and methods of TCM.

4 What is the opinion of the 'school of tonifying the Kidney' in the herbal literature?

The 'school of tonifying the Kidney' holds the opinion that the Kidney is the most important organ

in the body because the Yin, Yang, Qi and Essence of the Kidney are the principal substances of life and the Kidney determines the constitution and vitality of each individual. Moreover, the Yin, Yang, Qi and Essence of the Kidney are the origin of the Yin, Yang, Qi and Essence of the other organs, so the condition of the Kidney determines the condition of the whole body. This school therefore believes that the tonifying process should be started from the Kidney.

From study and practice, this school developed many very effective methods to treat Kidney deficiency based on the understanding of the relationship between Yin, Yang, Qi and Essence of the Kidney. A series of strategies was created. For instance, when treating Kidney-Yin deficiency, the practitioner will add in a small amount of herbs that tonify the Yang to a larger amount of herbs that tonify the Yin; the aim of this is to warm and activate the Yin in order to generate it sufficiently. Conversely, when treating Kidney-Yang deficiency, the practitioner adds some herbs that tonify the Yin with the herbs that tonify the Yang; this is because the Yin is regarded as the root of the Yang. When tonifying either the Yin or the Yang, the practitioner also uses a large amount of herbs that tonify the Kidney-Essence; this is because the Kidney-Essence is the fuel for the Yang and the substantial source of the Yin. When the Kidney-Essence is sufficient, the Yang acts on the Yin, and then generates the Kidney-Qi. This concept can be clearly seen in the formulas Zuo Gui Wan (*Restore the Left Kidney Pill*) and You Gui Wan (*Restore the Right Kidney Pill*), which were designed by the Taoist physician Zhang Jie Bin in the Ming dynasty.

As the Kidney is regarded as the root of life, this school has also invented many indirect methods of strengthening the other organs through tonifying the Kidney. For instance, when treating Spleen-Yang and Qi deficiency, the practitioner will use herbs that tonify the Kidney-Yang and Qi in order to warm and generate the Spleen-Yang and Qi. When treating a cough, shortness of breath and asthma, which are caused by Lung-Qi deficiency, the practitioner uses herbs that tonify the Kidney in order to grasp the Qi and regulate the breath. To treat chronic cough, thirst, a tendency to be hungry, dry eyes and blurred vision, caused by deficiency of the Lung-Yin, Stomach-Yin and Liver-Yin, the practitioner uses herbs that primarily tonify the Kidney-Yin in order to generate the Yin of these organs. To treat many emotional disorders, such as fear, anxiety or restlessness, or poor memory and inability to concentrate, the method of tonifying the Kidney is also often used.

Since the Kidney-Qi and Kidney-Essence determine the development of the body, the method of tonifying the Kidney plays an important role in the treatment of retardation in children, disorders of menstruation and learning difficulties in young people, infertility, menopausal syndrome in adults and degenerative disease in elderly people.

Since the Kidney-Qi and Kidney-Essence are inherited from the parents and do not increase after birth, some people have a passive attitude about the method of tonifying the Kidney; they think the Kidney-Qi and Kidney-Essence can only be consumed and the constitution cannot be changed as it depends on the Kidney condition. However, the school of tonifying the Kidney believes that, although the Kidney-Essence cannot easily be increased, it can be strong and sufficient if protected and used in the right way. Tonifying the Kidney is impossible to achieve in a short time, but people can use this idea to protect the Kidney in many ways over the whole lifetime. There are many ways to tonify and protect the Kidney, such as Chinese herbal therapy, Qi Gong exercise, Chinese dietary therapy and maintaining a healthy lifestyle. All of these can prevent disease, maintain health and lead to longevity. In this way, a person born with a poor constitution can live a happy and healthy life, and a person born with a robust constitution may live even longer than the average age at that time.

5 What are the differences between strong tonification and gentle tonification?

In strong tonification, either herbs that have a strong tonifying ability, or herbs that are gentle in action but in large dosage, are used to tonify severe weakness of the Qi, Blood, Yin or Yang of the body. This method can be generally divided into strong tonification of the Yang and Qi, and strong tonification of the Yin and Blood. Strong tonification of the Yang and Qi is especially used in critical conditions—for instance, in conditions where there is loss of a large amount of blood in a short time, or in myocardial infarction, when the blood pressure drops or is unstable. Because the substantial parts of the body, such as the Yin, Body Fluids, Blood and Essence, cannot be tonified in a very short time, first the

herbs that can strongly and quickly strengthen the Qi and rescue the Yang are used; in order to hold the Blood, the Yin and the Body Fluids, the herbs that tonify the Qi and Yang are administrated immediately by transfusion.

Strong tonification of the Yin and Blood is often used for severe weakness of the Blood and Essence, such as in conditions of advanced wasting in diabetes or starvation, and dyscrasia in advanced cancer. Strong tonification has a particular therapeutic value for treating young patients and patients whose Spleen and Stomach are not impaired as these herbs are rich, sweet and cloying, and they are not easily digested. The commonly used herbs for strong tonification are Ren Shen (*Ginseng radix*), Huang Qi (*Astragali radix*), Shu Di Huang (*Rehmanniae radix praeparata*), Huang Jing (*Polygonati rhizoma*) and E Jiao (*Asini corii colla*).

In gentle tonification, either herbs that have a gentle tonifying nature, or a small dosage of herbs that have a strong tonifying ability, are used to tonify the Qi, Blood, Yin and Yang gradually in order to treat Deficiency syndromes. This method is used much more often than strong tonification, as the Deficiency syndrome has a chronic process and chronic Deficiency syndromes are seen more often than acute cases in clinical practice.

Also, in chronic cases, all the organs and their functions are impaired, so the body cannot bear the strong tonifying herbs, which are sweet, rich and cloying and often bring about digestive disorders, or are harsh in action and may lead to new disturbances of the Yin and Yang, Qi and Blood. For example, patients who suffer from Qi deficiency will feel dryness in the nose, eyes and throat, and fullness in the chest and Stomach after using a large dosage of Ren Shen or Huang Qi because the herbs are heavy and generate Heat in the body. Patients who suffer from Blood deficiency may have ulcers in the mouth and get heavy menstruation or bleeding after using large amounts of Dang Gui (*Angelicae sinensis radix*) or Ren Shen because these herbs are warm and can activate the movement of the weakened Blood and Qi. Patients with dyscrasia can lose their appetite instead of putting on weight because the rich and sweet herbs are too heavy to be digested by a weak Spleen. A gentle method is thus more suitable for different chronic Deficiency syndromes. The commonly used herbs are Dang Shen (*Codonopsis radix*), Bai Zhu (*Atractylodis macrocephalae rhizoma*), Fu Ling (*Poria*), Dang Gui and Bai Shao Yao (*Paeoniae radix lactiflora*).

Gentle tonification can also be fulfilled by administration of patent herbal formulas, tablets, pills, syrups or herbal teas in order to meet the needs of the clinical practice.

6 What are the indications for herbs that tonify the Qi?

The herbs that tonify the Qi are used for conditions of Qi deficiency. Qi is a type of refined Essence produced by the internal organs. It also promotes the functions of these internal organs. According to its source, the place where it belongs and its function, Qi can be divided into different types, such as Original Qi, Nutritive Qi, Defensive Qi, gathering Qi, Qi of the Zang Fu organs or Qi of the meridians. Qi is able to warm and nourish the body, promote the physiological function of all organs of the body, and protect against the invasion of exogenous pathogenic factors. In a normal condition, Qi circulates smoothly and constantly in the body.

If the Qi is insufficient, it may manifest as either general weakness or specific weakness in a certain organ. The former shows in weakness of the constitution, an inability to endure intensive mental stress and physical exertion, a tendency to tire easily, and to fall ill often and then the disease develops quickly. It is often seen in children, elderly people, patients who are suffering from mild chronic disease or neurosis, and patients recovering from an operation or from disease. Qi deficiency may alternatively manifest in certain organs. For instance, Spleen-Qi deficiency manifests as a poor appetite, abdominal distension, loose stools or diarrhea, a feeling of heaviness in the limbs and fatigue; Lung-Qi deficiency manifests as shortness of breath, a low and weak voice, pallor and a tendency to sweat easily; Heart-Qi deficiency brings about palpitations, restlessness, tightness in the chest, perspiration, and a faint and irregular pulse; Kidney-Qi deficiency may cause retardation of development, a poor constitution, spermatorrhea, premature ejaculation, edema, enuresis, urinary incontinence, and weakness in the back and legs. In Qi deficiency conditions, the tongue is pale or slightly pale, the body of the tongue is flabby, with teeth marks in a severe case, and the coating is white, or white and sticky. The pulse is weak and soft, or deep and thready, especially at the region of the corresponding organ.

The herbs that tonify the Qi are very effective for improving the general condition and treating general weakness of the Qi. They can also tonify the Qi of a specific organ as the herbs enter different meridians and have specific functions for that organ. However, there are some exceptions. For instance, herbs that tonify the Kidney-Qi are just the herbs that tonify the Kidney-Essence, Yin and Yang because the Kidney-Qi is developed directly from these. Another example is the tonification of the Liver-Qi; since the Liver-Qi is directly generated by the Liver-Blood, the herbs that treat Liver-Qi deficiency are just the herbs that treat Liver-Blood deficiency.

7 What are the characteristics of the herbs that tonify the Qi?

The herbs that are able to tonify the Qi of the body have the following characteristic properties.

Sweet in taste

Most of herbs that tonify the Qi have a sweet taste. Sweetness has a nourishing, moistening and harmonizing nature, so is able to tonify the Qi, especially the substantial aspect of the Qi, in order to treat disorders caused by Qi deficiency. The therapeutic result of tonifying by sweet herbs is achieved from three approaches. First of all, sweetness is a suitable taste for Qi deficiency as, in the case of Qi deficiency, both the Qi and Yang are impaired. The syndrome shows as general weakness and coldness. If warm and pungent herbs are used to warm and activate the Qi and Yang, the condition of the patient can be improved in a short period of time. After a while, however, the symptoms reappear. Meanwhile, patients may complain of dryness in the nose, throat and mouth, constipation and even bleeding. This is because warmth and pungency can activate the function of the body, but do not tonify the substantial parts of it. Without supplementation of the substantial parts, such as the Yin, Body Fluids and Essence, the functional improvement does not last long. Warmth and pungency may consume the Yin and the Blood of the body, and bring about a side-effect of Dryness. In contrast, sweet herbs are neutral with respect to the Yin, Yang, Qi and Blood; they can tonify one party without injuring the others. Thus they are able not only to tonify the Qi, but also to nourish the Blood and Yin as well. As they do not give rise to a side-effect of Dryness, they are suitable for Qi deficiency and disharmony of the Qi and Blood, Yin and Yang. Secondly, sweetness enters the Spleen, the most important organ for Qi generation. The Spleen is located in the Middle Jiao, and connects with the Upper Jiao and Lower Jiao, so is very important for Qi transportation. Sweetness especially benefits the Spleen-Qi and strengthens its function, therefore spreading the Qi within the entire body. Thirdly, because sweetness remains working in one place and has no moving tendency, it may reduce the speed of an aggressive pathogenic process, moderate the harsh properties of herbs in a tonifying formula and slow the haste of other herbs so as to prevent the side-effects of these herbs.

Slightly warm in temperature

Most of the herbs that tonify the Qi are slightly warm in temperature. As Qi must constantly move, it needs not only the substantial part, which can be obtained from the sweet taste of the herbs, but also a moving capability, which can be increased by the warm nature of the herbs. When gentle warmth and sweetness coexist in one herb, the tonifying action shows clearly. This action is described as: '*the gentle Fire steams the sweet, and then the Qi is generated gradually*'. However, the herbs should be warm rather than hot because hot herbs consume the Yin and Qi. So there is also a saying: '*the gentle Fire generates the Qi and the strong Fire destroys the Qi*'.

Entering the Spleen and Lung meridians

Most of the herbs that tonify the Qi mainly enter the Spleen and Lung meridians. As the Spleen is the most important organ for producing the Qi, the herbs that enter the Spleen may effectively tonify the Qi of the whole body. Since the Lung can disperse and descend the Qi, it is an important organ for transporting and regulating the Qi. The herbs that enter the Lung meridian are effective for strengthening the function of the Lung and accelerating the Qi movement.

Bitter in taste

Some of the herbs that tonify the Qi have a bitter taste, which possesses a drying ability. When the Qi

is deficient in the body, and especially when the Spleen-Qi is deficient, the Qi may fail to transport Dampness and cause water or Dampness accumulation. Herbs that have bitter or bitter-warm properties may dry Dampness and strengthen the function of the Spleen as well as the other internal organs so as to treat Qi deficiency. Bai Zhu (*Atractylodis macrocephalae rhizoma*) is a good example.

Bland and neutral

Some of the herbs that tonify the Qi are bland and neutral. Blandness is able to leach out Dampness and promote urination. It is suitable for treating accumulation of Dampness that is caused by the Qi deficiency. Neutrality is an ideal temperature to treat disorders where Heat and Cold are complicated. Neutrality is easily combined with other tastes and temperature to treat Qi deficiency with the disharmony of the Blood, Yin and Yang. The commonly used herb is Fu Ling (*Poria*).

In addition, herbs that tonify the Qi may have some side-effects. These are mainly caused by their rich nature and the sweet taste, which place an extra burden on the Spleen and lead to Qi stagnation and Dampness accumulation. The manifestations of this are fullness of the epigastrium, distension of the abdomen and difficulty of bowel movement. To avoid this, in clinical practice, these tonifying herbs are often used with a small amount of herbs that promote Qi movement, such as Chen Pi (*Citri reticulatae pericarpium*) and Mu Xiang (*Aucklandiae radix*)**.

8 Ren Shen (*Ginseng radix*) and Huang Qi (*Astragali radix*) are the most important herbs for tonifying the Qi. What are their characteristics?

Ren Shen and Huang Qi are two strong herbs for tonifying the Qi. Both are sweet and slightly warm, and enter the Spleen and Lung meridians. Sweetness possesses a tonifying ability and the gentle warmth may gently strengthen the Yang, which further generates the Qi. They strongly tonify the Spleen-Qi, strengthen the Middle Jiao and promote the function of the Spleen to generate the Blood, Essence and Body Fluids. They can treat Spleen-Qi deficiency, which manifests as poor appetite, distension of the abdomen, loose stools, diarrhea and fatigue.

The Spleen, together with the Stomach, is regarded as the foundation of the life after birth. When the Spleen-Qi is strong enough, it can transport the Qi to the Lung so as to strengthen the Lung-Qi and the Defensive Qi. Both herbs are very effective for treating Lung-Qi deficiency, which manifests as shortness of breath, a weak voice, a tendency to catch cold and spontaneous sweating.

Ren Shen is particularly able to tonify the Original Qi and rescue the Yang and so is used for critical conditions where the Qi is severely injured and the Yang has collapsed. The patient may have shallow respiration, cold limbs, a pale face, profuse sweating and a very weak pulse. These conditions can be seen after severe vomiting or diarrhea, shock, fainting or losing a large amount of Blood. Because Ren Shen can strongly tonify the Original Qi, the principal Qi of the body, it can also tonify the Qi of all the internal organs—for instance, it tonifies the Heart-Qi, calms the Mind and therefore treats palpitations and restlessness. It can tonify the Spleen-Qi and promote the function of the Spleen. Moreover, it promotes the generation of the Blood and treats fatigue, insomnia and dizziness caused by Qi and Blood deficiency. It also promotes the generation of the Body Fluids and therefore treats profuse sweating and thirst caused by Qi and Yin deficiency.

Huang Qi is warmer than Ren Shen in temperature. As it does not tonify the Original Qi, it is not used in critical conditions or in Qi deficiency of all the internal organs. Huang Qi enters the Spleen and Lung meridians and its function focuses on the Spleen and the Lung. It can strongly tonify the Spleen-Qi and promote its function, strengthening the foundation of life so as to improve the patient's condition and strengthen the Qi in general. It is able to lift the Spleen-Qi and increase the strength of the muscles, which are controlled by the Spleen, and so it treats a prolapsed uterus, Stomach and rectum, as well as tiredness and heavy sensations in the body and limbs. Because it can tonify the Spleen-Qi and strengthen the muscles, it can promote the healing process in chronic ulceration, sores or wounding. It also strengthens the Spleen-Qi and controls the Blood, which must circulate in the blood vessels, and therefore can be used in bleeding conditions.

Huang Qi has another very important function—to tonify the Lung-Qi and stabilize the Exterior. Huang Qi can strongly tonify the Spleen-Qi, which can then further transport the Qi to the Lung; therefore it treats shortness of breath, and a low and weak voice, caused by the Lung-Qi deficiency. Furthermore, when the Spleen-Qi and the Lung-Qi are sufficient, the Defensive Qi is also strong; thus it can control the pores better and promote the Qi and Blood circulation on the surface of the body so as to strengthen the Exterior. This is why Huang Qi is often used to treat recurrent colds, spontaneous sweating and chronic sinusitis.

Ren Shen and Huang Qi have their own characteristic actions in tonifying the Qi. They are also characterized by their quick actions. In clinical practice, they can be used together to treat severe Qi deficiency. However, they can bring about some side-effects because of their rich and warm nature, especially in patients with deficiency of the Spleen and Stomach. If the patient complains of fullness in the Stomach or distension in the abdomen, herbs that promote the digestion should be used, such as Chen Pi (*Citri reticulatae pericarpium*) and Sha Ren (*Amomi xanthioidis fructus*).

9 What are the differences between the different products of Ren Shen (*Ginseng radix*)?

Ren Shen and its products are classified into many types according to the habitat, climate, the conditions of cultivation and the processing procedure. The properties and the functions of Ren Shen therefore vary vastly.

The type called 'Ye Shan Shen', or the 'wild mountain root', grows in the Chang Bai Mountain between China and Korea, and is regarded as the best quality of Ren Shen. Its function of tonifying the Qi is the strongest. Since the herb grows in the mountains for many years and is not easy to find, the price is very high and it is used only for very severe cases.

Most of the Ren Shen used today is cultivated. Its effect in tonifying the Qi is not as strong as that of the wild root. After it is collected, washed and then dried by wind or the sun, the product is called 'Sheng Shai Shen', or 'raw dried root'. It is sweet and neutral, and is effective for tonifying the Qi as well as nourishing the Yin. Its function is relatively strong for cultivated Ren Shen.

Alternatively, after the fresh Ren Shen is collected, washed and peeled, it may be steamed for

2–3 hours, and then dried. The color then becomes dark red or brown, and this product is called 'Hong Shen', or 'red root'. Its strength in the action of tonifying the Qi is similar to that of Sheng Shai Shen, but it is warm and sweet, so is often used for Qi and Yang deficiency. It is also used in winter for patients with Qi deficiency and elderly people.

If fresh Ren Shen is cured in rock candy, it is called 'Bai Shen', or 'white root'. This has a gentler action of tonifying the Qi compared with the other products.

'Xi Yang Shen' (*Panacis quinquefolii radix*), also called 'Hua Qi Shen', is sweet and cold in nature, and its function in tonifying the Qi is as strong as that of Sheng Shai Shen, but its action in nourishing the Yin is stronger than that of Sheng Shai Shen. As it can also clear Heat in the body, it is often used for the syndrome of deficiency of Qi and Yin with Empty-Fire, such as seen in diabetes and pulmonary tuberculosis.

Habitat is also important in the quality of Ren Shen. For instance, a product called 'Ji Lin Shen', because it is from Ji Lin province, which is located in the Chang Bai Mountain, is of good quality. Korean Ren Shen, which is also called 'Gao Li Shen', is warm and sweet, has a similar function to Hong Shen but is stronger for warming the Interior and tonifying the Qi. Although all the products of Ren Shen can tonify the Qi, from a clinical viewpoint it is necessary to make the proper choice from the different products to achieve the best effect.

10 Xi Yang Shen (*Panacis quinquefolii radix*), Sheng Shai Shen (raw dried *Ginseng radix*), Tai Zi Shen (*Pseudostellariae radix*) and Bei Sha Shen (*Glehniae radix*) are all able to tonify the Qi and Yin. What are the differences between their actions?

The syndrome of Qi and Yin deficiency can develop from different diseases. One of them is febrile disease, such as pneumonia, pulmonary tuberculosis and viral myocarditis. The Qi and Yin are consumed by Heat in the pathological process. The syndrome can also develop from chronic disease due to weak-

ness and disharmony of the Yin, Yang, Qi and Blood. For instance, in Waste and Thirsty syndrome (diabetes), the Yin of the Lung, Heart, Stomach, Liver and Kidney are all impaired. The symptoms of Qi and Yin deficiency are shortness of breath, tiredness, spontaneous sweating, thirst, palpitations, restlessness, insomnia, a reduced appetite, preference for drinking rather than eating, or getting hungry easily but not being willing to eat, dizziness, weakness in the back and spermatorrhea.

These four herbs are all able to tonify the Qi and Yin. They can be used for Qi and Yin deficiency of the Lung, Heart, Stomach and Kidney, but there are differences between their actions.

Xi Yang Shen is sweet, bitter and cold, and enters the Heart, Lung and Kidney meridians. It can tonify the Qi and generate Yin, and is the strongest among these four herbs. Since it is bitter and cold, it is able to clear Heat and reduce Fire, and is suitable for treating Qi and Yin deficiency with Excessive- or Empty-Fire. It can treat afternoon fever, irritability, warm palms, thirst, fatigue, hemoptysis, a shortened menstrual cycle or heavy menstruation.

Sheng Shai Shen, the raw, dried, and cultivated Ren Shen, is sweet and neutral. Its function is similar to that of Xi Yang Shen. To tonify the Qi and the Yin, it is as strong as Xi Yang Shen. However, this herb is not so cold and not bitter; therefore it cannot clear Heat and reduce Fire. If there is Heat in the syndrome, Xi Yang Shen is a better choice than Sheng Shai Shen.

Tai Zi Shen is slightly cold and bitter, and it enters the Spleen and Lung meridians. It can tonify the Qi and Yin of the Spleen and Lung but the function is weaker than that of Xi Yang Shen and Sheng Shai Shen. It must be used for a long period of time and in large dosage to treat Deficiency syndromes. However, its gentle and moderate nature is particularly suitable for patients with a rather weak constitution or only slight Yin deficiency. It is also used in patients who are in the recovery period of febrile diseases, in those who have a poor appetite, and are tired and thirsty, and for patients suffering from chronic diseases who cannot bear the strong tonifying herbs.

Bei Sha Shen is sweet and cold, and enters the Lung and Stomach meridians. The main function of the herb is to nourish the Yin and generate the Body Fluids. It has the function of tonifying the Qi but is very weak compared with the other three herbs. In clinical practice, if there is slight Qi deficiency in a Yin deficiency syndrome, this herb is a good choice.

11 What are the differences between Ren Shen (*Ginseng radix*) and Dang Shen (*Codonopsis radix*)?

Ren Shen is the most important herb for tonifying the Qi. It can tonify the Original Qi, therefore it is able to rescue collapsed Yang. It can also strongly tonify the Spleen-Qi, which is considered as the foundation of life and the source of Qi and Blood. However, although Ren Shen is an excellent herb for tonifying the Qi and promoting the functions of all the internal organs, it is very expensive if good quality products are required, therefore it is only used in severe cases. In most cases of Qi deficiency, and especially in chronic disorders, a large dosage of Dang Shen is often used as an effective substitution for Ren Shen.

Dang Shen is sweet and neutral, and enters the Spleen and Lung meridians. However, since it does not enter the Kidney meridian, it has no function in tonifying the Original Qi and so cannot be used in critical conditions. In acute Yang collapse condition, therefore, Ren Shen must be used. However, Dang Shen is effective for tonifying the Spleen-Qi and the Lung-Qi, and its action is much gentler than that of Ren Shen. The strong point of this herb is that it is not heavy and sticky, and does not generate Heat and Dryness in the body, so is more suitable for many chronic diseases with Spleen-Qi and Lung-Qi deficiency. It can also generate the Yin and Body Fluids, so is also used for deficiency of both Qi and Yin. In addition, a large dosage of Dang Shen (i.e. at least six times the dosage of Ren Shen) can be used as a substitute for Ren Shen in treating severe deficiency of the Spleen-Qi and Lung-Qi.

12 What are the differences in actions and applications between Huang Qi (*Astragali radix*) and Bai Zhu (*Atractylodis macrocephalae rhizoma*)?

Huang Qi and Bai Zhu are both commonly used for tonifying Qi and are also often used together. Both are sweet and warm, and enter the Spleen meridian. Both can strengthen the Middle Jiao and tonify the Spleen-Qi, therefore treating Spleen-Qi deficiency. They are also used together to strengthen the transportation function of the Spleen, eliminate Dampness and treat edema. Although the applications are similar, there are differences between their properties and actions.

Huang Qi is sweeter and warmer than Bai Zhu, and its action in tonifying the Spleen-Qi is stronger. Its specific action is to tonify the Qi, raise the Yang-Qi of the Spleen and increase the strength of muscles. It not only treats a poor appetite and indigestion, but also chronic diarrhea and prolapsed rectum, stomach, uterus or other internal organs. Furthermore, Huang Qi strengthens not only the muscles of the internal organs, but also those in the whole body, so it can be used for patients who complain of weakness and heaviness in the limbs and tiredness, such as seen in chronic fatigue syndrome. Moreover, since Huang Qi can improve the condition of the muscles, it is also able to promote the healing of wounds after operations or trauma.

As the Spleen controls the Blood circulating in the blood vessels, the ascending and tonifying function of Huang Qi can control the Blood; therefore this herb can be used in bleeding conditions caused by Spleen-Qi deficiency, such as seen in uterine bleeding, blood in the stools and purpura. It is also able to tonify the Spleen-Qi and transport the Dampness in time, so it can treat edema.

Bai Zhu is also sweet and warm, and can tonify the Spleen-Qi like Huang Qi; however, it is bitter in taste. Its effect in tonifying the Spleen-Qi is weaker than that of Huang Qi, and it has no function in raising the Spleen-Qi and controlling the Blood. However, its bitter and warm property can dry Dampness; therefore its characteristics are tonifying of the Spleen-Qi and transformation of Dampness. It can treat poor appetite, fullness in the Stomach, distension in the abdomen, diarrhea and heaviness of the limbs.

There are also some other differences between the two herbs. Huang Qi, and especially raw Huang Qi, enters the Lung meridian and can strengthen the Lung-Qi and the Defensive Qi. It is especially suitable for treating a deficiency of both the Spleen-Qi and Lung-Qi. In this condition the patient has a poor appetite, distension in the abdomen and loose stools, as well as spontaneous sweating, recurrent colds, shortness of breath and tiredness. Huang Qi can strengthen the Lung-Qi so as to regulate the water metabolism and treat edema, especially edema on the face and upper part of the body.

Bai Zhu does not enter the Lung meridian, and has little influence on the Lung-Qi and the Defensive Qi. However, it enters the Stomach meridian and can promote digestion and treat lack of appetite and fullness in the Stomach. It is often used for malnutrition in children. Furthermore, since it can regulate the whole function of the Middle Jiao, and it has no tendency to move upwards or downwards, it is often used to calm a restless fetus caused by Spleen-Qi deficiency in pregnant women.

As sinking of Spleen-Qi, weakness of the muscles and accumulation of Dampness often exist at the same time when the Spleen-Qi is weak, Huang Qi and Bai Zhu are often used together to treat those disorders.

13 What are the differences between raw Bai Zhu (Atractylodis macrocephalae rhizoma), Chao Bai Zhu (dry-fried Atractylodis macrocephalae rhizoma) and Jiao Bai Zhu (deep-dry-fried Atractylodis macrocephalae rhizoma)?

Bai Zhu, the very commonly used herb for tonifying the Spleen-Qi, can be processed in several ways to meet different clinical needs.

Raw Bai Zhu is the strongest of the products to tonify the Spleen-Qi, and it treats reduced appetite, indigestion, tiredness and a wan complexion.

When Bai Zhu is dry-fried, its action in drying Dampness is increased. It is especially effective for treating distension in the abdomen, loose stools and diarrhea.

When the color of the herb turns to deep brown after dry frying, it is then called 'Jiao Bai Zhu'. This enters the Stomach meridian particularly and has the strongest effect in strengthening the receiving, ripening and transporting functions of the Stomach

of the Bai Zhu products. It is very useful for treating a poor appetite, nausea, fullness in the Stomach and belching.

14 What are the differences in the functions of tonifying the Spleen-Qi and eliminating Dampness between Bai Zhu (Atractylodis macrocephalae rhizoma) and Fu Ling (Poria)?

Bai Zhu and Fu Ling both can tonify the Spleen-Qi and eliminate Dampness from the Middle Jiao. In clinical practice, they are often used together. However, there are differences between these two herbs.

Bai Zhu is warm and bitter, and its action in tonifying the Spleen-Qi is stronger than that of Fu Ling. At the same time, it can also strengthen the Stomach.

Fu Ling is neutral and bland, and it can gently tonify the Qi. It can be used with either warm or cold herbs to warm the Spleen-Yang, tonify the Spleen-Qi or eliminate Damp-Heat in the Middle Jiao. Fu Ling also has another function: it can tonify the Heart-Qi and therefore is used for calming the Mind. Because the function of Fu Ling is gentle and it has no strong taste, it can be used for a long period of time in chronic and mild syndromes of Qi deficiency of the Spleen and Heart. It is also used in Chinese food and biscuits as a health food supplement.

Both herbs can eliminate Dampness in the Middle Jiao, but they treat the same pathogenic factor by different approaches. Bai Zhu dries the Dampness in the Middle Jiao, as it is bitter and warm; Fu Ling promotes urination and leaches out Dampness from the Lower Jiao. Also, Bai Zhu can tonify the Spleen and calm the fetus, whereas Fu Ling is forbidden for use in pregnant women as its action has a descending tendency.

15 Bai Zhu (*Atractylodis macrocephalae rhizoma*), Shan Yao (*Dioscoreae rhizoma*) and Bai Bian Dou (*Dolichoris lablab semen*) are able to tonify the Spleen-Qi and stop diarrhea. What are the differences between their actions?

Bai Zhu, Shan Yao and Bai Bian Dou all enter the Spleen meridian. They have the function of tonifying the Spleen-Qi and are used for treating weakness of the Spleen-Qi and dysfunction of transportation and transformation of food and water in the Middle Jiao. They can also reduce accumulation of Dampness and stop diarrhea. However, these three herbs have their own characteristic properties and actions.

Bai Zhu is bitter and warm, and is an important herb for tonifying the Spleen-Qi and strengthening the function of the Spleen and Stomach. As Dampness easily accumulates when the Spleen-Qi is weak, this herb is particularly suitable for this situation as it is bitter and warm in nature and can dry the Dampness, therefore treating diarrhea as well as edema.

Shan Yao is neutral and sweet. Although its effect in tonifying the Spleen-Qi is not as strong as that of Bai Zhu, it can tonify either the Qi or the Yin, so it is especially suitable for treating deficiency of both Qi and Yin in the Middle Jiao. It also has a slightly astringent property, which is helpful for stopping diarrhea. Furthermore, this herb also enters the Lung and Kidney meridians, so is effective for tonifying and stabilizing the Qi and Yin of these organs. It can be used for patients suffering from a lack of appetite, fatigue, loose stools, shortness of breath, thirst and sweating.

Bai Bian Dao is sweet and slightly warm. Its action in tonifying the Spleen-Qi is the weakest of the three herbs, but it is neither dry nor moist, and is neutral and gentle. Unlike Bai Zhu, it can tonify the Spleen without the possibility of consuming the Yin and Body Fluids in the Middle Jiao; it is also unlike Shan Yao in that it can tonify the Spleen without the possibility of leaving Dampness in the Middle Jiao. It is especially suitable for treating chronic mild Qi deficiency of the Spleen and for use in the recovery period after a chronic disease when the condition of the patient is too weak to accept strong tonification.

These three herbs all stop diarrhea through different approaches. Bai Zhu dries Dampness in the Middle Jiao to stop diarrhea; Shan Yao stabilizes the Qi and Yin so as to stop diarrhea; Bai Bian Dou has both of these functions but is weaker in its action. It can also reduce Summer-Heat and treat diarrhea, vomiting and abdominal pain in influenza, acute gastroenteritis and heatstroke.

In clinical practice, Bai Zhu and Shan Yao are often used together to treat Qi deficiency of the Spleen and stop diarrhea, but Shan Yao should not be used if there is accumulation of Dampness in the Middle Jiao and the patient complains of distension in the abdomen. Bai Zhu should not be used if there is deficiency of the Yin or Body Fluids. Bai Bian Dou is used only for mild cases, or is administrated together with other herbs.

16 What are the characteristics of Gan Cao (*Glycyrrhizae radix*)?

Compared with other tonifying herbs, such as Huang Qi (*Astragali radix*) and Bai Zhu (*Atractylodis macrocephalae rhizoma*), the tonifying function of Gan Cao is weak. However, this herb has been studied and used to tonify the Qi since ancient times. In the book *Discussion on the Febrile Diseases* by Zhang Zhong Jing written 2000 years ago, Gan Cao is the most commonly used herb for tonifying the Qi and moistening Dryness, as well as for harmonizing the Yin and Yang. It was even used in critical conditions of collapse of Qi and Yang. Nowadays, although Gan Cao is not the first-line choice for treating Qi deficiency, it is still often used in combination with other tonifying herbs.

Gan Cao enters all the meridians, and is sweet and neutral in nature. According to the concept that the combination of sweetness, warmth and pungency in herbs gives an ability to tonify the Yang, and the combination of sweetness, cold and sourness in herbs gives an ability to nourish the Yin, Gan Cao is often used in combination with cold or warm herbs in order to tonify the Yin or the Yang respectively.

The moderate tonifying action is the most important characteristic of this herb. As sweetness may slow speed, release tension and alleviate the conflict of two or more parties in a pathological development, this herb can be used in critical conditions, such as Qi, Blood, Yin and Yang collapse.

The moderate nature of Gan Cao is also used in certain specific situations. For instance, it is very effective for treating cramp in the muscles caused by the Liver-Qi overcontrolling the Spleen. A large dosage of Gan Cao is excellent for tonifying the Qi and harmonizing its Qi movement. It can also treat Heart-Qi deficiency, which leads to a failure to promote the Blood circulation, and manifests as restlessness and palpitations, tightness in the chest and arrhythmia.

The moderate nature of Gan Cao is often useful in herbal combinations as well. In most formulas, Gan Cao plays the role of reducing the side-effects of harsh herbs, harmonizing herbs that move in different directions and work on different levels, and moderating quick actions of herbs to a steady and constant action.

There are differences between raw Gan Cao and toasted Gan Cao. The raw form is sweet and neutral and, besides the functions mentioned before, it is able to clear Heat and relieve toxicity. The toasted form is sweeter and slightly warm, it especially enters the Middle Jiao, and its function of tonifying and harmonizing the Qi is stronger than that of the raw form.

Although Gan Cao is often used in many formulas, its sweet property lacks a moving potential, and its use may lead to stagnation of Qi, retain Dampness and cause distension of the Stomach and abdomen. Therefore, patients with Dampness in the Middle Jiao should not use this herb in a large dosage. In addition, sweetness may worsen vomiting, and so patients with rebellious Stomach-Qi should not use this herb either.

17 What are the indications for the herbs that tonify the Blood?

Herbs that tonify the Blood are used for Blood deficiency. Blood is one of the principal substances of the body, and it is a type of refined Essence produced by the internal organs. It circulates smoothly and constantly in the body, nourishes and supports the internal organs, and maintains the functions and structures of the body. If the Blood is not sufficient, there are symptoms such as dry eyes, blurred vision,

stiffness of the muscles and joints, tingling or numbness in the muscles, dryness and itching of the skin, irregular menstruation and tiredness.

The mental state and activities of people are also dependent on sufficient Blood; if it is deficient, the patient may suffer from palpitations, restlessness, poor memory, inability to concentrate, insomnia and dream-disturbed sleep. Most patients with Blood deficiency have a pale or pallid complexion, a cracked, pale or delicate pink tongue and a thready and wiry, or thready and weak pulse.

The herbs that tonify the Blood can treat the Kidney-Essence deficiency as well. Because the Blood and Essence are the substantial parts of the body and can turn into each other in the body, herbs that tonify the Blood are often used for treating infertility, poor memory, blurred vision, deafness and retarded development in children.

In clinical practice, the syndrome of Blood deficiency is often caused by Blood loss, weak constitution and chronic disease, and can be seen in various anemias, menstrual disorders, malnutrition, hypotension, after an operation or after giving birth.

18 What are the characteristics of the herbs that tonify the Blood?

The herbs that tonify the Blood have the following characteristics.

Sweet and slightly warm

Since sweetness has a nourishing, moistening and harmonizing nature, and warmth (especially slight warmth) may activate and promote the functions of the internal organs, sweet-warm herbs can generate the Blood and tonify the Essence. They are especially suitable for treating patients who have not only Blood deficiency but also a mild Yang and Qi deficiency of the body. The commonly used herbs are Shu Di Huang (*Rehmanniae radix praeparata*), He Shou Wu (*Polygoni multiflori radix*), Dang Gui (*Angelicae sinensis radix*), Long Yan Rou (*Longanae arillus*) and Da Zao (*Jujubae fructus*).

Sweet and cold

Because sweetness can tonify the body, especially the substantial aspect of the body, and Cold can clear Heat, sweet-cold herbs can generate the Yin, Body Fluids and Blood. They are especially suitable for treating patients who have not only Blood deficiency but also a mild Yin deficiency with slight Empty-Heat in the Blood. The commonly used herbs are Bai Shao Yao (*Paeoniae radix lactiflora*) and Sang Shen (*Mori fructus*).

Entering the Heart, Liver, Kidney and Spleen meridians

Because the Heart governs the Blood and promotes the Blood circulation, the Liver stores and regulates the amount of Blood in circulation, the Kidney-Essence can turn into Blood and the Spleen can produce Blood from the Food-Essence, most of the herbs that tonify the Blood enter these meridians. For instance, Dang Gui (*Angelicae sinensis radix*) mainly enters the Heart and the Liver meridians, Gou Qi Zi (*Lycii fructus*) and Sang Shen enter the Liver and Kidney meridians and Long Yan Rou enters the Spleen meridian.

Tonifying the Blood and the Kidney-Essence

Many of the herbs that enter the Kidney and Liver meridians are able to tonify the Blood as well as the Kidney-Essence. Because the Blood and Essence both belong to the Yin, they are the substantial part of the body, and have a nourishing function. The Blood and Essence can turn into each other in the body. The herbs that can tonify both Blood and the Kidney-Essence are Shu Di Huang, Gou Qi Zi, He Shou Wu and Sang Shen.

19 What precautions should be observed when the herbs that tonify the Blood are used?

Most of the patients who suffer from the syndrome of Blood deficiency also have a slight deficiency of Yin or Yang according to the constitution and the duration of the disease. If there is Yin deficiency, the patient may feel warmth in the chest, thirst or dryness in the mouth and also suffer from constipation and restlessness. A thin tongue body with fresh red or pink color without a coating and a restless

and thready pulse are often present too. Herbs that are sweet and cold in nature should be used in this condition. If there is mild Yang deficiency, the patient is fearful of cold, has cold hands and feet, and feels tired. A dull pale tongue proper with a white coating and a deep, thready and slow pulse are often present. Herbs that are sweet and warm in nature should be used at this time.

Because of the relationship between the Qi and Blood, it is wise to choose a small amount of herbs that tonify the Qi in order to enhance the therapeutic result of tonifying the Blood, such as Huang Qi (*Astragali radix*) and Da Zao (*Jujubae fructus*).

Most of the herbs that tonify the Blood are rich and cloying in nature, so may place an extra burden on the Spleen and Stomach and cause a reduced appetite, distension in the abdomen and difficult bowel movement, especially in patients who suffer from digestive disorders; therefore herbs that regulate the Qi in the Middle Jiao should be used at the same time, such as Chen Pi (*Citri reticulatae pericarpium*), Ban Xia (*Pinelliae rhizoma*), Mu Xiang (*Aucklandiae radix*)** and Sha Ren (*Amomi xanthioidis fructus*).

20 What are the differences between Shu Di Huang (*Rehmanniae radix praeparata*) and He Shou Wu (*Polygoni multiflori radix*) in nourishing the Blood?

Both of these herbs enter the Kidney meridian, and are sweet and slightly warm in nature. They are able to tonify the Kidney-Essence and nourish the Blood. They treat weakness and stiffness in the back and knees, blurred vision, poor memory, disorders of menstruation, infertility, menopausal syndrome and sexual disorders caused by Kidney-Essence and Blood deficiency.

Shu Di Huang is the most important herb for tonifying the Blood as well as the Kidney-Essence, and its action is the strongest and quickest of the herbs that tonify the Blood. Comparing it with He Shou Wu, Shu Di Huang has a stronger effect in tonifying the Essence and Blood than does He Shou Wu, but it is also more cloying in nature, therefore it easily causes distension in the abdomen and a reduced appetite. It is often combined with

Sha Ren (*Amomi xanthioidis fructus*) to reduce this side-effect.

He Shou Wu is weaker in its tonifying actions than Shu Di Huang, but it is not cloying and does not disturb the Spleen and Stomach. It is therefore more suitable for treating a mild Blood deficiency syndrome and can also be used for a long period of time. It is one of the commonly used herbs in the Chinese diet for strengthening the Kidney and prolonging life. Furthermore, it can nourish the Kidney-Essence and keep the hair healthy, so is also used as an ingredient in herbal shampoo.

21 Why are Dang Gui (*Angelicae sinensis radix*) and Bai Shao Yao (*Paeoniae radix lactiflora*) often used together to tonify the Liver-Blood?

There are several ways of tonifying the Blood. One of them is through the approach of tonifying the Kidney, for instance by using Shu Di Huang (*Rehmanniae radix praeparata*) and He Shou Wu (*Polygoni multiflori radix*).

Another approach of tonifying the Blood is to tonify the Liver. In this method, the Blood is tonified directly. The first-line choice for this method is Dang Gui and Bai Shao Yao. The two herbs are often used together because they mutually accentuate each other.

Dang Gui is pungent, sweet and slightly warm. The sweet-warm property can tonify the Blood and the pungent-warm nature may promote its circulation. This matches the pathological changes of Blood weakness and the circulation dysfunction.

Bai Shao Yao is sour, bitter and slightly cold. Sourness and cold may generate the Blood and Yin and therefore reduce the shortage of the substantial part of the Blood. The bitter and cold properties can clear Heat and reduce Empty-Heat in the Blood, which is caused by Blood and Yin deficiency, and therefore allow the Blood to circulate in a moderate way.

When Dang Gui and Bai Shao Yao are used together, they can mutually harmonize the Blood circulation as one is warm, so can disperse and promote the Blood circulation, and the other is cold, so can moderate and stabilize the Blood circulation. Both can tonify the Blood but one focuses on promoting the function of the Liver and the other focuses on nourishing the substantial part of the Blood. Dang Gui belongs to the Yang herbs and Bai Shao Yao belongs to the Yin herbs. They match the physiological and pathological characteristics of the Liver and the Blood, so they are often used together.

22 How can Bai Shao Yao (*Paeoniae radix lactiflora*) soften the Liver?

The term to 'soften the Liver' means, in other words, to nourish the Liver-Blood and promote proper flow of the Liver-Qi. It is a treatment method that is based on the physiological and pathological characteristics of the Liver.

The Liver is regarded as a special organ in the body. It stores the Blood, which belongs to the Yin, but its function is characterized as promoting the free flow of Qi, which belongs to the Yang. The free flow of Liver-Qi is dependent on the support of sufficient Blood in the Liver. When the Liver-Blood is deficient, the Liver-Qi is stagnant, and such patients lose their usual amiable manner and show symptoms such as irritability, quick temper, insomnia and dream-disturbed sleep. In these circumstances it seems that the Liver becomes 'hard'. In the treatment of these symptoms, the main procedure is to nourish the Blood in order to turn the function of the Liver from hard to soft, so this method is called 'softening the Liver'. It is a much more effective method than that of simply spreading the Liver-Qi in the condition of the Blood deficiency.

Bai Shao Yao is the most commonly used herb to soften the Liver. It is sour, bitter and slightly cold. It is able to tonify the Yin and Blood of the Liver, and its cold and bitter nature can reduce Heat, which is caused by deficiency of Blood and stagnation of the Liver-Qi; therefore it can eliminate irritability. It is often used for treating hypertension, insomnia, hepatitis, cholecystitis, cholelithiasis, stress, depression, premenstrual syndrome, menopausal syndrome and glaucoma when the syndrome is Blood deficiency with stagnation of the Liver-Qi.

23 Which herbs can be used in the diet to tonify the Blood?

A tall building cannot be built in a day. To tonify the body, especially the substantial part of the body, is the same as setting up a tall building; it cannot be done in a short period of time. The Chinese people have a tradition of using diet to tonify the Blood and Essence, keep healthy and prolong life. Certain herbs are often used in the diet for recovery from operation or after giving birth, for elderly people, premature infants or people with a weak constitution or suffering from chronic disease.

The commonly used herbs are Long Yan Rou (*Longanae arillus*), Gou Qi Zi (*Lycii fructus*), Sang Shen (*Mori fructus*), Hei Zhi Ma (*Sesami semen nigricum*), Hu Tao Rou (*Juglandis semen*), Da Zao (*Jujubae fructus*), Gan Cao (*Glycyrrhizae radix*), Yi Tang (*Maltose*) and Feng Mi (*Mel*). They are mainly fruits or seeds, which are sweet and with a nice taste, and they are often used in sweets, cakes, drinks, tea, soup and porridge.

24 What are the causes of Yin deficiency? What are the indications for herbs that nourish the Yin?

Herbs that nourish the Yin treat the diseases and disorders caused by deficiency of the Yin and Body Fluids. There are several causes of deficiency of the Yin and Body Fluids of the internal organs. In some diseases, such as diabetes, hypertension, asthma and menopausal syndrome, the Yin is easily injured. Mental stress can also consume the Blood and Yin directly. Furthermore, most infectious diseases can cause internal Heat and also consume the Yin of the internal organs—for example, pneumonia, bronchitis, sinusitis, gastroenteritis and cystitis. Finally, certain dietary habits may consume the Yin of the body, such as drinking too much coffee and eating too much spicy food.

Since the Yin has the function of nourishing and moistening the body, Yin deficiency may manifest as Dryness and Empty-Heat. Yin deficiency exists particularly in the following Zang Fu organs.

When the Heart-Yin is not sufficient, insomnia, irritability, palpitations and night sweats are often present. When the Lung-Yin is deficient, the symptoms include a dry, hacking cough with scanty, thick and sticky sputum, thirst, and dryness in the nose and mouth. When the Stomach-Yin is deficient, there is often dryness in the mouth, severe thirst, a tendency to get hungry easily and constipation. When the Liver-Yin is deficient, there is often

dryness in the eyes, blurred vision, dizziness and tinnitus. When the Kidney-Yin is not sufficient, then dizziness, tinnitus, weakness in the back and legs, spermatorrhea, low-grade fever and warmth in the palms and soles of the feet are often present. If the Yin is deficient, patients have a thin and red tongue body without a coating, and a thready and rapid pulse.

25 What are the characteristics of the herbs that tonify the Yin?

The herbs that tonify the Yin have the following characteristics.

Sweet and cold

Sweetness has a tonifying and harmonizing ability, and Cold can clear Heat and protect the Yin. Sweet-cold herbs can generate the Yin and Body Fluids. Almost all the herbs that tonify the Yin are sweet and cold in nature.

Tonifying the thin-Yin or the thick-Yin

'Tonifying the thin-Yin' means tonifying the thin part of the Yin—that is, the Body Fluids. 'Tonifying the thick-Yin' means tonifying the Body Fluids, the Blood and the Essence. The former method is used for treating acute febrile disease, in which the Body Fluids are injured by Heat; it is also used in the process of some chronic diseases. The commonly used herbs are Bei Sha Shen (*Glehniae radix*), Mai Men Dong (*Ophiopogonis radix*), Nu Zhen Zi (*Ligustri lucidi fructus*), Han Lian Cao (*Ecliptae herba*) and Yu Zhu (*Polygonati odorati rhizoma*). The latter method is used in the late stage of febrile diseases or in the process of chronic diseases when the Liver-Blood and Kidney-Essence have also been injured. In these conditions, herbs that tonify the Blood and Essence, which are sweet and slightly warm in nature, are also used—for example, Shu Di Huang (*Rehmanniae radix praeparata*), Gou Qi Zi (*Lycii fructus*) and Hei Zhi Ma (*Sesami semen nigricum*). The sweet and cold herbs, which benefit the thick-Yin, are also used—for example, Bai Shao Yao (*Paeoniae radix lactiflora*), Shi Hu (*Dendrobii* caulis)**, Bai He (*Lilii bulbus*) and Tian Men Dong (*Asparagi radix*).

Rich and cloying in nature

All the herbs that tonify the Yin have the potential of staying in one place. The herbs that tonify the thick-Yin are rich and cloying. They should be used together with herbs that activate the Qi movement in order to avoid the side-effects to the Stomach and Spleen.

26 What are the differences in the function of tonifying the Yin between Tian Men Dong (*Asparagi radix*) and Mai Men Dong (*Ophiopogonis radix*)?

Tian Men Dong and Mai Men Dong are sweet, bitter and cold, and enter the Lung meridian. Both of them are able to nourish the Yin of the Lung and clear Heat. They both can be used for treating a dry cough and thirst. Since the Large Intestine and the Lung are externally–internally related, these two herbs can also be used for treating constipation caused by deficiency of the Body Fluids in the intestines.

Tian Men Dong is much colder and far more bitter than Mai Men Dong; therefore the action of nourishing the Yin and clearing Heat in the Lung is much stronger than that of Mai Men Dong. It is used for treating cough with thick sputum that is difficult to expectorate, and even hemoptysis. This herb also enters the Kidney meridian, so is able to nourish the Kidney-Yin as well, and can treat low-grade fever, warm palms and soles, and Wasting and Thirsty syndrome.

Mai Men Dong has the function of nourishing the Yin and clearing Heat in the Lung. Although it is weaker than Tian Men Dong, it is gentle and does not have a cloying nature. It is more suitable for mild cases of Yin deficiency and can also be used for a longer period of time without side-effects. Mai Men Dong does not enter the Kidney meridian, but the Heart and the Stomach meridians. It is an excellent herb for treating irritability, restlessness, insomnia and frequent sweating, which are caused by the Heart-Yin deficiency. It also treats severe thirst and a tendency to get hungry, which is caused by the Stomach-Yin deficiency. In the recovery period of a

febrile disease, since the Yin of the Lung, Heart and Stomach are all injured, Mai Men Dong is a better choice than Tian Men Dong.

27 Tian Men Dong (*Asparagi radix*), Mai Men Dong (*Ophiopogonis radix*), Bei Sha Shen (*Glehniae radix*), Bai He (*Lilii bulbus*) and Yu Zhu (*Polygonati odorati rhizoma*) are able to nourish the Lung-Yin and reduce Heat in the Upper Jiao. What are the differences between their actions?

All of these five herbs are sweet and cold in nature and enter the Lung meridian. They are able to nourish the Yin and clear Heat in the Lung. In clinical practice, they can be used together to increase the therapeutic effect. However, there are differences between their actions.

Tian Men Dong is the coldest one in the group; therefore its effect in clearing Heat and nourishing the Yin of the Lung is the strongest. It enters not only the Lung meridian, but also the Kidney meridian, and is especially useful in late stages of febrile diseases or some chronic diseases when the Lung-Yin and the Kidney-Yin are both injured. It treats not only dry cough with thick, scanty sputum and thirst, but also afternoon fever, warmth in the palms and soles of the feet, night sweating and coughing up of blood.

Mai Men Dong and Bei Sha Shen enter the Lung meridian, and their strength in nourishing the Yin of the Lung is the same. They also enter the Stomach meridian and can treat thirst, dry mouth and a poor appetite. They are very often used together in febrile disease or in the recovery period after febrile disease when the Yin has been injured by Heat. However, Mai Men Dong is bitter, so its action in reducing Heat is stronger than that of Bei Sha Shen. Moreover, it enters the Heart meridian, so if the patient suffers from restlessness, irritability and insomnia, which indicate Yin deficiency of the Heart, Mai Men Dong is more suitable than Bei Sha Shen. Mai Men Dong can gently tonify the Qi, so is used when Heat has consumed both the Yin and the Qi. In this situation, patients feel tired and have shortness of breath.

Bai He enters the Lung, Heart and Stomach meridians. Its effect in nourishing the Yin and clearing Heat is slightly weaker than that of Mai Men Dong. However, it also has a lubricating property and is able to regulate the Qi movement in the Upper Jiao. The strong point of this herb is that it can moisten the Lung-Yin and soothe the Lung-Qi. Since it also enters the Heart meridian, it is more suitable for situations in which the Heat injures the Yin and disturbs the Qi in the Upper Jiao. In this condition, patients suffer not only from a dry cough, coughing up of blood, and difficulty in expectorating scanty and thick sputum, but also from tight sensations in the chest, depression, grief and restless sleep, such as seen in the aftermath of febrile diseases and long-term emotional distress or stress.

Yu Zhu is sweet and neutral, moistens the Lung-Yin and reduces Dry-Heat. Its action is the weakest of this group, but it is gentle and does not have a cloying nature, so it can be used for a longer period of time. In addition, it can also be applied with herbs that release the Exterior where there is Yin deficiency in an Exterior syndrome; it can nourish the Yin but does not retain the exogenous pathogenic factors inside the body.

28 Shi Hu (*Dendrobii caulis*)**, Mai Men Dong (*Ophiopogonis radix*), Bei Sha Shen (*Glehniae radix*) and Yu Zhu (*Polygonati odorati rhizoma*) are able to nourish the Stomach-Yin and reduce Heat. What are the differences between their actions?

All of these four herbs are sweet and cold, enter the Stomach meridian and are able to nourish the Yin and reduce Heat. They are often used for treating thirst, heartburn and constipation.

Shi Hu is the coldest of the group and it is the strongest for nourishing the Stomach-Yin and reducing Heat. It is also slightly salty and enters the Kidney meridian, so is more suitable for treating

severe thirst, heartburn and nausea, such as seen in Wasting and Thirsty syndrome and in the aftermath of a febrile disease when the Stomach-Yin and the Kidney-Yin are both impaired. This herb is very cold and cloying, however, and easily disturbs the function of the Stomach and Spleen; therefore it should not be used where there is weakness of the Spleen or accumulation of Dampness in the Middle Jiao. Neither should it be used in the primary stage of febrile diseases because it may retain the exogenous pathogenic factor inside the body. Also, the dosage should be controlled carefully, as a large dosage of Shi Hu may inhibit the functions of the Heart and Lungs.

Mai Men Dong is slightly weaker than Shi Hu in its action of nourishing the Stomach-Yin, but it enters the Heart and the Lung meridians. It is therefore more suitable for treating syndromes of Heat spreading in the Upper Jiao and Middle Jiao.

Bei Sha Shen is weaker than Mai Men Dong in its action of nourishing the Yin and reducing Fire in the Stomach, so it is often combined with Mai Men Dong to treat thirst, heartburn, nausea and constipation.

Yu Zhu is the weakest of the group in its action, but it is very gentle and without any cloying side-effect. It can therefore be used for a long period of time for Stomach-Yin deficiency in a chronic disease or in the recovery period of febrile diseases. It can also be used in the primary stage of febrile disease if there is a slight Stomach-Yin deficiency.

29 Tian Men Dong (*Asparagi radix*), Shi Hu (*Dendrobii caulis*)**, Nu Zhen Zi (*Ligustri lucidi fructus*), Han Lian Cao (*Ecliptae herba*), Sheng Di Huang (*Rehmanniae radix*) and Xuan Shen (*Scrophulariae radix*) are able to nourish the Kidney-Yin. What are the differences between their actions?

These six herbs enter the Kidney meridian, and have the function of nourishing the Kidney-Yin and reducing Empty-Heat, but there are differences between their actions.

Tian Men Dong and Shi Hu are the coldest of the six herbs. They have the strongest effect in nourishing the Yin of the Kidney and so are used for severe Yin deficiency syndromes in chronic and febrile disease. Tian Men Dong is often used in Wasting and Thirsty syndrome and Shi Hu is especially effective for treating disorders of the eyes and vision caused by Kidney-Yin deficiency. However, they are very cold and have a cloying nature, so easily injure the function of the Spleen and Stomach; therefore they should not be used in patients with weakness of the Spleen and Stomach or accumulation of Dampness in the Middle Jiao. These two herbs can also retain the exogenous pathogenic factors within the body, so they should also not be used in the primary stage of febrile diseases.

Nu Zhen Zi and Han Lian Cao are sweet and cold, and enter the Liver and Kidney meridians. They can nourish the Yin without any cloying side-effects. They are suitable for treating dizziness, tinnitus, blurred vision, weakness in the back and knees and premature gray hair due to Liver-Yin and Kidney-Yin deficiency. Since they are not cloying in nature, and have gentle and steady actions, they can be used for a long period of time in chronic disease. Moreover, these two herbs are also suitable in conditions where the Blood is deficient and there is slight Heat in the Blood.

Comparing the two herbs, Nu Zhen Zi has a stronger action of nourishing the Yin than Han Lian Cao, and Han Lian Cao is more effective at reducing Heat than Nu Zhen Zi. They are often used together to enhance the therapeutic effect of each other.

Unlike the other four herbs, Sheng Di Huang and Xuan Shen not only tonify the Yin of the Kidney, but also cool the Blood. They are often used in bleeding conditions where Heat has injured the Yin and Blood. Compared with Xuan Shen, Sheng Di Huang has a stronger action in nourishing the Yin; Xuan Shen is bitter, salty and cold, and is more effective for reducing Heat and relieving Heat-toxin.

30 Shu Di Huang (*Rehmanniae radix praeparata*), He Shou Wu (*Polygoni multiflori radix*) and Gou Qi Zi (*Lycii fructus*) are called in some books 'the herbs that tonify the Kidney-Yin'. What are the differences of these herbs from the herbs that nourish the Yin discussed above?

These three herbs are sweet and warm, and they enter the Kidney and Liver meridians. They can tonify the Kidney-Essence and Liver-Blood. Since the Essence and Blood are the substantial parts of the body and belong to the Yin, they are also often called 'the herbs that tonify Yin'. In fact, they should be called 'the herbs that tonify the thick-Yin'. The herbs that nourish the Yin and reduce Heat that have been discussed above are the herbs that nourish the Body Fluids, and these should be called 'the herbs that nourish the thin-Yin' in order to avoid misunderstanding. In practice, however, because the syndrome of deficiency of the Kidney-Essence and Liver-Blood is related to the development of deficiency of Body Fluids in the internal organs, in a severe Yin deficient syndrome these two groups of herbs are often used together.

31 What are the indications for the herbs that tonify the Yang?

The herbs that tonify the Yang are able to treat the syndrome of Yang deficiency. Although all the internal organs contain Yin and Yang aspects and the syndrome of Yang deficiency may occur in all those organs, the Kidney-Yang is considered to be the root of the Yang of the internal organs. Therefore, the herbs that tonify the Yang especially focus on tonifying the Kidney-Yang.

The syndrome of Kidney-Yang deficiency often occurs in chronic disease and develops from Qi, Blood and Yin deficiency. Elderly people and people with a poor constitution stand more chance of developing this syndrome.

The main manifestations of Kidney-Yang deficiency are cold and soreness in the back, intolerance of cold, frequent urination, infertility, amenorrhea, irregular menstruation, impotence, enuresis, retardation in children and dementia in elderly people. If the Kidney-Yang is too weak to warm the Spleen-Yang, symptoms such as diarrhea and poor digestion may occur. If the Kidney-Yang is not able to warm the Heart-Yang and the Lung-Qi, patients may suffer from palpitations, restlessness, shortness of breath and edema. If the Kidney-Yang is too weak to house the will, one will lose one's goal in life, and depression and fear are often present. Patients with Yang deficiency often have a pale or purple tongue body with a white and moist coating and a very deep, slow and weak pulse.

32 What are the characteristics of the herbs that tonify the Yang?

The herbs that tonify the Yang often have the following characteristics.

Sweet and warm

Sweetness has a tonifying and harmonizing nature, and gentle warmth promotes the growth of Yang. Therefore, sweet-warm herbs are able to tonify the Yang and strengthen the Essence and Qi of the body. Almost all the herbs that tonify the Yang are sweet and warm.

Entering the Kidney and Spleen meridians

Most of the herbs that tonify the Yang enter the Kidney meridian because the Kidney-Yang is the root of the Yang of the other organs. Some herbs that tonify the Kidney also enter the Spleen meridian and tonify the Spleen-Yang—examples are Bu Gu Zhi (*Psoraleae fructus*) and Yi Zhi Ren (*Alpiniae oxyphyllae fructus*). Since the Spleen-Yang has the function of accelerating the transformation of food into Essence, Qi and Blood, these herbs are particularly effective for treating the syndrome of deficiency of the Kidney-Yang and Spleen-Yang.

Tonifying the Kidney-Yang as well as tonifying the Kidney-Essence and Liver-Blood

Because the Kidney-Yang is generated from the Kidney-Essence, the herbs that tonify the Kidney-Yang are based on their ability to tonify the Kidney-Essence. Almost all the herbs that tonify the Kidney-Yang can tonify the Kidney-Essence. Furthermore, since Kidney-Essence, Liver-Yin and Liver-Blood can change into each other, many herbs that tonify the Kidney-Yang also enter the Liver meridian and nourish the Liver-Yin and Blood—examples are Xian Ling Pi (*Epimedii herba*), Ba Ji Tian (*Morindae radix*), Du Zhong (*Eucomniae cortex*), Gou Ji (*Cibotii rhizoma*)**, Xu Duan (*Dipsaci radix*) and Tu Si Zi (*Cuscutae semen*).

33 What are the differences between warming the Yang and tonifying the Yang?

These are two methods of treatment. 'Warming the Yang' focuses on improving the function of the Yang—that is, to warm the Yang and spread it in order to activate its function of expelling Cold. The herbs that warm the Yang are all pungent and warm in nature, and their action is quick and strong—examples are Fu Zi (*Aconiti radix lateralis preparata*)*, Gan Jiang (*Zingiberis rhizoma*) and Wu Zhu Yu (*Evodiae fructus*). They are also called 'the herbs that warm the Interior and expel Cold'. Because of their hot and pungent nature, which may consume the Yin and further injure the Yang, they should not be used for too long or in large dosage.

'Tonifying the Yang' focuses on improving the quality and increasing the quantity of the Yang in order to strengthen its function. These herbs have a sweet and warm nature, and their action in expelling Cold is not quick, but steady and constant. The improvement of the Yang can be seen from the improved functioning of the internal organs, symptoms and constitutions. Herbs that are often used for this purpose are Ba Ji Tian (*Morindae radix*), Xian Ling Pi (*Epimedii herba*) and Tu Si Zi (*Cuscutae semen*).

34 What are the differences in warming and tonifying the Kidney-Yang between Xian Mao (*Curculinginis rhizoma*), Ba Ji Tian (*Morindae radix*) and Xian Ling Pi (*Epimedii herba*)?

These three herbs are pungent and warm. They all enter the Kidney meridian and are able to tonify the Kidney-Yang, strengthen the bones and tendons, and expel Wind, Dampness and Cold. They are often used for treating syndromes of Kidney-Yang deficiency, which can easily be found in menopausal syndrome, infertility, menstrual disorders, impotence and diseases in elderly people. They can also be used for treating Bi syndrome where there is Kidney-Yang deficiency, such as in rheumatic fever, rheumatoid arthritis and osteoarthritis.

Xian Mao is the most pungent and warm of the three herbs. It has a very strong action in expelling Cold and warming the Kidney-Yang. It is especially effective for treating cold limbs, intolerance of cold, cold sensations in the back and in the knees and impotence. Comparing Xian Mao with the other two herbs, it has little function in tonifying the Kidney-Yang. Since it is very pungent and warm, which may injure the Kidney-Yin, and is poisonous too, Xian Mao is used for only a short period of time. In small dosage it can be used in a group of herbs that tonify the Yang for a longer period of time.

Ba Ji Tian is sweet and slightly warm. It is an excellent herb for tonifying the Kidney-Yang because its warm-sweet nature will not bring about harsh, drying or cloying side-effects. Comparing Ba Ji Tian with the other two herbs, it is the best one for tonifying the Kidney-Yang and treating weakness of the legs and knees, chronic Bi syndrome and sexual disorders.

Xian Ling Pi can also tonify the Kidney-Yang and the action is less strong than that of Ba Ji Tian, but stronger than that of Xian Mao. It can also expel Cold and warm the Interior, and in this respect its function is less strong than that of Xian Mao but stronger than that of Ba Ji Tian. As the characteristic of this herb is to expel Wind-Dampness, it can treat numbness of the limbs. It can also stop coughing and relieve shortness of breath caused by Kidney-Yang deficiency.

35 What are the differences in the function of tonifying the Kidney and strengthening the bones between Du Zhong (*Eucomniae cortex*), Xu Duan (*Dipsaci radix*), Gou Ji (*Cibotii rhizoma*)** and Sang Ji Sheng (*Taxilli herba*)?

All of these four herbs enter the Liver and Kidney meridians. They have the function of tonifying the Kidney and Liver, and strengthening the bones and tendons. They are used for treating syndromes of Kidney and Liver deficiency, in which patients suffer from a weak, stiff and painful back and knees, and difficulty with walking for a long distance or standing for a long time. These herbs can be used alone or together in these situations.

Du Zhong has the strongest action in tonifying the Kidney of the four herbs. It also has a gentle action in regulating the Qi and Blood. It is often used for Kidney deficiency with symptoms of lower back pain and weakness, such as seen in chronic nephritis, chronic strain of the back and rheumatoid arthritis. It can also be used for prevention of miscarriage, bleeding or a weak and painful back during pregnancy caused by weakness of the Kidney.

Xu Duan has a similar function to that of Du Zhong, but it is weaker in tonifying the Kidney and stronger in regulating the Blood circulation. In Chinese, 'Xu' means 'connect' and 'Duan' means 'broken'. So it is very effective for strengthening the bones and tendons, and is often used for treating pain and stiffness in trauma, strain, wound and fracture, just as its name suggests. Like Du Zhong, it can also strengthen the Kidney and the back and prevent miscarriage.

Gou Ji is the warmest of the four herbs and can tonify the Kidney and Liver. Its function is similar to that of Xu Duan, but it is stronger in expelling Wind, Dampness and Cold, and regulating the Qi and Blood. It is used for pain and stiffness of the joints and muscles in chronic Bi syndrome. It can also warm and stabilize the Kidney-Qi and treat frequent urination. Unlike Du Zhong and Xu Duan, it has no function in preventing miscarriage.

Sang Ji Sheng is bitter, sweet and neutral. It is the weakest of the four herbs for tonifying the Kidney and Liver, and strengthening the bones and tendons. However, it can tonify the Blood, expel Wind and Dampness and is suitable for treating numbness of the muscles and stiffness of tendons caused by Blood deficiency and invasion of Wind and Dampness. Like Du Zhong and Xu Duan, it can strengthen the back and prevent miscarriage.

36 What are the differences in the function of tonifying the Kidney-Yang between Bu Gu Zhi (*Psoraleae fructus*), Tu Si Zi (*Cuscutae semen*), Sha Yuan Zi (*Astragali complanati semen*) and Rou Cong Rong (*Cistanchis herba*)**?

All of these four herbs enter the Kidney meridian and have the function of tonifying the Kidney-Yang. They are used for treating tinnitus, dizziness, cold and weakness in the back and knees, frequent urination, urinary incontinence, impotence and spermatorrhea caused by Kidney-Yang deficiency.

Bu Gu Zhi is very warm and pungent. It has a strong action in warming the Kidney-Yang and dispersing Cold. It can treat the symptoms mentioned above and particularly when the Cold is obvious. It is very often used for diarrhea due to Kidney-Yang deficiency. It is also able to warm the Fire of the Gate of Vitality (*Ming Men*) and grasp the Lung-Qi; therefore it treats shortness of breath caused by deficiencies of both the Lung and Kidney.

Tu Si Zi has the function of tonifying the Kidney and also stopping diarrhea. Unlike Bu Gu Zhi, it is not warm and pungent, but sweet and neutral. It is not warm, dry or cloying, so is excellent for tonifying either the Kidney-Yin or the Kidney-Yang. It is also often used for treating Kidney-Essence deficiency, which results in weakness of the back and knees, blurred vision and a poor memory. In addition, it has the ability to strengthen and stabilize the Kidney-Essence; therefore it is used for treating infertility, habitual miscarriage, copious leukorrhea and nocturnal emission.

Sha Yuan Zi has a similar function to Tu Si Zi but is warmer and stronger in stabilizing the Kidney-Essence. It can tonify the Kidney-Essence and Yang, so is used for both Kidney-Essence and Kidney-Yang deficiency. Moreover, it can brighten the eyes, and so is effective for treating blurred vision. Comparing it with Tu Si Zi, it has no function in stopping diarrhea, but can stabilize the Essence and treat infertility, habitual miscarriage and nocturnal emission.

In Chinese, 'Cong Rong' means 'calm', 'unhurried'. As described in the name, Rou Cong Rong is sweet and warm, and it warms the Kidney without the potential of drying, nourishes the Essence without any cloying property, and tonifies the body without a harsh action. It can strengthen the Kidney-Yang and Essence; therefore it treats weakness of the Bones and tendons. It can also moisten the intestines and treat constipation when the Yang is too weak to transport the feces and the Yin is too weak to moisten the intestines.

References

Li Dong Yuan 1976, First published in 1249 Discussion on the Spleen and Stomach (Pi Wei Lun). People's Health Publishing House, Beijing

Zhang Zhong Jing 1963 Discussion on the febrile diseases (Shang Han Lun). People's Medical Publishing House, Beijing

Comparisons of strength and temperature in herbs that tonify

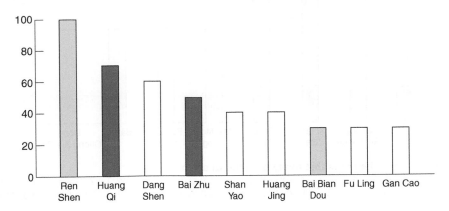

Fig. 14.1 • Comparison of the herbs that tonify the Qi.
Ren Shen (*Ginseng radix*), Huang Qi (*Astragali radix*), Dang Shen (*Codonopsis radix*), Bai Zhu (*Atractylodis macrocephalae rhizoma*), Shan Yao (*Dioscoreae rhizoma*), Huang Jing (*Polygonati rhizoma*), Bai Bian Dou (*Dolichoris lablab semen*), Fu Ling (*Poria*), Gan Cao (*Glycyrrhizae radix*).

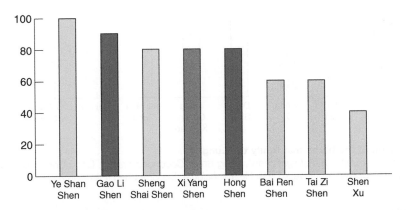

Fig. 14.2 • Comparison of the different Ren Shen products.
Ye Shan Shen (wild mountain *Ginseng radix*), Gao Li Shen (Korean *Ginseng radix*), Sheng Shai Shen (raw dried *Ginseng radix*), Xi Yang Shen (*Panacis quinquefolii radix*), Hong Shen (red *Ginseng radix*), Bai Ren Shen (white *Ginseng radix*), Tai Zi Shen (*Pseudostellariae radix*), Shen Xu (*Ginseng fibrosa*).

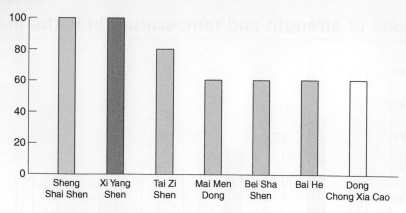

Fig. 14.3 • Comparison of the herbs that tonify both the Qi and Yin.
Sheng Shai Shen (raw dried *Ginseng radix*), Xi Yang Shen (*Panacis quinquefolii radix*), Tai Zi Shen (*Pseudostellariae radix*), Mai Men Dong (*Ophiopogonis radix*), Bei Sha Shen (*Glehniae radix*), Bai He (*Lilii bulbus*), Dong Chong Xia Cao (*Cordyceps sinensis*).

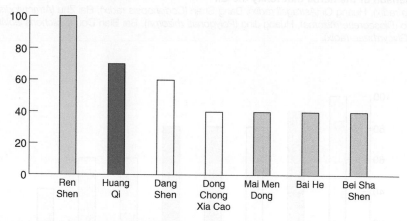

Fig. 14.4 • Comparison of the herbs that tonify the Lung-Qi.
Ren Shen (*Ginseng radix*), Huang Qi (*Astragali radix*), Dang Shen (*Codonopsis radix*), Dong Chong Xia Cao (*Cordyceps sinensis*), Mai Men Dong (*Ophiopogonis radix*), Bai He (*Lilii bulbus*), Bei Sha Shen (*Glehniae radix*).

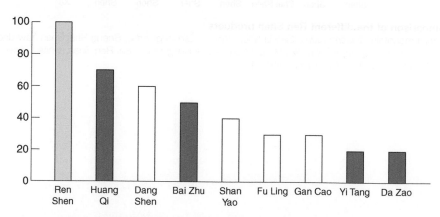

Fig. 14.5 • Comparison of the herbs that tonify the Spleen-Qi.
Ren Shen (*Ginseng radix*), Huang Qi (*Astragali radix*), Dang Shen (*Codonopsis radix*), Bai Zhu (*Atractylodis macrocephalae rhizoma*), Shan Yao (*Dioscoreae rhizoma*), Fu Ling (*Poria*), Gan Cao (*Glycyrrhizae radix*), Yi Tang (*Maltose*), Da Zao (*Jujubae fructus*).

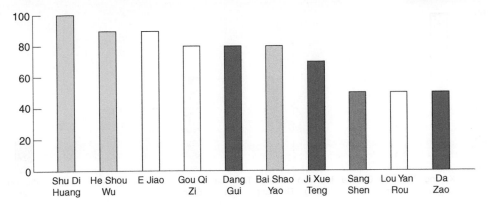

Fig. 14.6 • Comparison of the herbs that tonify the Blood.
Shu Di Huang (*Rehmanniae radix praeparata*), He Shou Wu (*Polygoni multiflori radix*), E Jiao (*Asini corii colla*), Gou Qi Zi (*Lycii fructus*), Dang Gui (*Angelicae sinensis radix*), Bai Shao Yao (*Paeoniae radix lactiflora*), Ji Xue Teng (*Spatholobi caulis et radix*), Sang Shen (*Mori fructus*), Long Yan Rou (*Longanae arillus*), Da Zao (*Jujubae fructus*).

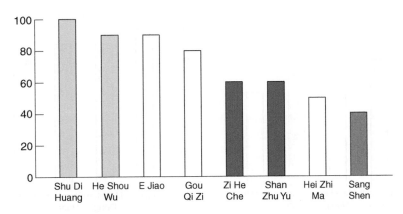

Fig. 14.7 • Comparison of the herbs that tonify the Kidney-Essence and the Liver-Blood.
Shu Di Huang (*Rehmanniae radix praeparata*), He Shou Wu (*Polygoni multiflori radix*), E Jiao (*Asini corii colla*), Gou Qi Zi (*Lycii fructus*), Zi He Che (*Placenta hominis*), Shan Zhu Yu (*Corni fructus*), Hei Zhi Ma (*Sesami semen nigricum*), Sang Shen (*Mori fructus*).

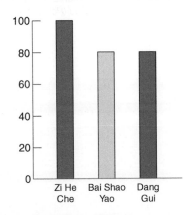

Fig. 14.8 • Comparison of the herbs that tonify the Liver-Blood.
Zi He Che (*Placenta hominis*), Bai Shao Yao (*Paeoniae radix lactiflora*), Dang Gui (*Angelicae sinensis radix*).

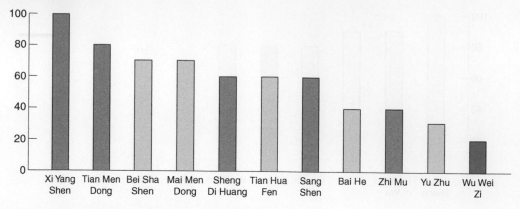

Fig. 14.9 • Comparison of the herbs that nourish the Lung-Yin.
Xi Yang Shen (*Panacis quinquefolii radix*), Tian Men Dong (*Asparagi radix*), Bei Sha Shen (*Glehniae radix*), Mai Men Dong (*Ophiopogonis radix*), Sheng Di Huang (*Rehmanniae radix*), Tian Hua Fen (*Trichosanthis radix*), Sang Shen (*Mori fructus*), Bai He (*Lilii bulbus*), Zhi Mu (*Anemarrhenae rhizoma*), Yu Zhu (*Polygonati odorati rhizoma*), Wu Wei Zi (*Schisandrae fructus*).

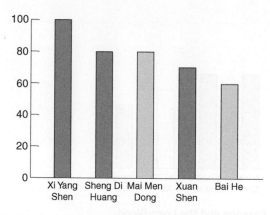

Fig. 14.10 • Comparison of the herbs that nourish the Heart-Yin.
Xi Yang Shen (*Panacis quinquefolii radix*), Sheng Di Huang (*Rehmanniae radix*), Mai Men Dong (*Ophiopogonis radix*), Xuan Shen (*Scrophulariae radix*), Bai He (*Lilii bulbus*).

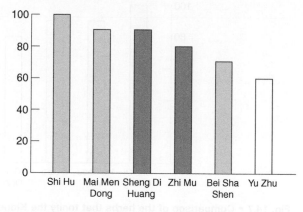

Fig. 14.11 • Comparison of the herbs that nourish the Stomach-Yin.
Shi Hu (*Dendrobii caulis*)**, Mai Men Dong (*Ophiopogonis radix*), Sheng Di Huang (*Rehmanniae radix*), Zhi Mu (*Anemarrhenae rhizoma*), Bei Sha Shen (*Glehniae radix*), Yu Zhu (*Polygonati odorati rhizoma*).

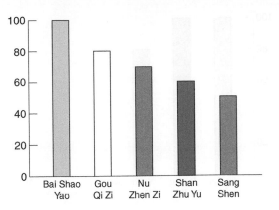

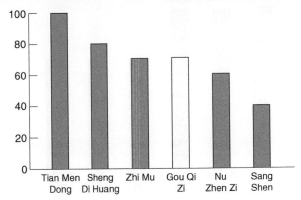

Fig. 14.12 • Comparison of the herbs that nourish the Liver-Yin.
Bai Shao Yao (*Paeoniae radix lactiflora*), Gou Qi Zi (*Lycii fructus*), Nu Zhen Zi (*Ligustri lucidi fructus*), Shan Zhu Yu (*Corni fructus*), Sang Shen (*Mori fructus*).

Fig. 14.13 • Comparison of the herbs that nourish the Kidney-Yin.
Tian Men Dong (*Asparagi radix*), Sheng Di Huang (*Rehmanniae radix*), Zhi Mu (*Anemarrhenae rhizoma*), Gou Qi Zi (*Lycii fructus*), Nu Zhen Zi (*Ligustri lucidi fructus*), Sang Shen (*Mori fructus*).

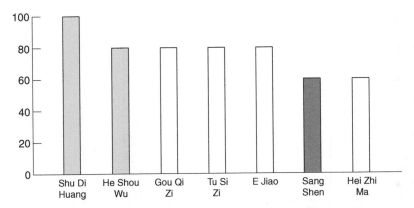

Fig. 14.14 • Comparison of the herbs that tonify the Kidney-Yin and the Kidney-Essence.
Shu Di Huang (*Rehmanniae radix praeparata*), He Shou Wu (*Polygoni multiflori radix*), Gou Qi Zi (*Lycii fructus*), Tu Si Zi (*Cuscutae semen*), E Jiao (*Asini corii colla*), Sang Shen (*Mori fructus*), Hei Zhi Ma (*Sesami semen nigricum*).

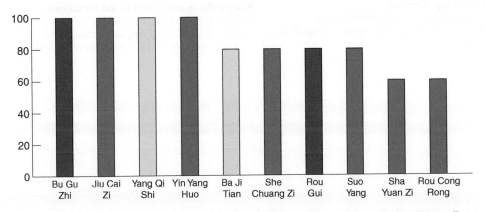

Fig. 14.15 • Comparison of the herbs that strengthen the Kidney-Yang and tonify the Kidney-Essence.
Bu Gu Zhi (*Psoraleae fructus*), Jiu Cai Zi (*Allii tuberosi semen*), Yang Qi Shi (*Actinolitum*), Yin Yang Huo (*Epimedii herba*), Ba Ji Tian (*Morindae radix*), She Chuang Zi (*Cnidii fructus*), Rou Gui (*Cinnamomi cassiae cortex*), Suo Yang (*Cynomorii caulis*), Sha Yuan Zi (*Astragali complanati semen*), Rou Cong Rong (*Cistanchis herba*)**.

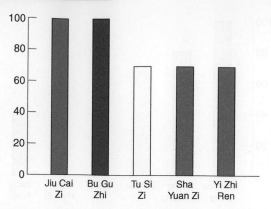

Fig. 14.16 • Comparison of the herbs that strengthen the Kidney-Yang, tonify and stabilize the Kidney-Essence.
Jiu Cai Zi (*Allii tuberosi semen*), Bu Gu Zhi (*Psoraleae fructus*), Tu Si Zi (*Cuscutae semen*), Sha Yuan Zi (*Astragali complanati semen*), Yi Zhi Ren (*Alpiniae oxyphyllae fructus*).

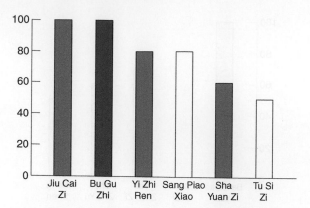

Fig. 14.17 • Comparison of the herbs that tonify the Kidney and stabilize the function of the Bladder.
Jiu Cai Zi (*Allii tuberosi semen*), Bu Gu Zhi (*Psoraleae fructus*), Yi Zhi Ren (*Alpiniae oxyphyllae fructus*), Sang Piao Xiao (*Mantidis oötheca*), Sha Yuan Zi (*Astragali complanati semen*), Tu Si Zi (*Cuscutae semen*).

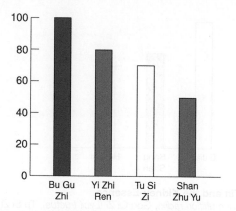

Fig. 14.18 • Comparison of the herbs that tonify the Kidney-Yang and stop diarrhea.
Bu Gu Zhi (*Psoraleae fructus*), Yi Zhi Ren (*Alpiniae oxyphyllae fructus*), Tu Si Zi (*Cuscutae semen*), Shan Zhu Yu (*Corni fructus*).

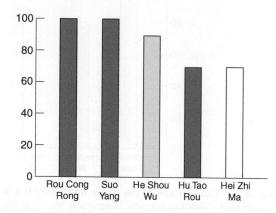

Fig. 14.19 • Comparison of the herbs that tonify the Kidney-Yang and moisten the intestines.
Rou Cong Rong (*Cistanchis herba*)**, Suo Yang (*Cynomorii caulis*), He Shou Wu (*Polygoni multiflori radix*), Hu Tao Rou (*Juglandis semen*), Hei Zhi Ma (*Sesami semen nigricum*).

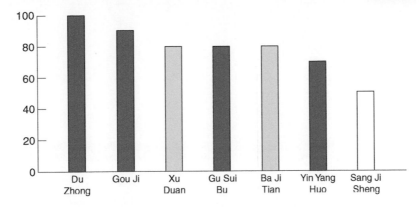

Fig. 14.20 • Comparison of the herbs that tonify the Kidney and strengthen the bones.
Du Zhong (*Eucomniae cortex*), Gou Ji (*Cibotii rhizoma*)**, Xu Duan (*Dipsaci radix*), Gu Sui Bu (*Drynariae rhizoma*), Ba Ji Tian (*Morindae radix*), Yin Yang Huo (*Epimedii herba*), Sang Ji Sheng (*Taxilli herba*).

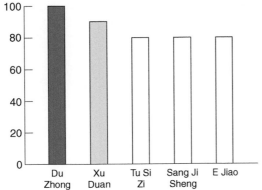

Fig. 14.21 • Comparison of the herbs that tonify the Kidney and calm the fetus.
Du Zhong (*Eucomniae cortex*), Xu Duan (*Dipsaci radix*), Tu Si Zi (*Cuscutae semen*), Sang Ji Sheng (*Taxilli herba*), E Jiao (*Asini corii colla*).

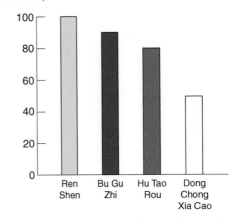

Fig. 14.22 • Comparison of the herbs that tonify the Kidney-Qi and stabilize the Lung-Qi.
Ren Shen (*Ginseng radix*), Bu Gu Zhi (*Psoraleae fructus*), Hu Tao Rou (*Juglandis semen*), Dong Chong Xia Cao (*Cordyceps sinensis*).

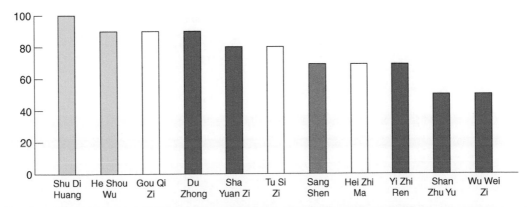

Fig. 14.23 • Comparison of the herbs that tonify the Kidney and improve the memory.
Shu Di Huang (*Rehmanniae radix praeparata*), He Shou Wu (*Polygoni multiflori radix*), Gou Qi Zi (*Lycii fructus*), Du Zhong (*Eucomniae cortex*), Sha Yuan Zi (*Astragali complanati semen*), Tu Si Zi (*Cuscutae semen*), Sang Shen (*Mori fructus*), Hei Zhi Ma (*Sesami semen nigricum*), Yi Zhi Ren (*Alpiniae oxyphyllae fructus*), Shan Zhu Yu (*Corni fructus*), Wu Wei Zi (*Schisandrae fructus*).

Chapter Fifteen

15

Astringent herbs

收涩药

1 What are the indications for and characteristics of the astringent herbs?

The astringent herbs have the function of stabilizing the Essence, Body Fluids and Qi. They treat abnormal discharge of the essential substances of the body through excessive sweating, vomiting, urination, spermatorrhea and diarrhea. They can also treat abnormal consumption of the Qi from excessive coughing, shortness of breath, asthma and palpitations. They are sometimes used to stabilize the structure of organs and keep them from slipping from their proper positions in the condition of Qi deficiency, such as seen in prolapse of the rectum or uterus.

The cause of abnormal discharge of the essential substances is Qi deficiency. When the internal organs are very weak, the Qi is not strong enough to keep the Essence and Body Fluids in the body and to keep the organ in its proper place and position, so this disorder occurs. Elderly people and those with chronic disease or a very weak constitution are more likely to have this disorder. The herbs that stabilize abnormal discharge of the essential substances focus on treating the manifestations; however, they have little influence on the organ itself and do not treat the cause, so they should be used together with herbs that treat the causes.

Most of the herbs that stabilize the Qi, Essence and Body Fluids are sour or astringent. Sourness has a contracting ability and an inwards-moving tendency. Herbs with an astringent property are able to prevent or reverse the abnormal leakage of the Qi, Essence and Body Fluids. Of these herbs, some particularly stabilize the Lung-Qi; others are effective at stabilizing the Heart-Qi or the Kidney-Essence, or binding up the intestines.

2 What precautions should be observed in the use of astringent herbs?

In clinical practice, the astringent herbs should be used with caution. First of all, as mentioned above, since these herbs treat only the manifestations, they should be combined with herbs that treat the causes of the disorders. To treat chronic conditions, astringent herbs should be used with herbs that tonify the Qi in order to treat the abnormal discharge completely. In acute conditions—such as in excessive sweating and diarrhea—the astringent herbs can be used alone; however, when the condition is stabilized the appropriate tonifying herbs should then be used immediately.

Secondly, astringent herbs should be used only in Deficiency syndromes. They are prohibited for use in Excess syndromes or syndromes in which Deficiency and Excess coexist—for instance, where there is Dampness, Phlegm and Heat. This is because these herbs are able to stabilize the Essence and Body Fluids, so they can also retain pathogenic factors within the body.

There are many factors that can cause abnormal discharge of the Body Fluids and Essence, therefore correct differentiation of the syndrome is required.

The astringent herbs are prohibited for use in the following syndromes: diarrhea caused by Damp-Heat in the intestines, excessive urination or spermatorrhea caused by Damp-Heat in the Lower Jiao, shortness of breath due to accumulation of Phlegm, or excessive sweating due to Excessive- or Deficient-Heat in the body.

3 Which herbs can stabilize the Lung-Qi and Lung-Yin and how should one prescribe them in clinical practice?

The commonly used herbs that particularly stabilize the Lung-Qi are Wu Wei Zi (*Schisandrae fructus*), Wu Mei (*Mume fructus*), He Zi (*Chebulae fructus*) and Bai Guo (*Ginkgo semen*). The herbs that stabilize the Lung-Qi can be used to relieve thirst and shortness of breath, and are used in the treatment of asthma, pulmonary pneumonia, pulmonary emphysema, acute and chronic bronchitis, cough and hyperventilation.

There are herbs that can especially stabilize the Exterior, which is governed by the Lung, and stop sweating. These are Ma Huang Gen (*Ephedrae radix*)* and Nuo Dao Gen Xu (*Oryzae glutinosae radix et rhizoma*).

If there is Lung-Qi deficiency, Ren Shen (*Ginseng radix*), Mai Men Dong (*Ophiopogonis radix*), Bei Sha Shen (*Glehniae radix*) and Nan Sha Shen (*Adenophorae radix*) are often used as well to tonify the Qi and nourish the Yin.

If there is Liver-Qi stagnation at the same time, Chai Hu (*Bupleuri radix*), Zhi Ke (*Aurantii fructus*) and Xiang Fu (*Cyperi rhizoma*) are often added.

Herbs that direct the Lung-Qi to descend and transform Phlegm should be added to ensure that the astringent herbs do not obstruct the Lung-Qi and retain the Phlegm—examples are Qian Hu (*Peucedani radix*) and Pi Pa Ye (*Eriobotryae folium*).

4 Which herbs can stabilize the Heart-Qi and how should one prescribe them in clinical practice?

The herbs that are particularly effective for stabilizing the Heart-Qi are Wu Wei Zi (*Schisandrae fructus*), Fu Xiao Mai (*Tritici fructus germinatus*), Mu Li (*Ostrea concha*) and Long Gu (*Mastodi fossilium ossis*). These herbs are used to treat palpitations, restlessness, spontaneous sweating, night sweats and insomnia. In clinical practice, they are used in the treatment of arrhythmia, tachycardia, hyperventilation and insomnia.

Of these herbs, Mu Li is particularly effective for treating night sweats, whereas Fu Xiao Mai and Long Gu can treat both night sweating and spontaneous sweating.

If there is Qi deficiency, Huang Qi (*Astragali radix*) should be added to strengthen the action of stabilizing the Exterior and stopping spontaneous sweating.

In the syndrome of Heart-Qi deficiency, the astringent herbs should be prescribed together with Dang Shen (*Codonopsis radix*), Suan Zao Ren (*Ziziphi spinosae semen*) and Mai Men Dong to nourish the Yin and Blood of the Heart and calm the Mind.

5 Which herbs can bind up the intestines and stop diarrhea and how should one prescribe them in clinical practice?

The herbs that bind up the intestines and stop diarrhea are Wu Mei (*Mume fructus*), Wu Bei Zi (*Chinensis galla*), Ying Su Ke (*Papaveris somniferi pericarpium*), Qian Shi (*Euryalis semen*), Rou Dou Kou (*Myristicae semen*), He Zi (*Chebulae fructus*), Chi Shi Zhi (*Halloysitum rubrum*), Lian Zi (*Nelumbinis semen*) and Jin Ying Zi (*Rosae laevigatae fructus*).

They are used to treat chronic diarrhea and heavy diarrhea, from which the body becomes very weak. Poor appetite, tiredness, cold limbs and shortness of breath are generally present too. In clinical practice, they are used in the treatment of colitis, chronic enteritis, dysentery and allergy if there are no Excess pathogenic factors.

If there is Spleen-Qi deficiency, Huang Qi (*Astragali radix*), Bai Zhu (*Atractylodis macrocephalae rhizoma*), Fu Ling (*Poria*) and Bai Bian Dou (*Dolichoris lablab semen*) can be used simultaneously. If there is Spleen-Yang deficiency, Gan Jiang (*Zingiberis rhizoma*) can be added in with the herbs that tonify the Spleen-Qi.

6 Which herbs can stabilize the Bladder and treat frequent urination and incontinence?

The substances that are particularly effective for stabilizing the Bladder are Qian Shi (*Euryalis semen*), Jin Ying Zi (*Rosae laevigatae fructus*), Sang Piao Xiao (*Mantidis oötheca*), Shan Zhu Yu (*Corni fructus*) and Yi Zhi Ren (*Alpiniae oxyphyllae fructus*).

These substances are used to stop frequent micturition, excessive production of urine, incontinence of urine and enuresis in Kidney-Qi deficiency. In clinical practice, these herbs are often used together with herbs that tonify the Kidney-Qi and Kidney-Yang—for instance, Ren Shen (*Ginseng radix*) and Tu Si Zi (*Cuscutae semen*).

7 Which herbs can stabilize the Kidney-Essence and how should one prescribe them in clinical practice?

The substances that particularly stabilize the Kidney-Essence are Shan Zhu Yu (*Corni fructus*), Wu Wei Zi (*Schisandrae fructus*) and Wu Zei Gu (*Sepiae seu sepiellae os*), Qian Shi (*Euryalis semen*), Fu Pen Zi (*Rubi fructus*), Lian Zi (*Nelumbinis semen*) and Lian Xu (*Nelumbinis stamen*).

These herbs are used in the treatment of frequent night urination, enuresis, impotence, spermatorrhea and premature ejaculation in Kidney-Yang or Kidney-Qi deficiency. They can be used together with herbs that tonify the Kidney-Yang and Kidney-Qi such as Sha Yuan Zi (*Astragali complanati semen*), Tu Si Zi (*Cuscutae semen*), Rou Gui (*Cinnamomi cassiae cortex*) and Ren Shen (*Ginseng radix*).

Comparisons of strength and temperature in astringent herbs

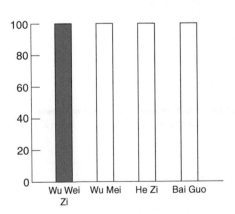

Fig. 15.1 • Comparison of the herbs that stabilize the Lung-Qi.
Wu Wei Zi (*Schisandrae fructus*), Wu Mei (*Mume fructus*), He Zi (*Chebulae fructus*), Bai Guo (*Ginkgo semen*).

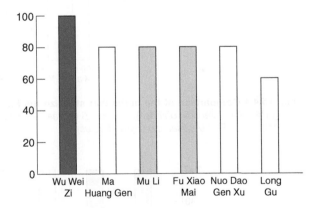

Fig. 15.2 • Comparison of the herbs that stop sweating.
Wu Wei Zi (*Schisandrae fructus*), Ma Huang Gen (*Ephedrae radix*)*, Mu Li (*Ostrea concha*), Fu Xiao Mai (*Tritici fructus germinatus*), Nuo Dao Gen Xu (*Oryzae glutinosae radix et rhizoma*), Long Gu (*Mastodi fossilium ossis*).

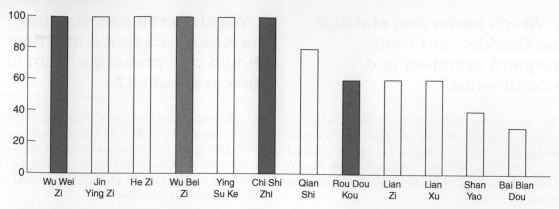

Fig. 15.3 • Comparison of the herbs that restrain leakage from the intestines and stop diarrhea.
Wu Wei Zi (*Schisandrae fructus*), Jin Ying Zi (*Rosae laevigatae fructus*), He Zi (*Chebulae fructus*), Wu Bei Zi (*Chinensis galla*), Ying Su Ke (*Papaveris somniferi pericarpium*), Chi Shi Zhi (*Halloysitum rubrum*), Qian Shi (*Euryalis semen*), Rou Dou Kou (*Myristicae semen*), Lian Zi (*Nelumbinis semen*), Lian Xu (*Nelumbinis stamen*), Shan Yao (*Dioscoreae rhizoma*), Bai Bian Dou (*Dolichoris lablab semen*).

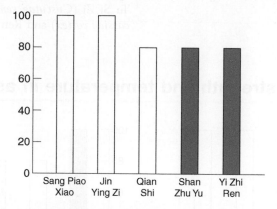

Fig. 15.4 • Comparison of the herbs that stabilize the Bladder and treat incontinence and enuresis.
Sang Piao Xiao (*Mantidis oötheca*), Jin Ying Zi (*Rosae laevigatae fructus*), Qian Shi (*Euryalis semen*), Shan Zhu Yu (*Corni fructus*), Yi Zhi Ren (*Alpiniae oxyphyllae fructus*).

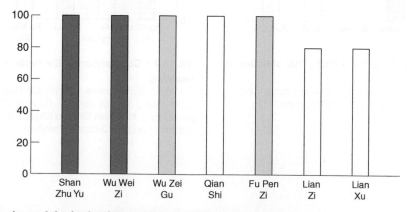

Fig. 15.5 • Comparison of the herbs that stabilize the Kidney-Essence.
Shan Zhu Yu (*Corni fructus*), Wu Wei Zi (*Schisandrae fructus*), Wu Zei Gu (*Sepiae seu sepiellae os*), Qian Shi (*Euryalis semen*), Fu Pen Zi (*Rubi fructus*), Lian Zi (*Nelumbinis semen*), Lian Xu (*Nelumbinis stamen*).

Chapter Sixteen

16

Substances that sedate the Spirit and calm the Mind

安神药

1 What are the indications for the substances that sedate the Spirit and calm the Mind?

The substances that sedate the Spirit and calm the Mind are able to treat restlessness, anxiety, palpitations, irritability, insomnia and emotional distress. The symptoms are directly caused by disturbance of the Heart, which is the residence of the Spirit, and determines the emotional, mental and spiritual features of the individual. The syndrome of Heart-Spirit disturbance can primarily be subdivided into the syndromes of Excessive-Heat and Blood deficiency.

In the Excessive-Heat syndrome, the symptoms have a pronounced and aggressive feature. Rage and stress may, in a very short time, cause Liver-Qi stagnation, Liver-Fire blazing upwards or Liver-Yang rising that influence the Heart immediately. Meanwhile, the Heart-Yin can be directly injured by Heat in many infectious diseases, which in Chinese medicine are considered as febrile diseases. Some chronic diseases often consume the Heart-Yin too. All these factors cause the Heart-Fire to blaze up, which disturbs the Spirit and leads to anxiety, irritability, palpitations, difficulty in falling asleep and dream-disturbed sleep.

In the syndrome of Blood deficiency, the symptoms have a mild and chronic feature. Since the state of the Heart-Spirit is based on sufficient Blood, when there is Blood deficiency there are symptoms such as restlessness and fear without any reason, emotional distress, palpitations, frequent sweating or night sweats, dream-disturbed sleep or frequent waking up at night. The tongue body is usually pale or delicate red with a thin white coating and the pulse is often thready, weak and restless.

In clinical practice, the syndromes are often more complicated. The Excess is often complicated with the Deficiency, and all the outlined symptoms may be present simultaneously. Therefore it may be necessary to sedate the Spirit, reduce Fire or direct the Liver-Yang to descend, as well as tonify the Blood and Yin of the body.

2 What are the characteristics of the substances that sedate the Spirit and calm the Mind? What precautions should be observed when using them?

The substances that sedate the Spirit and calm the Mind can be divided into two groups. One group focuses on sedating the Spirit; these substances can control the symptoms quickly. They are mainly used in acute situations and especially in an Excessive syndrome. A second group deals with the causes and the manifestations of the syndrome; these substances have the function of tonifying the Blood and Yin, reducing the Heat from the Heart and calming the Mind. They are used for a chronic or mild syndrome.

The substances that sedate the Spirit and calm the Mind have the following characteristics.

Entering the Heart, Liver and Kidney meridians

The five internal organs are connected with the seven emotions. Of these emotions, the symptoms of restlessness with anxiety, difficulty in falling asleep and palpitations are linked with the Heart; irritability, insomnia and dream-disturbed sleep are linked with the Liver; restlessness and fear with anxiety are linked with the Kidney. Most of the substances that sedate the Spirit and calm the Mind enter the Heart, Liver and Kidney meridians; therefore they control the disorders from different aspects.

Many mineral substances

Mineral substances in TCM are considered to have a descending nature because they are heavier in weight and more solid than the herbs. Heaviness can sedate the Spirit, descend the Yang and Fire, and control fear. They are often used for treating acute or Excessive conditions. The commonly used substances are Ci Shi (*Magnetitum*), Zhen Zhu (*Margarita usta*), Zhen Zhu Mu (*Concha margaritifera usta*), Zi Shi Ying (*Fluoritum*), Hu Po (*Succinum*), Long Gu (*Mastodi fossilium ossis*) and Mu Li (*Ostrea concha*).

Cold and salty

Since most of the acute cases of mental disturbance are caused by Excessive- or Empty-Fire, a cold and salty substance is able to reduce and purge the Fire and protect the Yin of the body. These substances are effective for treating disorders with obvious Heat signs. The commonly used substances are Mu Li, Ci Shi, Zhen Zhu, Zhen Zhu Mu and Bai Zi Ren (*Platycladi semen*).

Sweet

Sweetness has a capacity of moderating, tonifying and moistening. Some substances that are used for acute and severe cases are sweet in taste too. They can moderate the conflict and reduce the speed of the pathological progress of the disorder; Zhen Zhu and Zhen Zhu Mu are examples.

In chronic or mild cases, the sweet herbs are often used to tonify the Blood of the Heart and Liver, and moisten the Dryness that is caused by Yin and Blood deficiency. The commonly used herbs are Suan Zao Ren (*Ziziphi spinosae semen*), Bai Zi Ren, He Huan Pi (*Albiziae cortex*) and Ye Jiao Teng (*Polygoni multiflori caulis*).

In clinical practice, one should be aware that the mineral substances control the symptoms of the disorder rather than treat the cause, so they should not be used for a prolonged period of time. When the condition of the patient has improved, the substances that treat the cause of the disorder should then be used.

Furthermore, mineral substances are heavy on the Stomach, and may cause indigestion, stomach pain and constipation; therefore they should be used together with other herbs that protect the Stomach. If the patient complains of such symptoms after taking these substances, or feels sleepy during the day, the dosage should be reduced, and may even need to be used only in the evening. In addition, the mineral substances have a descending tendency, so pregnant women should not use them, or use them with caution.

3 Ci Shi (*Magnetitum*), Zhen Zhu (*Margarita usta*), Zhen Zhu Mu (*Concha margaritifera usta*) and Hu Po (*Succinum*) are all used for disturbance of the Heart-Spirit. What are the differences between them?

All four of these substances are able to treat restlessness, palpitations with anxiety, insomnia, convulsions and epilepsy due to disturbance of the Heart-Spirit. In clinical practice, they are used to sedate the Spirit, and are particularly effective in treating acute and Excessive disorders. However, there are some differences between their actions.

Ci Shi is pungent, salty and cold. It is the strongest of the four substances for sedating the Spirit. Since it enters the Liver and Kidney meridians, it is more suitable to treat disturbance of the Spirit which is directly caused or influenced by the Liver and Kidney, with symptoms such as palpitations and restlessness with fear, dream-disturbed sleep and ease of waking up at night. It is a heavy and solid substance and is also able to stabilize the Kidney-Qi and Essence and direct the Liver-Yang to descend. Therefore it is also used for deafness, tinnitus, shortness of breath or asthma, dizziness, headache and blurred vision.

Zhen Zhu is sweet, salty and cold; its action of sedating the Heart-Spirit is more moderate than that of Ci Shi. It enters the Heart and Liver meridians and works more directly on the disorders of the Heart. It is good at clearing Fire of the Heart and Liver, and is used to treat restlessness, anxiety, palpitations, irritability, difficulty in falling asleep, epilepsy and febrile convulsions. It can also treat blurred vision, such as in cataract due to Heat in the Liver and Heart.

Zhen Zhu Mu is the pearl shell. Like Zhen Zhu, it is cold and salty, and enters the Heart and Liver meridians. It also has the function of clearing Heat from the Heart and Liver, and sedating the Spirit, but its action is weaker than that of Zhen Zhu. However, it is more effective for subduing the Liver-Yang and treating dizziness, headache and tinnitus, and is more suitable for use when the patient suffers from Liver-Yang rising syndrome and also complains of palpitations, irritability and insomnia.

Hu Po is sweet and neutral, and enters primarily the Heart and Liver meridians. It enters the Blood level of the Heart and Liver, and is particularly effective for sedating the Spirit and removing congealed Blood. In clinical practice, it is used for patients with Heart diseases when the Blood is not circulating properly, and at the same time the patient has palpitations and restlessness, such as is seen in coronary heart disease. It is also used for febrile convulsions and epilepsy.

4 What are the differences in function between Long Gu (*Mastodi fossilium ossis*) and Long Chi (*Mastodi fossilia dentis*)?

Long Gu and Long Chi are different parts of fossil fragments and both have the function of sedating the Heart-Spirit. However, there are differences between them.

Long Gu is sweet, neutral and astringent, and enters the Heart, Liver and Kidney meridians. Its action in sedating the Spirit is not as strong as that

of Long Chi, but it can also control fear as it works on the Kidney. Long Gu has two further functions that Long Chi does not. First, it can anchor the Liver-Yang to treat Liver-Yang rising, which manifests as dizziness, tinnitus, headache and dream-disturbed sleep. Secondly, it can stabilize the leakage of the Essence and Body Fluids. If a patient suffers from Liver-Yang rising, as well as palpitations, anxiety with fear, insomnia and night sweating, Long Gu is more suitable than Long Chi.

Long Chi is cold and enters the Heart and Liver meridians. It is heavier than Long Gu and its descending property is stronger and quicker than that of Long Gu. Long Chi is very effective for sedating the Heart-Spirit and calming the Mind, and is used to treat manic–depressive psychosis, hysteria, anxiety, irritability and insomnia.

5 What are the differences between Long Gu (*Mastodi fossilium ossis*) and Mu Li (*Ostrea concha*) in the function of calming the Mind?

Long Gu and Mu Li both have the function of pacifying the Liver and calming the Mind. They are both astringent substances and are also able to stabilize the Essence and Body Fluids. Both can be used to treat insomnia, irritability, dizziness, night sweating and spermatorrhea.

However, compared with Mu Li, Long Gu has a stronger effect in sedating the Heart-Spirit and calming the Mind. It is sweet and neutral, and is more effective in treating insomnia, restlessness, palpitations and dream-disturbed sleep.

Mu Li is salty and cold, has a stronger effect in reducing Heat in order to calm the Mind, and is more effective for treating night sweats and restlessness with anxiety. Mu Li also has another function— that of softening hardness and dissipating Phlegm. If the mental disorder is caused by Phlegm-Heat with symptoms of night sweating, insomnia and irritability, such as seen in schizophrenia, manic–depressive psychosis, hepatocirrhosis and hepatic coma, Mu Li is more suitable than Long Gu. In clinical practice, however, Long Gu and Mu Li are often used together to strengthen the function of pacifying the Liver and calming the Mind so as to be able to treat more complaints.

6 What are the differences in treating insomnia between Suan Zao Ren (*Ziziphi spinosae semen*), Bai Zi Ren (*Platycladi semen*), Ye Jiao Teng (*Polygoni multiflori caulis*), He Huan Pi (*Albiziae cortex*) and Yuan Zhi (*Polygalae radix*)?

These five are all commonly used herbs to treat insomnia. Except for Yuan Zhi, they are all sweet herbs. They can tonify the body and calm the Mind, and are particularly suitable for treating long-term insomnia due to disorders of the internal organs. However, each herb has its own characteristics, so the applications of each are also different.

Suan Zao Ren is sweet and sour; it enters primarily the Liver meridian, and secondarily the Heart meridian. Sweetness can tonify the Liver and Heart-Blood, and sourness can stabilize the Blood and the Qi. It is the most commonly used herb to tonify the Liver-Blood and calm the Mind. It is particularly effective for treating restlessness and irritability with no reason, restless sleep, dream-disturbed sleep and nightmares.

Bai Zi Ren primarily enters the Heart meridian, and enters the Liver meridian secondarily. It is sweet and has a moistening nature. It is an excellent herb for nourishing the Heart-Blood and calming the Mind. It also has the function of stopping sweating and is more suitable for treating difficulty in falling asleep, restlessness and palpitations, a tendency to become nervous easily and sweating. Since the mental state and sleeping are related to Heart and Liver, Suan Zao Ren and Bai Zhi Ren are often used together.

Ye Jiao Teng is the vine of the same plant as He Shou Wu (*Polygoni multiflori radix*). Like He Shou Wu, it also has the function of tonifying the Blood. It is sweet and neutral, and enters the Heart and Liver meridians. It is able to tonify the Blood and calm the Mind, as well as open the meridians and collaterals. It is especially suitable for treating conditions in which the Blood is too weak to circulate properly and causes restless sleep, dream-disturbed sleep and insomnia, together with an uneasy sensation in all muscles during and after sleep.

He Huan Pi is sweet and neutral, and enters the Heart, Spleen and Lung meridians. It regulates the Qi in the chest and calms the Mind. It is especially suitable for treating patients who suffer from depression as well as insomnia, with symptoms such as sadness, grief, tightness in the chest and reduced appetite.

Yuan Zhi is pungent and bitter, and enters the Heart and Kidney meridians. Pungency has a dispersing nature and bitterness has a descending property, so the herb is good at removing Phlegm and improving the Qi connection between the Heart and Kidney so that the Mind is calmed and sleep improves. It is suitable for treating palpitations, forgetfulness, poor concentration and insomnia. In clinical practice, this herb should be used with caution because when the dosage is too high, it can irritate the gastric mucosa and cause nausea, and it can also increase the secretion of the respiratory tract.

7 Dang Gui (*Angelicae sinensis radix*), Bai Shao Yao (*Paeoniae radix lactiflora*), Bai He (*Lilii bulbus*), Fu Ling (*Poria*), Sheng Di Huang (*Rehmanniae radix*) and Mai Men Dong (*Ophiopogonis radix*) can all calm the Mind. What are the differences between them?

Dang Gui and Bai Shao Yao are a pair of herbs that tonify the Blood. Although they have no function in calming the Mind in themselves, they are effective for nourishing the Blood of the Heart and Liver, and are often used with Suan Zao Ren (*Ziziphi spinosae semen*) and Bai Zi Ren (*Platycladi semen*) to treat insomnia due to Blood deficiency.

Bai He is sweet and bland, slightly cold, and enters the Lung and Heart meridians. It is particularly effective for moistening the Lung-Yin and nourishing the Heart-Yin. It is also able to calm the Mind. It is often used together with He Huan Pi (*Albiziae cortex*) to treat insomnia with depression due to Lung-Yin and Heart-Yin deficiency and Liver-Qi stagnation.

Fu Ling is sweet, neutral and bland, and enters the Heart, Spleen and Bladder meridians. It has the functions of tonifying the Spleen-Qi and Heart-Qi, and calming the Mind. It is often used together with other herbs to tonify the Qi and Blood to calm the mind.

Sheng Di Huang and Mai Men Dong are both sweet and cold, and enter the Heart meridian. They can nourish the Yin and reduce Heat. They are also often used together with Ci Shi (*Magnetitum*), Zhen Zhu Mu (*Concha margaritifera usta*), Long Gu

(*Mastodi fossilium ossis*) and Mu Li (*Ostrea concha*) to treat insomnia due to Excessive- or Empty-Heat in the Blood that disturbs the Heart-Spirit.

Although these six herbs do not directly calm the Mind, or are not strong enough to calm the Mind alone, they are able to treat the causes of the disorder. They can form some very good combinations with other herbs that calm the Mind to enhance their functions.

Comparisons of strength and temperature in substances that sedate the Spirit and calm the Mind

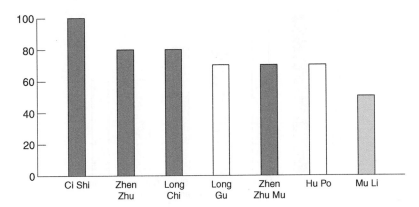

Fig. 16.1 • Comparison of the substances that directly calm the Mind.
Ci Shi (*Magnetitum*), Zhen Zhu (*Margarita usta*), Long Chi (*Mastodi fossilia dentis*), Long Gu (*Mastodi fossilium ossis*), Zhen Zhu Mu (*Concha margaritifera usta*), Hu Po (*Succinum*), Mu Li (*Ostrea concha*).

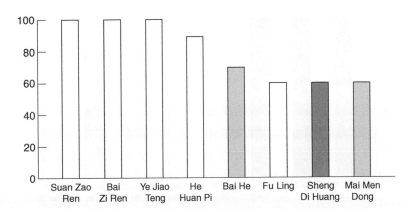

Fig. 16.2 • Comparison of the herbs that nourish the Heart, calm the Mind and improve sleep.
Suan Zao Ren (*Ziziphi spinosae semen*), Bai Zi Ren (*Platycladi semen*), Ye Jiao Teng (*Polygoni multiflori caulis*), He Huan Pi (*Albiziae cortex*), Bai He (*Lilii bulbus*), Fu Ling (*Poria*), Sheng Di Huang (*Rehmanniae radix*), Mai Men Dong (*Ophiopogonis radix*).

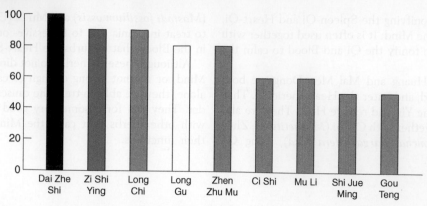

Fig. 16.3 • Comparison of the substances that anchor the Liver-Yang and calm the Mind.
Dai Zhe Shi (*Haematitum*), Zi Shi Ying (*Fluoritum*), Long Chi (*Mastodi fossilia dentis*), Long Gu (*Mastodi fossilium ossis*), Zhen Zhu Mu (*Concha margaritifera usta*), Ci Shi (*Magnetitum*), Mu Li (*Ostrea concha*), Shi Jue Ming (*Haliotidis concha*), Gou Teng (*Uncariae ramulus cum uncis*).

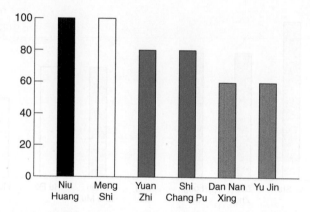

Fig. 16.4 • Comparison of the substances that transform Phlegm and settle the Spirit.
Niu Huang (*Bovis calculus*)**, Meng Shi (*Lapis micae seu chloriti*)*, Yuan Zhi (*Polygalae radix*), Shi Chang Pu (*Acori graminei rhizoma*), Dan Nan Xing (*Pulvis arisaemae cum felle bovis*), Yu Jin (*Curcumae radix*).

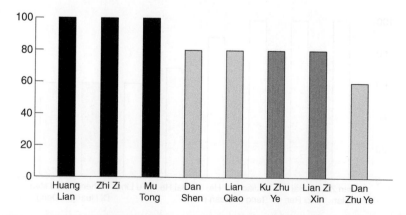

Fig. 16.5 • Comparison of the herbs that clear Excessive-Heat from the Heart and calm the Mind.
Huang Lian (*Coptidis rhizoma*), Zhi Zi (*Gardeniae fructus*), Mu Tong (*Mutong caulis*)*, Dan Shen (*Salviae miltiorrhizae radix*), Lian Qiao (*Forsythiae fructus*), Ku Zhu Ye (*Bambusae amarae folium*), Lian Zi Xin (*Nelumbinis plumula*), Dan Zhu Ye (*Lophatheri herba*).

Chapter Seventeen

Herbs that subdue the Liver-Yang and extinguish Liver-Wind

平肝熄风药

1 What are the pathological changes and manifestations in the syndromes of Liver-Yang rising and Liver-Wind?

The syndrome of Liver-Yang rising is caused by Liver-Yin deficiency. It is often seen in people over 50 years old or who are suffering from certain chronic diseases that injure the Liver-Yin. As soon as the Liver-Yin fails to control the Liver-Yang, the Yang rises. The manifestations are dizziness with a slightly tight sensation in the head, headache, blurred vision and tinnitus. In a severe case, there is irritability, dream-disturbed sleep and a distending pain in the hypochondriac region and the patient prefers a quiet and relaxing environment. If the Liver-Yang and Heat disturb the Stomach, patients may have a red face, a dry and bitter taste in the mouth, nausea or belching. The tongue body is red, or red only on the border, and the coating is thin, dry and yellow. The pulse is thready and wiry, or thready, wiry and rapid. In clinical practice, this syndrome is often seen in hypertension, menopausal syndrome, neurotinnitus, nervous deafness and glaucoma.

If the Liver-Yang is not controlled with proper treatment, it may turn to Liver-Wind, especially in those with a Yang constitution, or in conditions of rage, high stress, eating too much spicy food or taking certain medications. At that moment, the Liver-Yang rises rapidly and stirs up the Wind. This is called 'Liver-Yang stirs up the Wind' or 'Liver-Yang turns to Wind'. Since the Liver controls all the tendons, the symptoms of Liver-Wind are character-ized by tremors or spasms of the limbs, severe dizziness, nausea, vomiting, tingling or numbness of the limbs, and loss of balance in standing or walking. In severe cases, Liver-Wind may disturb the normal circulation of Qi and Blood, and rebellious Qi and Blood, as well as Fire and Phlegm, attack the head, block the meridians and cover the Mind. The patient may suddenly lose consciousness and afterwards will have hemiplegia and deviation of the eyes and mouth. In this case, the tongue body is red, the coating is yellow and dry, or yellow and sticky, and the pulse is wiry, forceful and rapid. In clinical practice, this syndrome is often seen in epilepsy, convulsions in infectious disease, severe cases of hypertension and glaucoma, facial paralysis, facial spasms and cerebrovascular accident and its sequelae.

2 What are the treatment principles for the syndromes of Liver-Yang rising and Liver-Wind? What precautions should be observed in their treatment?

Since the syndrome of Liver-Yang rising is the result of Liver-Yin deficiency, one of the treatment principles is to nourish the Liver-Yin so as to control the Liver-Yang, and this is especially necessary in the mild, chronic cases of Liver-Yang rising. However, because the Liver-Yang has already left its original place, the Lower Jiao, it is not so easy to get it to return to its place quickly by means of nourishing the Yin. So a second principle of the treatment is to anchor the Yang and sedate the Liver so as to build up a new balance between the Liver-Yin and Liver-Yang, especially in acute cases. In a severe case of Liver-Yang rising, the procedure of anchoring the Yang should be carried out at once so as to stop the development of the pathological changes and prevent the occurrence of Liver-Wind syndrome.

If the Liver-Wind has already been stirred up by the suddenly rising Liver-Yang, the treatment principles mentioned above are not enough to handle the Wind, so methods that strongly direct the Liver-Yang to descend, pacify the Liver and extinguish Wind should be applied immediately.

In the treatment of Liver-Yang rising or Liver-Wind, it is important to make a clear differentiation of the stage of the disorder and the primary and secondary steps of treatment. If a patient has family history of hypertension, is over 50 years old and feels quite stressed, and the blood pressure is slightly higher than normal, treatment should be given to nourish the Liver-Yin and calm the Liver-Yang. If, at certain moments, such as in the springtime, when under high stress or in a rage, the patient's blood pressure rises quickly, and there are all the obvious symptoms of Liver-Yang rising, then the treatment to anchor the Yang and sedate the Liver should be given immediately. If the patient not only has the symptoms of Liver-Yang rising, but also feels tingling in the fingers or limbs, and loses balance in walking, then treatment to extinguish Liver-Wind and anchor the Yang must be given immediately.

To treat patients with a syndrome of Liver-Yang rising and Liver Wind, it is also important to advise the patient to avoid all the factors that may contribute to the Liver-Yang rising, such as herbs that move upwards and outwards, alcohol, spicy food, stress and rage.

3 What are the characteristics of the substances that anchor the Liver-Yang and extinguish Liver-Wind? What precautions should be observed when these substances are prescribed?

The substances that sedate and anchor the Liver-Yang and extinguish Liver-Wind are used for acute and subacute conditions of Liver-Yang rising or Liver-Wind and they have the following characteristics.

Mineral substances

In TCM, mineral substances are considered to have a descending tendency because they are heavy in weight. They can direct the Liver-Yang downwards and are also able to bring down the Liver-Wind and rebellious Qi and Blood, which have been stirred up by the rapidly rising Liver-Yang. The commonly used substances are Shi Jue Ming (*Haliotidis concha*), Long Gu (*Mastodi fossilium ossis*), Mu Li (*Ostrea concha*), Ci Shi (*Magnetitum*), Zhen Zhu Mu (*Concha margaritifera usta*) and Dai Zhe Shi (*Haematitum*).

Sedating the Heart-Spirit and calming the Mind

Since the Liver is the mother organ of the Heart, Liver-Yang rising may cause Heart-Fire blazing. In most of the cases of Liver-Yang rising there are also symptoms of Heart-Fire disturbance, such as restlessness, anxiety, irritability, insomnia, a bitter taste in the mouth and a red face. The substances that bring down the Liver-Yang are also able to sedate the Heart-Spirit and calm the Mind—examples are Ci Shi, Long Gu, Mu Li and Zhen Zhu Mu.

Usage of worms for opening the collaterals and extinguishing Wind and relieving spasms

It is considered in TCM that worms are able to get into the small collaterals because they have the habit of drilling holes or passing through cracks. Worms that enter the Liver meridian can open meridians and collaterals so as to extinguish Wind and relieve spasms. The worms used are Di Long (*Pheretima*), Jiang Can (*Bombyx batrycatus*), Quan Xie (*Scorpio*)* and Wu Gong (*Scolopendra*)*.

In clinical practice, it is important to know the precautions and contraindications for the usage of these substances. Since the mineral substances are heavy in weight, they are also heavy on the Stomach. For patients who have a weakness in the Middle Jiao, the mineral substances should be used in a smaller dosage, shorter treatment course or combined with other herbs that protect the Stomach. Since they are heavy on the Stomach and can strongly direct the Liver-Yang downwards, they are used only in the acute and subacute conditions. In the syndrome of Liver-Yin deficiency with Liver-Yang rising, the treatment should be based on tonifying the Yin and pacifying the Liver-Yang. In addition, Dai Zhe Shi, Quan Xie and Wu Gong are poisonous substances, so the dosages should be controlled carefully. Lastly, these mineral substances should not be used by pregnant women.

4 Shi Jue Ming (*Haliotidis concha*), Zhen Zhu Mu (*Concha margaritifera usta*), Ci Shi (*Magnetitum*), Long Gu (*Mastodi fossilium ossis*) and Dai Zhe Shi (*Haematitum*) can all be used for the syndromes of Liver-Yang rising and Liver-Wind. What are the differences between them?

These five herbs are all mineral substances and are commonly used for the syndrome of Kidney-Yin and Liver-Yin deficiency and Liver-Yang rising with Liver-Wind. However, there are some differences between their functions.

Shi Jue Ming is salty and slightly cold, and enters the Kidney and Liver meridians. Saltiness and Cold possess reducing and descending capacities and a heavy mineral substance is considered to have a downward-moving tendency. Shi Jue Ming is able to direct the Liver-Yang strongly downwards, clear the Liver-Fire and therefore extinguish the Liver-Wind. It is commonly used to treat the syndromes of Liver-Yang rising and Liver-Wind. In clinical practice, it can treat headache, dizziness, blurred vision, irritability, dream-disturbed sleep and tingling or numbness of the fingers and limbs, such as seen in hypertension. It is also able to brighten the eyes and treat disorders of the eyes due to Liver-Yang rising and Liver-Fire, such as blurred vision, hypopsia, asthenopia, optic atrophy, glaucoma, primary cataract, conjunctivitis and Bitot's spot.

Zhen Zhu Mu is salty and cold, and enters the Heart and Liver meridians. Compared with Shi Jue Ming, it has the same function of descending the Liver-Yang and Liver-Wind, and it can be used for the same disorders, but the action of this substance is weaker. However, the strong point of this substance is that it can calm the Mind as it enters the Heart meridian and clear the Heat there. In clinical practice, if the patient complains of restless sleep, insomnia and palpitations, as well as the symptoms of Liver-Yang rising, then Zen Zhu Mu is the better choice.

Ci Shi is pungent, salty and cold, and enters the Liver and Kidney meridians. It is as strong as Shi Jue Ming in directing the Liver-Yang downwards, but is less strong in calming the Liver-Wind, so is less effective for treating headache, dizziness, tingling of the fingers or numbness of the limbs. However, Ci Shi is able to calm the Wind caused by Heart-Fire, such as seen in convulsions due to high fever in children. Meanwhile, it has a strong action in strengthening and stabilizing the Kidney-Qi and Essence, and is used for treating tinnitus, deafness and hypopsia, as well as shortness of breath. Compared with Zhen Zhu Mu, Ci Shi has a stronger action in calming the Mind, and settling and tranquilizing the Heart-Spirit, so is used not only in insomnia and restlessness, but also in phobia, anxiety and manic–depressive psychosis.

Long Gu is sweet, astringent and neutral, and enters the Heart, Liver and Kidney meridians. It is a very good substance for directing the Liver-Yang downwards and calming Liver-Wind. Since it is sweet and neutral, and is less irritating to the Stomach, it can be used for a longer period of time—for instance, in hypertension. It is also often combined with other substances that direct the Liver-Yang downwards, and which are very cold and heavy—for instance, Dai Zhe Shi and Ci Shi.

Long Gu makes the action of bringing down the Liver-Yang sufficient, so the dosages of the other substances that are too cold and salty can be reduced. Like Zhen Zhu Mu and Ci Shi, Long Gu can also be used to calm the Mind and control anxiety. Because it is an astringent substance, it is able to stabilize the Body Fluids and Essence, so is more suitable for treatment in menopause when the patient has hypertension, emotional disorders, sleep disorders, hot flushes and night sweating.

Dai Zhe Shi is bitter and cold, and enters the Liver and Pericardium meridians. It is an important substance for directing the Yang downwards. It is also the strongest of these five substances for bringing down the Liver-Yang and extinguishing the

Wind. It can intensively and quickly direct the Yang, Wind, Fire, Phlegm, Qi and Blood downwards, so it is often used for acute situations—for instance, when the blood pressure rises rapidly, or the patient has a cerebrovascular accident or some severe infectious disease. Symptoms that may be present include severe headache with heavy and distending sensations, tinnitus, stiffness of the neck, dizziness and loss of balance in walking, belching, nausea, vomiting, stifling in the chest and fullness in the Stomach and hypochondriac region, nose bleeding or vomiting of Blood. However, since Dai Ze Shi is a heavy, cold and bitter substance, can easily injure the Stomach, and contains a tiny amount of arsenic, it cannot be used in large dosages or for a long period of time.

5 What are the differences between Tian Ma (*Gastrodiae rhizoma*)** and Gou Teng (*Uncariae ramulus cum uncis*) in the function of extinguishing Liver-Wind?

Tian Ma and Gou Teng both are sweet, enter the Liver meridian, and are able to pacify the Liver and extinguish the Liver-Wind. They are used to treat dizziness, headache, convulsions, tremor and spasm caused by Liver-Wind. They are often used together to accentuate each other's therapeutic actions. However, they have some individual characteristics in both nature and function, so the clinical applications are also different.

Tian Ma is sweet and neutral, and has a moderate and moist nature. The characteristic of this herb is that it can extinguish internal Wind as well as expel external Wind. In clinical practice, it is good at treating dizziness and headache due to deficiency of the Liver-Yin and Blood. It is also used to treat dizziness with nausea and vomiting caused by disturbance of Wind-Phlegm. If it is combined with the herbs that cool the Liver, it is effective for calming spasm and convulsions from high fever; if it is used together with the herbs that promote Qi movement and Blood circulation, it can treat stiff, painful, numb and tingling limbs, such as seen in Bi syndrome or the sequelae of cerebrovascular accident.

Since it is so often used in different types of Wind syndrome, it has acquired the name 'grass of settling Wind'.

Gou Teng is sweet and cold. Although it is not so widely used as Tian Ma for treating various Wind syndromes, it has an obvious strong function of clearing and reducing Liver-Heat, no matter whether Excess-Heat or Empty-Heat; therefore it can calm Wind. It is used to treat dizziness, headache, tinnitus, irritability, and red and irritated eyes. Because it enters the Pericardium meridian, it is also very effective for treating convulsions in children when high fever is present that is caused by Liver-Fire and Heart-Fire.

6 Quan Xie (*Scorpio*)*, Wu Gong (*Scolopendra*)* and Di Long (*Pheretima*) are all able to extinguish Liver-Wind, relieve spasms and control tremor. What are the differences between them?

Quan Xie, Wu Gong and Di Long are all able to extinguish Liver-Wind, relieve spasms, control tremor, open the meridians and stop pain. They are used in the treatment of convulsions, epilepsy, tetanus, hemiplegia, facial paralysis, facial spasm and chronic arthritis.

Quan Xie and Wu Gong are pungent and poisonous; both are able to extinguish Liver-Wind, release spasm, open the meridians and stop pain. The functions of these two substances are almost the same, but Wu Gong is the stronger. In clinical practice, Quan Xie is more suitable for treating tremor due to Liver-Wind and Heat. It is also effective in opening up the collaterals, relieving pain and reducing the speed of deformation and stiffness of the joints. Wu Gong is warm and more pungent, can intensively relieve spasms, and is more suitable for severe spasms with internal Cold. It can also remove the toxin from poisonous snakebites, sores and carbuncles. Although there are differences between Quan Xie and Wu Gong, they are often used together because these two substances can strongly enhance each other's actions; therefore the dosage of each substance can be reduced as they are poisonous.

Di Long is salty and cold; its action in extinguishing the Wind is weaker than that of either Quan Xie or Wu Gong, but its effect in clearing Liver-Heat is the strongest of the three. In clinical practice, it is more suitable for treating convulsions, tremor with irritability or fever. When it is used together with Tian Ma (*Gastrodiae rhizoma*)** and Quan Xie, it becomes more effective. Moreover, Di Long particularly enters the collaterals, and is able to break up obstructions, so is used for Bi syndrome and hemiplegia when the limbs are stiff, weak, numb and painful.

7 Di Long (*Pheretima*) and Jiang Can (*Bombyx batrycatus*) can both extinguish Wind and are used for facial paralysis and facial spasm. What are the differences between them?

Di Long and Jiang Can both can effectively open up collaterals and relieve spasms. In clinical practice, they are often used for facial paralysis and facial spasms. However, Di Long is salty and cold, and is good at clearing Heat, controlling Liver-Wind, relieving spasms and stopping pain, whereas Jiang Can is neutral and pungent, and is able to remove Phlegm obstruction from the collaterals so can relieve spasms, numbness and paralysis. Because they treat facial paralysis or spasms by different approaches, they are often used together in clinical practice.

8 Jiang Can (*Bombyx batrycatus*), Bai Ji Li (*Tribuli fructus*), Chan Tui (*Cicadae periostracum*) and Jing Jie (*Schizonepetae herba*) are all able to relieve itching and treat itchy skin lesions or rashes. What are the differences between them?

These four herbs are effective for relieving itching because they are pungent and light, and are able to expel Wind-Heat. They are often used for skin diseases such as urticaria, eczema, neurodermatitis and pruritus; they can be also used for treating some allergic disorders such as hay fever or some infectious diseases with pathological changes on the skin, such as chickenpox, rubella and measles.

Of these four substances, Chan Tui and Jing Jie are particularly often used in cases caused by external Wind, such as infectious diseases of children and allergies.

Jiang Can and Bai Ji Li are able not only to expel external Wind, but also to extinguish internal Wind, the Liver-Wind. They are more suitable for use when the patient has Liver-Yin and Blood deficiency, and disturbance of the Liver-Wind, such as seen in pruritus in elderly people, skin diseases starting or worsening in stressful situations, itchy rashes in the evening, in the night or after menstruation, and chronic skin diseases. Since external Wind and internal Wind often coexist—for instance, the itch may not only be worse in the above conditions, but also when the weather changes, after taking spicy food or during cold infections—therefore substances that expel external Wind and those that extinguish internal Wind can be used together.

Comparisons of strength and temperature in herbs that sedate the Liver-Yang and extinguish Liver-Wind

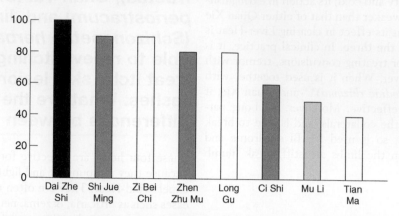

Fig. 17.1 ● Comparison of the substances that anchor the Liver-Yang.
Dai Zhe Shi (*Haematitum*), Shi Jue Ming (*Haliotidis concha*), Zi Bei Chi (*Erosaria caputserpentis*), Zhen Zhu Mu (*Concha margaritifera usta*), Long Gu (*Mastodi fossilium ossis*), Ci Shi (*Magnetitum*), Mu Li (*Ostrea concha*), Tian Ma (*Gastrodiae rhizoma*)**.

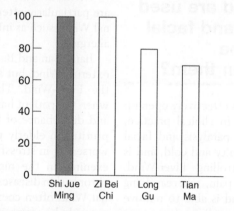

Fig. 17.2 ● Comparison of the herbs that extinguish Liver-Wind and subdue the Liver-Yang.
Shi Jue Ming (*Haliotidis concha*), Zi Bei Chi (*Erosaria caputserpentis*), Long Gu (*Mastodi fossilium ossis*) and Tian Ma (*Gastrodiae rhizoma*)**.

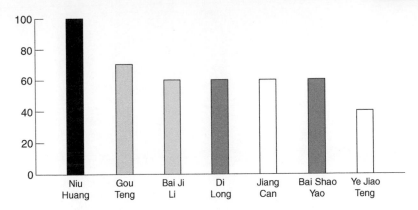

Fig. 17.3 • Comparison of the herbs that cool the Liver or disperse Liver-Heat and extinguish Wind.
Niu Huang (*Bovis calculus*)**, Gou Teng (*Uncariae ramulus cum uncis*), Bai Ji Li (*Tribuli fructus*), Di Long (*Pheretima*), Jiang Can (*Bombyx batrycatus*), Bai Shao Yao (*Paeoniae radix lactiflora*), Ye Jiao Teng (*Polygoni multiflori caulis*).

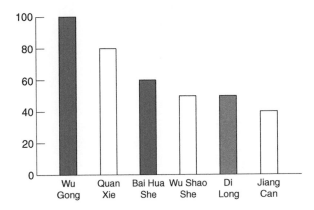

Fig. 17.4 • Comparison of the substances that open the collaterals and extinguish Wind.
Wu Gong (*Scolopendra*)*, Quan Xie (*Scorpio*)*, Bai Hua She (*Agkistrodon acutus*)*, Wu Shao She (*Zaocys*), Di Long (*Pheretima*), Jiang Can (*Bombyx batrycatus*).

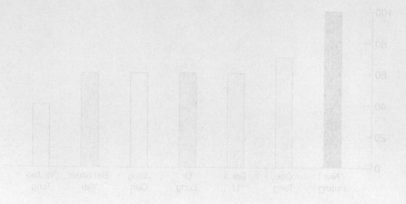

Appendix 1

Daily dosages for individual crude herbs above 6–9 grams

Note

Standard dosages for individual herbs

- Generally speaking, the most common dosage for most crude herbs in Chinese texts is about 3–9 grams orally per day.
- Modern concentrated herbal powder is six times stronger than crude herb, thus the common dosage for most single herbs is 0.5–1.5 grams per day.
- According to my own experience, this dosage can be reduced to 0.2–0.5 gram.
- The specifying exceptions of the dosages for individual herbs can be summarized in the following list.

Less than 0.1 g

Bing Pian (*Borneol*)
She Xiang (*Moschus*)**
Tan Xiang (*Santali albi lignum*)

Dosage up to 1 g

Zhen Zhu (*Margarita usta*)
Zhu Sha (*Cinnabaris*)*

Dosage up to 3 g

Bai Fu Zi (*Typhonii rhizoma praeparatum*)
Cao Dou Kou (*Alpiniae katsumadai semen*)
Ding Xiang (*Caryophylli flos*)
Hu Po (*Succinum*)

Lu Rong (*Cervi cornu*)**
Ma Bo (*Lasiosphaera*)
Mang Chong (*Tabanus*)*
Quan Xie (*Scorpio*)*
Wu Gong (*Scolopendra*)*
Xi Xin (*Asari herba*)*
Zhe Chong (*Eupolyphaga seu opisthoplatia*)*

Dosage up to 6 g

Ai Ye (*Artemisiae argyi folium*)
Bai Dou Kou (*Amomi fructus rotundus*)
Bo He (*Menthae herba*)
Chen Xiang (*Aquilariae lignum*)
Deng Xin Cao (*Junci medulla*)
Fan Xie Ye (*Sennae folium*)
Gao Liang Jiang (*Alpiniae officinari rhizoma*)
Ge Jie (*Gecko*)**
He Zi (*Chebulae fructus*)
Hua Jiao (*Zanthoxyli fructus*)
Huang Lian (*Coptidis rhizoma*)
Ling Yang Jiao (*Antelopis cornu*)**
Mu Tong (*Mutong caulis*)*
Qing Dai (*Indigo naturalis*)
Rou Gui (*Cinnamomi cassiae cortex*)
Sha Ren (*Amomi xanthioidis fructus*)
Sheng Ma (*Cimicifugae rhizoma*)
Tan Xiang (*Santali albi lignum*)
Wu Wei Zi (*Schisandrae fructus*)
Wu Zhu Yu (*Evodiae fructus*)
Xi Yang Shen (*Panacis quinquefolii radix*)
Yi Zhi Ren (*Alpiniae oxyphyllae fructus*)
Yue Ji Hua (*Rosae chinensis flos*)
Zi He Che (*Placenta hominis*)

Dosage up to 12 g

Bai Tou Weng (*Pulsatilla radix*)
Chi Shao Yao (*Paeoniae radix rubra*)
Da Huang (*Rhei rhizoma*)
Huang Qin (*Scutellariae radix*)
Mai Ya (*Hordei fructus germinatus*)
Mu Dan Pi (*Moutan cortex*)
Pi Pa Ye (*Eriobotryae folium*)
Zhi Mu (*Anemarrhenae rhizoma*)

Dosage up to 15 g

Bai Ji (*Bletillae tuber*)**
Ba Ji Tian (*Morindae radix*)
Bai Mao Gen (*Imperatae rhizoma*)
Bai Zhu (*Atractylodis macrocephalae rhizoma*)
Bei Sha Shen (*Glehniae radix*)
Ce Bai Ye (*Platycladi cacumen*)
Che Qian Zi (*Plantaginis semen*)
Da Jì (*Cirsii japonici herba seu radix*)
Da Zao (*Jujubae fructus*)
Dan Shen (*Salviae miltiorrhizae radix*)
Dan Zhu Ye (*Lophatheri herba*)
Dang Gui (*Angelicae sinensis radix*)
Dang Shen (*Codonopsis radix*)
Di Ding (*Violae herba*)
Di Fu Zi (*Kochiae fructus*)
Di Yu (*Sanguisorbae radix*)
Du Zhong (*Eucommiae cortex*)
Gou Ji (*Cibotii rhizoma*)**
Gou Teng (*Uncariae ramulus cum uncis*)
Hai Zao (*Sargassum*)
He Huan Pi (*Albiziae cortex*)
Hua Shi (*Talcum*)
Huai Hua (*Sophorae flos*)
Kun Bu (*Eckloniae thallus*)
Lai Fu Zi (*Raphani semen*)
Lian Qiao (*Forsythiae fructus*)
Lian Zi (*Nelumbinis semen*)
Lu Gen (*Phragmitis rhizoma*)
Ma Chi Xian (*Portulacae herba*)
Mang Xiao (*Natrii sulfas*)
Nu Zhen Zi (*Ligustri lucidi fructus*)
Pu Gong Ying (*Taraxaci herba*)
Qian Shi (*Euryalis semen*)
Shan Zha (*Crataegi fructus*)
Shan Zhu Yu (*Corni fructus*)
Shen Qu (*Massa medicata fermentata*)
Tian Hua Fen (*Trichosanthis radix*)
Tian Men Dong (*Asparagi radix*)
Tu Si Zi (*Cuscutae semen*)

Xiao Ji (*Cirsii herba*)
Xuan Shen (*Scrophulariae radix*)
Yin Yang Huo (*Epimedii herba*)
Yu Zhu (*Polygonati odorati rhizoma*)

Dosage up to 20 g

Bai Bian Dou (*Dolichoris lablab semen*)
Bai Zi Ren (*Platycladi semen*)
Chi Shi Zhi (*Halloysitum rubrum*)
He Shou Wu (*Polygoni multiflori radix*)
Huang Jing (*Polygonati rhizoma*)
Huang Qi (*Astragali radix*)
Mai Men Dong (*Ophiopogonis radix*)
Rou Cong Rong (*Cistanchis herba*)
Sha Yuan Zi (*Astragali complanati semen*)
Suan Zao Ren (*Ziziphi spinosae semen*)
Xu Duan (*Dipsaci radix*)

Dosage up to 30 g

Bai He (*Lilii bulbus*)
Bai Shao Yao (*Paeoniae radix lactiflora*)#
Bian Xu (*Polygoni avicularis herba*)
Bie Jia (*Trionycis carapax*)**
Ci Shi (*Magnetitum*)
Chi Xiao Dou (*Phaseoli semen*)
Dai Zhe Shi (*Haematitum*)#
Feng Mi (*Mel*)
Fu Xiao Mai (*Tritici fructus germinatus*)
Gua Lou (*Trichosanthis fructus*)
Gui Ban (*Testudinis carapax*)**
Han Lian Cao (*Ecliptae herba*)
Hei Zhi Ma (*Sesami semen nigricum*)
Hu Tao Rou (*Juglandis semen*)
Huo Ma Ren (*Cannabis semen*)
Ji Xue Teng (*Spatholobi caulis et radix*)
Long Gu (*Mastodi fossilium ossis*)
Lü Dou (*Phaseoli radiati semen*)
Mu Li (*Ostrea concha*)
Ou Jie (*Nelumbinis nodus rhizomatis*)
Qu Mai (*Dianthi herba*)
Sang Ji Sheng (*Taxilli herba*)
Shan Yao (*Dioscoreae rhizoma*)
Sheng Di Huang (*Rehmanniae radix*)
Shi Jue Ming (*Haliotidis concha*)
Shu Di Huang (*Rehmanniae radix praeparata*)
Tai Zi Shen (*Pseudostellariae radix*)
Ye Jiao Teng (*Polygoni multiflori caulis*)
Yi Mu Cao (*Leonuri herba*)
Yi Yi Ren (*Coicis semen*)
Yin Chen Hao (*Artemisiae scopariae herba*)

Yu Xing Cao (*Houttuyniae herba cum radice*)
Zao Xin Tu (*Terra flava usta*)
Zi Zhu Cao (*Callicarpae folium*)

Dosage up to 60 g

Fei Zi (*Torreyae semen*)
Jin Qian Cao (*Lysimachiae herba*)
Jin Yin Hua (*Lonicerae flos*)
Long Yan Rou (*Longanae arillus*)#

Shi Wei (*Pyrrosiae folium*)#
Xian He Cao (*Agrimoniae herba*)
Xiao Mai (*Tritici fructus*)
Yi Tang (*Maltose*)
Zhu Li (*Bambusae succus*)

Dosage up to 120 g

Nan Gua Zi (*Curcubitae semen*)

#Occasional large dosage.

Appendix 2

Commonly used herbal combinations and their applications

Mutual accentuation (Xiang Xu)

In this type of combination, two or more herbs with similar functions are used together to increase the therapeutic effect and achieve a safer and more effective therapeutic result than the use of a larger dosage of a single herb.

Combinations of releasing the Exterior syndrome

To expel Wind and release the Exterior syndrome

- Jing Jie (*Schizonepetae herba*): Expels Wind from the superficial region;
- Fang Feng (*Saposhnikoviae radix*): Expels Wind from skin, subcutaneous region.

To expel Wind-Heat and treat Wind-Heat in the Upper Jiao

- Sang Ye (*Mori folium*): Expels Wind-Heat in the Lung and Liver;
- Ju Hua (*Chrysanthemi flos*): Expels Wind-Heat in the Liver and Lung.

To expel Wind-Heat and relieve itch

- Chan Tui (*Cicadae periostracum*): Expels Wind, clears Heat of the superficial region;
- Bo He (*Menthae herba*): Expels Wind-Heat from the Upper Jiao.

To treat Wind-Heat in the Lung

- Jin Yin Hua (*Lonicerae flos*): Expels Wind-Heat and removes Heat-toxin;
- Lian Qiao (*Forsythiae fructus*): Expels Heat from the Heart and removes Heat-toxin.

To expel Wind, Damp and Cold and treat the Bi syndrome

- Qiang Huo (*Notopterygii rhizoma*): Expels Wind-Damp-Cold in the upper body;
- Du Huo (*Angelicae pubescentis radix*): Expels Wind-Damp-Cold in the lower body.

Combinations of clearing internal Heat

To reduce excess Heat in the Stomach and Lung

- Shi Gao (*Gypsum*): Clears excess Heat of Stomach and Lung, increases Body Fluid;
- Zhi Mu (*Anemarrhenae rhizoma*): Clears Heat and nourishes Yin of the Kidney, Stomach and Lung.

To clear Heat in the San Jiao

- Huang Qin (*Scutellariae radix*): Clears Heat in the Upper Jiao;
- Huang Lian (*Coptidis rhizoma*): Clears Heat in the Middle Jiao;
- Huang Bai (*Phellodendri cortex*): Clears Heat in the Lower Jiao.

Combinations of tonifying the Qi, Essence, Yin and Yang

To tonify and stabilize the Spleen-Qi

- Huang Qi (*Astragali radix*): Tonifies the Spleen-Qi and ascends the Qi;
- Shan Yao (*Dioscoreae rhizoma*): Tonifies the Spleen-Qi and stabilizes Essence.

To tonify and stabilize the Qi and Essence in the Middle Jiao

- Shan Yao (*Dioscoreae rhizoma*): Tonifies the Spleen-Qi and stabilizes Essence;
- Bai Bian Dou (*Dolichoris lablab semen*): Tonifies the Spleen-Qi, stabilizes Essence and removes Dampness.

To tonify the Spleen-Qi and dry Dampness in the Middle Jiao

- Bai Zhu (*Atractylodis macrocephalae rhizoma*): Tonifies the Spleen-Qi and dries Dampness;
- Fu Ling (*Poria*): Tonifies the Spleen-Qi and drains Dampness.

To treat Kidney-Yin and Essence deficiency

- Sheng Di Huang (*Rehmanniae radix*): Nourishes Kidney-Yin and reduces Empty-Heat;
- Shu Di Huang (*Rehmanniae radix praeparata*): Nourishes Kidney-Yin, Blood and Essence.

To moisten the intestine and promote bowel movement

- Dang Gui (*Angelicae sinensis radix*): Tonifies Blood and moistens the intestine;
- Rou Cong Rong (*Cistanchis herba*): Tonifies the Kidney-Yang and Kidney-Essence and moistens the intestine.

To nourish the Yin

- Tian Men Dong (*Asparagi radix*): Nourishes the Kidney-Yin and Lung-Yin;
- Mai Men Dong (*Ophiopogonis radix*): Nourishes the Heart-Yin, Stomach-Yin and Lung-Yin.

To tonify the Kidney-Yang and expel Wind, Damp and Cold

- Xian Mao (*Curculiginis rhizoma*): Warms the Kidney-Yang, expels Wind, Damp and Cold;
- Xian Ling Pi (*Epimedii herba*): Tonifies the Kidney-Yang, expels Wind, Damp and Cold;
- Ba Ji Tian (*Morindae radix*): Tonifies the Kidney-Yang, expels Wind, Damp and Cold.

Combinations of regulating Qi

To regulate Qi and remove Phlegm in the Stomach and Lung

- Chen Pi (*Citri reticulatae pericarpium*): Regulates Qi in the Stomach, Spleen and Lung;
- Ban Xia (*Pinelliae rhizoma*): Soothes Stomach-Qi, removes Phlegm from Stomach and Lung.

To regulate the Qi and relieve distending pain in the abdomen

- Mu Xiang (*Aucklandiae radix*)**: Regulates Qi in Spleen and Liver;
- Sha Ren (*Amomi xanthioidis fructus*): Regulates Qi in Spleen and intestine.

To reduce distension in the Stomach and hypochondriac region

- Qing Pi (*Citri reticulatae viride pericarpium*): Regulates the Qi of the Liver;
- Chen Pi (*Citri reticulatae pericarpium*): Regulates the Qi of the Spleen and Stomach.

To promote Qi movement and remove Phlegm

- Zhi Shi (*Aurantii fructus immaturus*): Descends the Qi in the intestine and removes Phlegm;
- Hou Po (*Magnoliae cortex*): Descends the Qi in the Lung, Spleen and intestine, removes Phlegm.

To reduce Qi, water and food stagnation in the abdomen

- Da Fu Pi (*Arecae pericarpium*): Promotes Qi movement and drains water in the abdomen;

- Bing Lang (*Arecae semen*): Promotes Qi movement and digestion, promotes bowel movement.

Combinations of breaking up congealed Blood

To relieve pain due to Blood stagnation

- Pu Huang (*Typhae pollen*): Promotes Blood circulation, dissolves congealed Blood;
- Wu Ling Zhi (*Trogopterori faeces*): Dissolves congealed Blood.

To remove congealed Blood and stop pain

- Tao Ren (*Persicae semen*): Promotes Blood circulation, breaks up congealed Blood;
- Hong Hua (*Carthami flos*): Promotes Blood circulation and dissolves congealed Blood.

To dissolve and break up congealed Blood, stop pain and applied in trauma

- Ru Xiang (*Olibanum*): Promotes Qi and Blood circulation, removes congealed Blood;
- Mo Yao (*Myrrhae*): Removes congealed Blood and softens the hardness.

To break up congealed Blood and treat palpable mass

- E Zhu (*Curcumae rhizoma*): Promotes Qi and Blood circulation, removes congealed Blood;
- San Leng (*Sparganii rhizoma*): Removes congealed Blood and softens the hardness.

Other combinations

To reduce fullness of Stomach, nausea and vomiting due to Dampness in the Middle Jiao

- Huo Xiang (*Agastachis herba*): Aromatically transforms Dampness in the Middle Jiao;
- Pei Lan (*Eupatorii herba*): Aromatically transforms Dampness in the Middle Jiao.

To calm the Mind and treat restlessness and insomnia

- Bai Zi Ren (*Platycladi semen*): Calms the Mind and improves sleep;
- Suan Zao Ren (*Ziziphi spinosae semen*): Nourishes the Liver-Blood, improves sleep.

To calm the Mind by descending the Liver-Yang

- Long Gu (*Mastodi fossilium ossis*): Descends the Liver-Yang, calms the Mind;
- Mu Li (*Ostrea concha*): Descends the Liver-Yang, clears Heat and calms the Mind.

To calm the Mind by sedating the Heart-Spirit

- Ci Shi (*Magnetitum*): Descends the Liver-Yang, sedates the Heart-Spirit and calms the Mind;
- Zhen Zhu Mu (*Concha margaritifera usta*): Sedates the Heart-Spirit, clears Heat and calms the Mind.

To soften hardness, remove Phlegm and therefore treat mass, such as tumor

- Hai Zao (*Sargassum*): Removes Phlegm and softens hardness;
- Kun Bu (*Eckloniae thallus*): Removes Phlegm and softens hardness.

To treat concentration disorder, anxiety and confusion due to Damp-Phlegm covering the Mind

- Shi Chang Pu (*Acori graminei rhizoma*): Aromatically transforms Damp-Phlegm, opens the orifices;
- Yuan Zhi (*Polygalae radix*): Removes Phlegm from Heart meridian and associates the Heart with the Kidney.

To expel Wind and open the meridians and collaterals

- Bai Hua She (*Agkistrodon acutus*)*: Expels Wind;
- Wu Shao She (*Zaocys*): Expels Wind.

Mutual enhancement (Xiang Shi)

This type of combination involves two herbs which have different functions—the first directly targets the pathological condition and the second increases the therapeutic effect of the first.

To clear Heat in the Lower Jiao

- Zhi Mu (*Anemarrhenae rhizoma*): Nourishes Yin of the Kidney and clears Heat in the Lower Jiao;
- Huang Bai (*Phellodendri cortex*): Reduces Empty-Heat in the Lower Jiao.

To nourish the Kidney-Yin

- Nu Zhen Zi (*Ligustri lucidi fructus*): Nourishes Kidney-Yin and clears Heat;
- Han Lian Cao (*Ecliptae herba*): Clears Heat of the Kidney and Liver, nourishes the Yin.

To stimulate the Kidney-Yang, expel Cold and warm the Interior

- Fu Zi (*Aconiti radix lateralis preparata*)*: Stimulates Yang, warms the Interior, expels Cold;
- Rou Gui (*Cinnamomi cassiae cortex*): Warms the Interior, stimulates Blood, expels Cold and enhances the function of Fu Zi.

To expel Wind-Cold sufficiently in the Exterior

- Ma Huang (*Ephedrae herba*)*: Stimulates the Yang and Qi of the Lung and Bladder meridians, induces sweating and releases the Exterior;
- Gui Zhi (*Cinnamomi cassiae ramulus*): Stimulates the Yang and Qi in Blood, promotes Blood circulation and enhances the function of Ma Huang.

To warm the Middle Jiao, treat abdominal pain and diarrhea due to Cold in the Middle Jiao

- Gan Jiang (*Zingiberis rhizoma*): Warms the Spleen-Yang, expels Cold;

- Fu Zi (*Aconiti radix lateralis preparata*): Stimulates Yang, warms the Interior, expels Cold and enhances the function of Gan Jiang.

To regulate the Lung-Qi and relieve wheezing

- Ma Huang (*Ephedrae herba*)*: Disperses and ascends the Lung-Qi;
- Xing Ren (*Armeniacae semen*): Disperses and descends the Lung-Qi and transforms Phlegm, particularly enhances the descending function of Ma Huang.

Mutual enhancement (Xiang Shi)/Mutual counteraction (Xiang Wei)

In this type of combination, the first herb treats the main disorder and its dosage and function are larger and stronger than those of the second (and third) herbs. The second (and third) herbs serve to reduce the side-effects and to moderate the speed and the temperature of the first.

This type of combination is widely used to correct the side-effects of a particular herb, to prolong the action of a herb in a steady way, to moderate the movement of Qi and to harmonize the internal organs.

Moreover, some special strategies have been developed from this type of combination to attain efficient therapeutic effects. For example, upward-moving and downward-moving herbs, and dispersing and restraining herbs, may be used at the same time. The first herb treats the disorder and the second herb—which has different or opposite properties, directional tendency and functions—serves as its assistant. In this way, it keeps the action of the first herb steady and moderate.

To ascend the Yang and strengthen the Exterior

- Huang Qi (*Astragali radix*): Strengthens and stabilizes the Defensive Qi;
- Fang Feng (*Saposhnikoviae radix*): Disperses the Wind from the Exterior.

To strengthen the Heart-Qi, treat restlessness and palpitations

- Ren Shen (*Ginseng radix*): Tonifies the Heart-Qi;
- Wu Wei Zi (*Schisandrae fructus*): Stabilizes the Heart-Qi.

To tonify the Blood and Essence

- Shu Di Huang (*Rehmanniae radix praeparata*): Tonifies the Blood and Essence;
- Sha Ren (*Amomi xanthioidis fructus*): Promotes the Qi movement and removes the sticky nature of Shu Di Huang.

To moderately drain Heat accumulation in the intestine

- Da Huang (*Rhei rhizoma*): Drains Heat and purges the intestine;
- Zhi Gan Cao (*Glycyrrhizae radix preparata*): Moderates the harsh nature and the speed of Da Huang.

To steadily warm the Interior

- Fu Zi (*Aconiti radix lateralis preparata*)*: Strongly moves the Qi, spreads the Yang and disperses the internal Cold;
- Zhi Gan Cao (*Glycyrrhizae radix preparata*): Moderates the harsh nature and the speed of Fu Zi.

To relieve the Cold-type wheezing

- Xi Xin (*Asari herba*)*: Disperses the Lung-Qi, warms the Interior;
- Sheng Jiang (*Zingiberis rhizoma recens*): Warms the Stomach and disperses the Cold and congested water;
- Wu Wei Zi (*Schisandrae fructus*): Stabilizes the Lung-Qi.

To treat excessive Heat in the Stomach

- Huang Lian (*Coptidis rhizoma*): Descends and clears the Fire from the Stomach;
- Sheng Ma (*Cimicifugae rhizoma*): Ascends and disperses the constrained Qi and Fire in the Stomach.

To reduce constrained Fire in the Spleen

- Shi Gao (*Gypsum*): Descends the Fire from Spleen and Stomach;
- Fang Feng (*Saposhnikoviae radix*): Disperses constrained Heat and Qi.

Sedating the Liver-Yang

To harmonize the Qi movement in the process of descending the Liver-Yang

- Dai Zhe Shi (*Haematitum*) and Shi Jue Ming (*Haliotidis concha*): Descend Liver-Yang;
- Qing Hao (*Artemisiae annuae herba*) and Mai Ya (*Hordei fructus germinatus*): Ascend suppressed Qi from the Middle Jiao.

To calm the Mind and treat restlessness and insomnia

- Long Gu (*Mastodi fossilium ossis*) and Mu Li (*Ostrea concha*): Sedate the Spirit and calm the Mind;
- Chai Hu (*Bupleuri radix*): Ascends and spreads the Liver-Qi.

To treat constipation and distension in the abdomen

- Da Huang (*Rhei rhizoma*): Purges the intestines and moves stool;
- Jie Geng (*Platycodi radix*): Ascends the Lung-Qi to accelerate the Qi downward moving in the Large Intestine.

To treat irritability due to constraint of Qi and Heat in the chest

- Zhi Zi (*Gardeniae fructus*): Descends Heat in the chest;
- Dan Dou Chi (*Sojae semen praeparatum*): Disperses Heat in the chest.

Combinations to treat complicated syndromes or disorders

This type of combination is based on two or more herbs, each of which partly fulfills the therapeutic role. They are equally important and work as one unit, even though the herbs have very different properties and functions. Together they treat a condition that a single herb would not be able to deal with.

To tonify the Blood and regulate the circulation

- Dang Gui (*Angelicae sinensis radix*): Warms the Blood, tonifies the Blood and promotes its circulation;
- Bai Shao Yao (*Paeoniae radix lactiflora*): Cools the Blood, tonifies the Blood and stabilizes the Blood circulation.

To stimulate Blood circulation

- Dang Gui (*Angelicae sinensis radix*): Warms the Blood, tonifies the Blood and promotes its circulation;
- Chuan Xiong (*Chuanxiong rhizoma*): Promotes Blood circulation.

To activate the Blood circulation and spread the warmth in the body

- Dang Gui (*Angelicae sinensis radix*): Warms the Blood, tonifies the Blood and promotes its circulation;
- Gui Zhi (*Cinnamomi cassiae ramulus*): Warms the Blood and stimulates the circulation.

To harmonize the Ying and Wei (Qi and Blood)

- Gui Zhi (*Cinnamomi cassiae ramulus*): Disperses the Defensive Qi;
- Bai Shao Yao (*Paeoniae radix lactiflora*): Nourishes the Nutritive Qi.

To tonify the Yin, soften the Liver and ease muscular cramp

- Bai Shao Yao (*Paeoniae radix lactiflora*): Sour and Cold, nourishes the Yin and the Blood, softens the Liver;
- Zhi Gan Cao (*Glycyrrhizae radix preparata*): Sweet and warm, together with Bai Shao Yao generates and stabilizes the Yin.

To harmonize the Liver-Qi

- Chai Hu (*Bupleuri radix*): Disperses and ascends the Qi of the Liver and Gall Bladder;
- Bai Shao Yao (*Paeoniae radix lactiflora*): Nourishes the Liver-Yin and Blood, softens the Liver.

To protect the Middle Jiao and promote digestion

- Sheng Jiang (*Zingiberis rhizoma recens*): Warms the Stomach, promotes digestion;
- Da Zao (*Jujubae fructus*): Tonifies the Qi and Blood, strengthens the Middle Jiao.

To regulate the Lung-Qi, clear the Heat and relieve shortness of breath

- Ma Huang (*Ephedrae herba*)*: Disperses the Lung Qi, opens the obstruction of the Lung;
- Shi Gao (*Gypsum*): Descends the Lung-Qi and clears the Heat of the Lung.

To treat pain due to Qi and Blood stagnation, especially in hypochondriac regions and the lateral sides of the abdomen

- Chuan Lian Zi (*Toosendan fructus*): Drains the Liver-Heat and Qi, reduces Qi stagnation;
- Yan Hu Suo (*Corydalidis rhizoma*): Promotes Blood circulation and reduces pain.

To reduce the Heat in the Blood and promote Blood circulation

- Mu Dan Pi (*Moutan cortex*): Reduces the Empty-Heat in the Blood;
- Chi Shao Yao (*Paeoniae radix rubra*): Reduces the excess Heat in the Blood.

To promote digestion

- Mai Ya (*Hordei fructus germinatus*): Adds the digestion of starch food;
- Shen Qu (*Massa medicata fermentata*): Adds the digestion of cereals and alcohol;
- Shan Zha (*Crataegi fructus*): Adds the digestion of meat and fat.

To purge the Heat accumulation in the intestine

- Da Huang (*Rhei rhizoma*): Stimulates the intestine, drains Heat, purges the accumulation in the intestine;
- Mang Xiao (*Natrii sulfas*): Increases the fluid in the intestine, softens feces, drains Heat.

To open the San Jiao, separate Damp-Heat in the San Jiao

- Xing Ren (*Armeniacae semen*): Disperses the Lung-Qi, opens the Upper Jiao;
- Bai Dou Kou (*Amomi fructus rotundus*): Promotes the Qi movement, transforms Dampness and opens the Middle Jiao;
- Yi Yi Ren (*Coicis semen*): Promotes urination, drains Damp-Heat and clears the Lower Jiao.

To expel Wind-Heat from the Lung, descend the Lung-Qi and relieve wheezing

- Sang Ye (*Mori folium*): Disperses Wind-Heat;
- Sang Bai Pi (*Mori cortex*): Clears Heat and descends Qi of the Lung.

To regulate the function of the Lung and remove Phlegm

- Jie Geng (*Platycodi radix*): Ascends the Lung-Qi, eliminates Phlegm and stops cough;
- Xing Ren (*Armeniacae semen*): Descends the Lung-Qi, eliminates Phlegm and stops cough.

Regulating the Qi in the Middle Jiao and promoting digestion

- Bai Zhu (*Atractylodis macrocephalae rhizoma*): Strengthens the Spleen-Qi and promotes the function of transportation and transformation of the Spleen;
- Zhi Shi (*Aurantii fructus immaturus*): Descends the Qi in the intestine and removes the accumulation of food, Phlegm and Qi.

To regulate the Stomach, treat nausea and poor appetite, especially under stress

- Ban Xia (*Pinelliae rhizoma*): Disperses stagnation of Stomach-Qi and accumulation of Phlegm;
- Huang Qin (*Scutellariae radix*): Clears Heat that is caused by the accumulations in the Stomach.

To eliminate Dampness and treat edema

- Cang Zhu (*Atractylodis rhizoma*): Disperses and dries Dampness;
- Huang Bai (*Phellodendri cortex*): Clears Heat and dries Dampness in the Lower Jiao.

To reduce distension in the chest and abdomen

- Zhi Ke (*Aurantii fructus*): Disperses the Qi and opens the chest;
- Zhi Shi (*Aurantii fructus immaturus*): Descends the Qi in the intestine.

To associate the Heart and Kidney and treat insomnia

- Huang Lian (*Coptidis rhizoma*): Reduces the excessive Heat from the Heart;
- Rou Gui (*Cinnamomi cassiae cortex*): Strengthens the Kidney-Yang and warms the vital Fire.

To eliminate Blood stasis in the chest

- Chai Hu (*Bupleuri radix*) and Jie Geng (*Platycodi radix*): Ascend and disperse Qi;
- Zhi Ke (*Aurantii fructus*): Broadens the chest, activates Qi movement;
- Chuan Niu Xi (*Cyathulae radix*): Directs the Blood downwards.

To enter the Yin level and return to the Qi level in order to eliminate Heat at the Yin level in febrile disease

- Qing Hao (*Artemisiae annuae herba*): Enters the Yin level by the guidance of Bie Jia, brings the Heat to the Qi level and disperses it;
- Bie Jia (*Trionycis carapax*)**: Enters the Yin level and clears Heat there, moves out to the Qi level under the guidance of Qing Hao.

Commonly used Chinese words in herbal names

Color

Hong/Chi/Dan/Zhu—red

Hong Hua (*Carthami flos*)
Chi Shao Yao (*Paeoniae radix rubra*)
Dan Shen (*Salviae miltiorrhizae radix*)
Zhu Sha (*Cinnabaris*)*

Huang—yellow

Huang Bai (*Phellodendri cortex*)
Huang Lian (*Coptidis rhizoma*)
Huang Qi (*Astragali radix*)
Huang Qin (*Scutellariae radix*)
Da Huang (*Rhei rhizoma*)
Pu Huang (*Typhae pollen*)
Sheng Di Huang (*Rehmanniae radix*)

Bai—white

Bai Guo (*Ginkgo semen*)
Bai Ji (*Bletillae tuber*)**
Bai Mao Gen (*Imperatae rhizoma*)
Bai Shao Yao (*Paeoniae radix lactiflora*)
Bai Xian Pi (*Dictamni cortex*)
Bai Zhi (*Angelicae dahuricae radix*)

Qing—green

Qing Dai (*Indigo naturalis*)
Qing Hao (*Artemisiae annuae herba*)
Qing Pi (*Citri reticulatae viride pericarpium*)

Hei/Xuan/Wu—black

Hei Zhi Ma (*Sesami semen nigricum*)
Xuan Shen (*Scrophulariae radix*)
He Shou Wu (*Polygoni multiflori radix*)
Wu Mei (*Mume fructus*)

Zi—purple

Zi Cao (*Arnebiae/Lithospermi radix*)
Zi Su Ye (*Perillae folium*)

Jin—gold

Jin Yin Hua (*Lonicerae flos*)
Jin Ying Zi (*Rosae laevigatae fructus*)
Yu Jin (*Curcumae radix*)
Ji Nei Jin (*Gigeriae galli endothelium corneum*)

Yin—silver

Yin Chai Hu (*Stellariae radix*)
Yin Xing/Bai Guo (*Ginkgo semen*)
Jin Yin Hua (*Lonicerae flos*)

Part of plant or medical substances

Pi/Ke—skin, peel, bark, shell

Bai Xian Pi (*Dictamni cortex*)
Chen Pi (*Citri reticulatae pericarpium*)
Da Fu Pi (*Arecae pericarpium*)
He Huan Pi (*Albiziae cortex*)

Qing Pi (*Citri reticulatae viride pericarpium*)
Sang Bai Pi (*Mori cortex*)
Sheng Jiang Pi (*Zingiberis rhizoma recens cortex*)
Hai Ge Ke (*Meretricis/Cyclinae concha*)
Zhi Ke (*Aurantii fructus*)

Hua—flower

Hong Hua (*Carthami flos*)
Huai Hua (*Sophorae flos*)
Jin Yin Hua (*Lonicerae flos*)
Ju Hua (*Chrysanthemi flos*)
Mei Gui Hua (*Rosae flos*)

Guo/Shi—fruit

Bai Guo (*Ginkgo semen*)
Qian Shi (*Euryalis semen*)
Zhi Shi (*Aurantii fructus immaturus*)

Zi/Ren—seed or fruit

Bai Zi Ren (*Platycladi semen*)
Che Qian Zi (*Plantaginis semen*)
He Zi (*Chebulae fructus*)
Lian Zi (*Nelumbinis semen*)
Nu Zhen Zi (*Ligustri lucidi fructus*)
Ting Li Zi (*Lepidii/Descurainiae semen*)
Tu Si Zi (*Cuscutae semen*)
Huo Ma Ren (*Cannabis semen*)
Sha Ren (*Amomi xanthioidis fructus*)
Suan Zao Ren (*Ziziphi spinosae semen*)
Tao Ren (*Persicae semen*)
Xing Ren (*Armeniacae semen*)
Yi Zhi Ren (*Alpiniae oxyphyllae fructus*)

Shen—root (used only in TCM)

Dan Shen (*Salviae miltiorrhizae radix*)
Dang Shen (*Codonopsis radix*)
Ku Shen (*Sophorae flavescentis radix*)
Ren Shen (*Ginseng radix*)
Xuan Shen (*Scrophulariae radix*)

Zhi—twig

Gui Zhi (*Cinnamomi cassiae ramulus*)
Sang Zhi (*Mori ramulus*)

Teng—vine

Hai Feng Teng (*Piperis caulis*)
Ji Xue Teng (*Spatholobi caulis et radix*)

Luo Shi Teng (*Trachelospermi caulis*)
Ye Jiao Teng (*Polygoni multiflori caulis*)

Cao—grass, herbal plant

Gan Cao (*Glycyrrhizae radix*)
Qian Cao Gen (*Rubiae radix*)
Yi Mu Cao (*Leonuri herba*)
Yu Xing Cao (*Houttuyniae herba cum radice*)
Zi Cao (*Arnebiae/Lithospermi radix*)

Ye—leaf

Da Qing Ye (*Isatidis folium*)
Dan Zhu Ye (*Lophatheri herba*)
Pi Pa Ye (*Eriobotryae folium*)
Sang Ye (*Mori folium*)
Zi Su Ye (*Perillae folium*)

Gu—bone

Bu Gu Zhi (*Psoraleae fructus*)
Gu Sui Bu (*Drynariae rhizoma*)
Long Gu (*Mastodi fossilium ossis*)

Rou—meat, fruit without peel and seed

Long Yan Rou (*Longanae arillus*)
Rou Cong Rong (*Cistanchis herba*)**
Rou Gui (*Cinnamomi cassiae cortex*)

Shi—stone, rock

Ci Shi (*Magnetitum*)
Dai Zhe Shi (*Haematitum*)
Hai Fu Shi (*Pumex*)
Shi Gao (*Gypsum*)
Shi Jue Ming (*Haliotidis concha*)

Smell

Xiang—aroma

An Xi Xiang (*Benzoinum*)
Chen Xiang (*Aquilariae lignum*)
Ding Xiang (*Caryophylli flos*)
Huo Xiang (*Agastachis herba*)
Mu Xiang (*Aucklandiae radix*)**
Ru Xiang (*Olibanum*)
She Xiang (*Moschus*)**
Su He Xiang (*Styrax*)
Tan Xiang (*Santali albi lignum*)
Xiao Hui Xiang (*Foeniculi fructus*)

Taste

Gan—sweet

Gan Cao (*Glycyrrhizae radix*)

Ku—bitter

Ku Shen (*Sophorae flavescentis radix*)

Xin—pungent

Xi Xin (*Asari herba*)*
Xin Yi (*Magnoliae flos*)

Suan—sour

Suan Zao Ren (*Ziziphi spinosae semen*)

Substances used for processing herbs

Yan—salt

(Yan) Zhi Huang Bai (salt-processed *Phellodendri cortex*)
(Yan) Zhi Zhi Mu (salt-processed *Anemarrhenae rhizoma*)

Jiu—wine, alcohol

Jiu Zhi Da Huang (alcohol-fried *Rhei rhizoma*)

Cu—vinegar

Cu Chao Chai Hu (vinegar-fried *Bupleuri radix*)

Mi—honey

(Mi) Zhi Pi Pa Ye (honey-fried *Eriobotryae folium*)
(Mi) Zhi Gan Cao (honey-fried *Glycyrrhizae radix*)

Sheng—raw, unprocessed

Sheng Di Huang (*Rehmanniae radix*)
Sheng Huang Qi (raw *Astragali radix*)
Sheng Shi Gao (raw *Gypsum*)

Processing of herbs

Zhi—processed

Zhi Gan Cao (processed *Glycyrrhizae radix*)
Zhi Huang Qi (processed *Astragali radix*)
Zhi Xiang Fu (processed *Cyperi rhizoma*)

Chao—dry frying

Chao Bai Zhu (dry-fried *Atractylodis macrocephalae rhizoma*)

Chao Jiao—dry frying or baking until the herb becomes dark brown in color

Jiao Mai Ya (dry-fried *Hordei fructus germinatus*)
Jiao Shan Zha (dry-fried *Crataegi fructus*)
Jiao Shen Qu (dry-fried *Massa medicata fermentata*)

Duan—calcined

Duan Long Gu (calcined *Mastodi fossilium ossis*)
Duan Mu Li (calcined *Ostrea concha*)

Herbs named with functions or appearance

Bai Tou Weng (*Pulsatilla radix*): Old man (with) white hair
Bu Gu Zhi (*Psoraleae fructus*): Essence that strengthens bones
Chen Xiang (*Aquilariae lignum*): Heavy and aromatic (wood)
Di Long (*Pheretima*): Earth dragon
Fo Shou (*Citri sarcodactylis fructus*): Buddha's hand
Gou Ji (*Cibotii rhizoma*)**: Dog spine
Gu Sui Bu (*Drynariae rhizoma*): Tonic for broken bone
Ji Nei Jin (*Gigeriae galli endothelium corneum*): The inner golden (layer) of chicken
Ji Xue Teng (*Spatholobi caulis et radix*): Vine with a color of chicken blood
Jiang Can (*Bombyx batrycatus*): Rigid (dead) silkworm
Shen Jin Cao (*Lycopodii herba*): Grass that stretches tendons
Tou Gu Cao (*Tuberculate speranskia herba*): Grass that penetrates bones
Xu Duan (*Dipsaci radix*): Connecting the broken (parts)
Yi Mu Cao (*Leonuri herba*): Grass that benefits the mother
Yu Xing Cao (*Houttuyniae herba cum radice*): Grass with fish smell

Appendix 4

Pinyin names of herbs with Latin (pharmaceutical) equivalents

A Wei (*Resina ferulae asafoetida*)
Ai Ye (*Artemisiae argyi folium*)
An Xi Xiang (*Benzoinum*)

Ba Dou (*Crotonis fructus*)*
Ba Ji Tian (*Morindae radix*)
Bai Bian Dou (*Dolichoris lablab semen*)
Bai Bu (*Stemonae radix*)
Bai Cao Shuang (*Fuligo plantae*)
Bai Dou Kou (*Amomi fructus rotundus*)
Bai Fu Zi (*Typhonii rhizoma praeparatum*)*
Bai Guo (*Ginkgo semen*)
Bai He (*Lilii bulbus*)
Bai Hua She (*Agkistrodon acutus*)*
Bai Ji (*Bletillae tuber*)**
Bai Ji Li (*Tribuli fructus*)
Bai Jiang Cao (*Patriniae herba*)
Bai Jie Zi (*Sinapis albae semen*)
Bai Lian (*Ampelopsitis radix*)
Bai Mao Gen (*Imperatae rhizoma*)
Bai Qian (*Cynanchi stauntonii radix*)
Bai Shao Yao (*Paeoniae radix lactiflora*)
Bai Shen (white *Ginseng radix*)
Bai Tou Weng (*Pulsatilla radix*)
Bai Wei (*Cynanchi atrati radix*)
Bai Xian Pi (*Dictamni cortex*)
Bai Zhi (*Angelicae dahuricae radix*)
Bai Zhu (*Atractylodis macrocephalae rhizoma*)
Bai Zi Ren (*Platycladi semen*)
Ban Bian Lian (*Lobelia chinensis herba*)
Ban Lan Gen (*Isatidis/Baphicacanthis radix*)
Ban Mao (*Mylabris*)*
Ban Xia (*Pinelliae rhizoma*)
Bei Sha Shen (*Glehniae radix*)
Bei Wu Jia Pi (*Periploca sepium bunge*)

Bi Ba (*Piperis longi fructus*)
Bi Cheng Qie (*Litseae fructus*)
Bi Xie (*Dioscoreae hypoglaucae rhizoma*)
Bian Xu (*Polygoni avicularis herba*)
Bie Jia (*Trionycis carapax*)**
Bing Lang (*Arecae semen*)
Bing Pian (*Borneol*)
Bo He (*Menthae herba*)
Bu Gu Zhi (*Psoraleae fructus*)

Can Sha (*Bombycis mori excrementum*)
Cang Er Zi (*Xanthii fructus*)
Cang Zhu (*Atractylodis rhizoma*)
Cao Dou Kou (*Alpiniae katsumadai semen*)
Cao Guo (*Tsaoko fructus*)
Cao Wu (*Aconiti kusnezoffii radix*)*
Ce Bai Ye (*Platycladi cacumen*)
Chai Hu (*Bupleuri radix*)
Chan Tui (*Cicadae periostracum*)
Chang Shan (*Dichroae febrifugae radix*)
Chao Jing Jie (dry-fried *Schizonepetae herba*)
Che Qian Zi (*Plantaginis semen*)
Chen Pi (*Citri reticulatae pericarpium*)
Chen Xiang (*Aquilariae lignum*)
Chi Fu Ling (*Poriae cocos rubrae*)
Chi Shao Yao (*Paeoniae radix rubra*)
Chi Shi Zhi (*Halloysitum rubrum*)
Chi Xiao Dou (*Phaseoli semen*)
Chou Wu Tong (*Clerodendri folium*)
Chuan Bei Mu (*Fritillariae cirrhosae bulbus*)
Chuan Lian Zi (*Toosendan fructus*)
Chuan Mu Tong (*Clematidis armandii caulis*)
Chuan Mu Xiang (*Vladimirae radix*)
Chuan Niu Xi (*Cyathulae radix*)
Chuan Shan Jia (*Manitis squama*)**

Chuan Wu (*Aconiti carmichaeli radix*)*
Chuan Xiong (*Chuanxiong rhizoma*)
Ci Shi (*Magnetitum*)
Cong Bai (*Allii fistulosi bulbus*)

Da Fu Pi (*Arecae pericarpium*)
Da Huang (*Rhei rhizoma*)
Da Jǐ (*Knoxiae radix*)*
Da Jì (*Cirsii japonici herba seu radix*)
Da Qing Ye (*Isatidis folium*)
Da Zao (*Jujubae fructus*)
Dai Zhe Shi (*Haematitum*)
Dan Dou Chi (*Sojae semen praeparatum*)
Dan Nan Xing (*Pulvis arisaemae cum felle bovis*)
Dan Shen (*Salviae miltiorrhizae radix*)
Dan Zhu Ye (*Lophatheri herba*)
Dang Gui (*Angelicae sinensis radix*)
Dang Gui Wei (*Angelicae sinensis radix extremitas*)
Dang Shen (*Codonopsis radix*)
Deng Xin Cao (*Junci medulla*)
Di Ding (*Violae herba*)
Di Fu Zi (*Kochiae fructus*)
Di Gu Pi (*Lycii cortex*)
Di Long (*Pheretima*)
Di Yu (*Sanguisorbae radix*)
Ding Xiang (*Caryophylli flos*)
Dong Chong Xia Cao (*Cordyceps sinensis*)
Dong Gua Zi (*Benincasae semen*)
Dong Kui Zi (*Malvae semen*)
Du Huo (*Angelicae pubescentis radix*)
Du Zhong (*Eucomniae cortex*)
Duan Shi Gao (calcined *Gypsum*)

E Jiao (*Asini corii colla*)
E Zhu (*Curcumae rhizoma*)

Fan Xie Ye (*Sennae folium*)
Fang Feng (*Saposhnikoviae radix*)
Fei Zi (*Torreyae semen*)
Feng Mi (*Mel*)
Fo Shou (*Citri sarcodactylis fructus*)
Fu Ling (*Poria*)
Fu Ling Pi (*Poriae cocos cortex*)
Fu Pen Zi (*Rubi fructus*)
Fu Shen (*Poriae cocos pararadicis*)
Fu Xiao Mai (*Tritici fructus germinatus*)
Fu Zi (*Aconiti radix lateralis preparata*)*

Gan Cao (*Glycyrrhizae radix*)
Gan Jiang (*Zingiberis rhizoma*)
Gan Qi (*Toxicodendri resina*)
Gan Sui (*Euphorbiae kansui radix*)*

Gao Ben (*Ligustici sinensis radix*)
Gao Li Shen (Korean *Ginseng radix*)
Gao Liang Jiang (*Alpiniae officinari rhizoma*)
Ge Gen (*Puerariae radix*)
Ge Jie (*Gecko*)**
Gou Ji (*Cibotii rhizoma*)**
Gou Qi Zi (*Lycii fructus*)
Gou Teng (*Uncariae ramulus cum uncis*)
Gu Sui Bu (*Drynariae rhizoma*)
Gu Ya (*Oryzae fructus germinatus*)
Gua Di (*Pedicellus cucumeris*)
Gua Lou (*Trichosanthis fructus*)
Gua Lou Gen (*Trichosanthis radix*)
Gua Lou Pi (*Trichosanthis pericarpium*)
Gua Lou Ren (*Trichosanthis semen*)
Guan Mu Tong (*Aristolochia manshurensis caulis*)*
Guan Zhong (*Dryopteridis rhizoma*)
Guang Fang Ji (*Aristolochiae radix*)*
Gui Ban (*Testudinis carapax*)**
Gui Zhi (*Cinnamomi cassiae ramulus*)

Hai Feng Teng (*Piperis caulis*)
Hai Fu Shi (*Pumex*)
Hai Ge Ke (*Meretricis/Cyclinae concha*)
Hai Jin Sha (*Lygodii spora*)
Hai Tong Pi (*Erythrinae cortex*)
Hai Zao (*Sargassum*)
Han Fang Ji (*Stephaniae tetrandrae radix*)
Han Lian Cao (*Ecliptae herba*)
He Geng (*Nelumbinis ramulus*)
He Huan Hua (*Albiziae flos*)
He Huan Pi (*Albiziae cortex*)
He Shi (*Carpesii fructus*)
He Shou Wu (*Polygoni multiflori radix*)
He Ye (*Nelumbinis folium*)
He Zi (*Chebulae fructus*)
Hei Zhi Ma (*Sesami semen nigricum*)
Hong Hua (*Carthami flos*)
Hong Shen (red *Ginseng radix*)
Hong Teng (*Sargentodoxae caulis*)
Hou Po (*Magnoliae cortex*)
Hou Po Hua (*Magnoliae officinalis flos*)
Hu Gu (*Tigris os*)**
Hu Huang Lian (*Picrorhizae rhizoma*)
Hu Lu Ba (*Trigonellae semen*)
Hu Po (*Succinum*)
Hu Tao Rou (*Juglandis semen*)
Hu Zhang (*Polygoni cuspidati rhizoma*)
Hua Jiao (*Zanthoxyli fructus*)
Hua Rui Shi (*Ophicalcitum*)
Hua Shi (*Talcum*)

Huai Hua (*Sophorae flos*)
Huai Jiao (*Sophorae fructus*)
Huai Niu Xi (*Achyranthis bidentatae radix*)
Huang Bai (*Phellodendri cortex*)
Huang Jing (*Polygonati rhizoma*)
Huang Lian (*Coptidis rhizoma*)
Huang Qi (*Astragali radix*)
Huang Qin (*Scutellariae radix*)
Huang Yao Zi (*Dioscoreae bulbiferae rhizoma*)
Huo Ma Ren (*Cannabis semen*)
Huo Xiang (*Agastachis herba*)

Ji Nei Jin (*Gigeriae galli endothelium corneum*)
Ji Xue Teng (*Spatholobi caulis et radix*)
Jiang Can (*Bombyx batrycatus*)
Jiang Huang (*Curcumae longae rhizoma*)
Jie Geng (*Platycodi radix*)
Jin Qian Cao (*Lysimachiae herba*)
Jin Yin Hua (*Lonicerae flos*)
Jin Ying Zi (*Rosae laevigatae fructus*)
Jing Jie (*Schizonepetae herba*)
Jing Jie Sui (*Schizonepetae flos*)
Jing Tian San Qi (*Sedi aizoon herba*)
Jiu Cai Zi (*Allii tuberosi semen*)
Ju He (*Aurantii semen*)
Ju Hong (*Citri erythrocarpae pars rubra epicarpii*)
Ju Hua (*Chrysanthemi flos*)
Ju Luo (*Citri reticulatae fructus retinervus*)
Ju Ye (*Citri reticulatae folium*)
Ju Ye San Qi (*Gynura segetum*)
Jue Ming Zi (*Cassiae semen*)

Ku Lian Pi (*Meliae cortex*)
Ku Shen (*Sophorae flavescentis radix*)
Ku Zhu Ye (*Bambusae amarae folium*)
Kuan Dong Hua (*Tussilaginis farfarae*)
Kun Bu (*Eckloniae thallus*)

Lai Fu Zi (*Raphani semen*)
Lei Gong Teng (*Tripterygii wilfordii caulis*)*
Lei Wan (*Omphalia*)
Li Lu (*Veratri nigri radix et rhizoma*)
Li Zhi He (*Litchi semen*)
Lian Qiao (*Forsythiae fructus*)
Lian Fang (*Nelumbinis receptaculum*)
Lian Xu (*Nelumbinis stamen*)
Lian Zi (*Nelumbinis semen*)
Lian Zi Xin (*Nelumbinis plumula*)
Ling Xiao Hua (*Campsitis flos*)
Ling Yang Jiao (*Antelopis cornu*)**
Long Chi (*Mastodi fossilia dentis*)
Long Dan Cao (*Gentianae radix*)

Long Gu (*Mastodi fossilium ossis*)
Long Yan Rou (*Longanae arillus*)
Lü Dou (*Phaseoli radiati semen*)
Lu Gen (*Phragmitis rhizoma*)
Lu Hui (*Aloe folii extractus*)
Lu Lu Tong (*Liquidambaris fructus*)
Lu Rong (*Cervi cornu*)**
Lu Ti Cao (*Pyrola rotundifolia*)
Luo Shi Teng (*Trachelospermi caulis*)

Ma Bo (*Lasiosphaera*)
Ma Chi Xian (*Portulacae herba*)
Ma Huang (*Ephedrae herba*)*
Ma Huang Gen (*Ephedrae radix*)
Ma Qian Zi (*Strychni semen*)*
Mai Men Dong (*Ophiopogonis radix*)
Mai Ya (*Hordei fructus germinatus*)
Man Jing Zi (*Viticis fructus*)
Mang Chong (*Tabanus*)*
Mang Xiao (*Natrii sulfas*)
Mei Gui Hua (*Rosae flos*)
Meng Shi (*Lapis micae seu chloriti*)*
Mi Meng Hua (*Buddlejae flos*)
Mo Yao (*Myrrhae*)
Mu Dan Pi (*Moutan cortex*)
Mu Fang Ji (*Aristolochiae fangchi radix*)
Mu Gua (*Chaenomelis fructus*)
Mu Li (*Ostrea concha*)
Mu Tong (*Mutong caulis*)*
Mu Xiang (*Aucklandiae radix*)**

Nan Gua Zi (*Curcubitae semen*)
Nan Sha Shen (*Adenophorae radix*)
Nan Wu Jia Pi (*Acanthopanacis cortex*)
Nao Yang Hua (*Rhododendron molle flos*)*
Niu Bang Zi (*Arctii fructus*)
Niu Huang (*Bovis calculus*)**
Nu Zhen Zi (*Ligustri lucidi fructus*)
Nuo Dao Gen Xu (*Oryzae glutinosae radix et rhizoma*)

Ou Jie (*Nelumbinis nodus rhizomatis*)

Pao Jiang (quick-fried *Zingiberis rhizoma preparatum*)
Pei Lan (*Eupatorii herba*)
Pi Pa Ye (*Eriobotryae folium*)
Pu Gong Ying (*Taraxaci herba*)
Pu Huang (*Typhae pollen*)

Qian Cao Gen (*Rubiae radix*)
Qian Hu (*Peucedani radix*)

Qian Nian Jian (*Homalomenae rhizoma*)
Qian Niu Zi (*Pharbitidis semen*)*
Qian Shi (*Euryalis semen*)
Qiang Huo (*Notopterygii rhizoma*)
Qin Jiao (*Gentianae macrophyllae radix*)
Qin Pi (*Fraxini cortex*)
Qing Dai (*Indigo naturalis*)
Qing Feng Teng (*Sinomenii caulis*)
Qing Hao (*Artemisiae annuae herba*)
Qing Mu Xiang (*Aristolochia debilis*)*
Qing Pi (*Citri reticulatae viride pericarpium*)
Qing Xiang Zi (*Celosiae semen*)
Qu Mai (*Dianthi herba*)
Quan Xie (*Scorpio*)*

Ren Shen (*Ginseng radix*)
Ren Shen Lu (*Ginseng cervix*)
Rou Cong Rong (*Cistanchis herba*)**
Rou Dou Kou (*Myristicae semen*)
Rou Gui (*Cinnamomi cassiae cortex*)
Ru Xiang (*Olibanum*)

San Leng (*Sparganii rhizoma*)
San Qi (*Notoginseng radix*)
Sang Bai Pi (*Mori cortex*)
Sang Ji Sheng (*Taxilli herba*)
Sang Piao Xiao (*Mantidis oötheca*)
Sang Shen (*Mori fructus*)
Sang Ye (*Mori folium*)
Sang Zhi (*Mori ramulus*)
Sha Ren (*Amomi xanthioidis fructus*)
Sha Yuan Zi (*Astragali complanati semen*)
Shan Dou Gen (*Sophorae tonkinensis radix*)
Shan Yang Jiao (*Naemorhedis cornu*)
Shan Yao (*Dioscoreae rhizoma*)
Shan Zha (*Crataegi fructus*)
Shan Zhu Yu (*Corni fructus*)
Shang Lu (*Phytolaccae radix*)
She Chuang Zi (*Cnidii fructus*)
She Gan (*Belamcandae rhizoma*)
She Xiang (*Moschus*)**
Shen Jin Cao (*Lycopodii herba*)
Shen Qu (*Massa medicata fermentata*)
Shen Xu (*Ginseng fibrosa*)
Sheng Di Huang (*Rehmanniae radix*)
Sheng Jiang (*Zingiberis rhizoma recens*)
Sheng Jiang Pi (*Zingiberis rhizoma recens cortex*)
Sheng Jiang Zhi (*Zingiberis rhizoma recens succus*)
Sheng Ma (*Cimicifugae rhizoma*)
Sheng Shai Shen (raw dried *Ginseng radix*)
Sheng Shi Gao (raw *Gypsum*)
Shi Chang Pu (*Acori graminei rhizoma*)

Shi Di (*Kaki diospyri calyx*)
Shi Gao (*Gypsum*)
Si Gua Luo (*Luffae fructus*)
Shi Hu (*Dendrobii caulis*)**
Shi Jue Ming (*Haliotidis concha*)
Shi Jun Zi (*Quisqualis fructus*)
Shi Liu Pi (*Granati pericarpium*)
Shi Wei (*Pyrrosiae folium*)
Shi Yan (*Sal*)
Shu Di Huang (*Rehmanniae radix praeparata*)
Shui Niu Jiao (*Bubali cornu*)
Shui Zhi (*Hirudo*)
Song Jie (*Pini nodi lignum*)
Su He Xiang (*Styrax*)
Su Mu (*Sappan lignum*)
Su Zi (*Perillae fructus*)
Suan Zao Ren (*Ziziphi spinosae semen*)
Suo Yang (*Cynomorii caulis*)

Tai Zi Shen (*Pseudostellariae radix*)
Tan Xiang (*Santali albi lignum*)
Tao Ren (*Persicae semen*)
Tian Hua Fen (*Trichosanthis radix*)
Tian Ma (*Gastrodiae rhizoma*)**
Tian Men Dong (*Asparagi radix*)
Tian Nan Xing (*Arisaematis rhizoma*)
Tian Xian Zi (*Hyoscyamus niger semen*)*
Tian Zhu Huang (*Bambusae concretio silicea*)
Ting Li Zi (*Lepidii/Descurainiae semen*)
Tong Cao (*Tetrapanacis medulla*)
Tou Gu Cao (*Tuberculate speranskia herba*)
Tu Fu Ling (*Smilacis glabrae rhizoma*)
Tu Si Zi (*Cuscutae semen*)

Wa Leng Zi (*Arcae concha*)
Wang Bu Liu Xing (*Vaccariae semen*)
Wei Sheng Jiang (roasted *Zingiberis rhizoma recens*)
Wei Ling Xian (*Clematidis radix*)
Wu Bei Zi (*Chinensis galla*)
Wu Gong (*Scolopendra*)*
Wu Jia Pi (*Acanthopanacis cortex*)
Wu Ling Zhi (*Trogopterori faeces*)
Wu Mei (*Mume fructus*)
Wu Shao She (*Zaocys*)
Wu Tou (*Aconiti radix*)*
Wu Wei Zi (*Schisandrae fructus*)
Wu Yao (*Linderae radix*)
Wu Ye Mu Tong (*Akebiae caulis*)
Wu Yi (*Ulmi fructus praeparatus*)
Wu Zei Gu (*Sepiae seu sepiellae os*)
Wu Zhu Yu (*Evodiae fructus*)

Xi Gua Cui Yi (*Citrulli exocarpium*)
Xi Jiao (*Rhinoceri cornu*)**
Xi Xian Cao (*Sigesbeckiae herba*)
Xi Xin (*Asari herba*)*
Xi Yang Shen (*Panacis quinquefolii radix*)
Xia Ku Cao (*Prunellae spica*)
Xian He Cao (*Agrimoniae herba*)
Xian Ling Pi (*Epimedii herba*)
Xian Mao (*Curculinginis rhizoma*)
Xiang Fu (*Cyperi rhizoma*)
Xiang Ru (*Moslae herba*)
Xiang Yuan (*Citri fructus*)
Xiao Hui Xiang (*Foeniculi fructus*)
Xiao Ji (*Cirsii herba*)
Xie Bai (*Allii macrostemi bulbus*)
Xin Yi (*Magnoliae flos*)
Xing Ren (*Armeniacae semen*)
Xu Duan (*Dipsaci radix*)
Xuan Fu Hua (*Inulae flos*)
Xuan Ming Fen (*Mirabilitum purum*)
Xuan Shen (*Scrophulariae radix*)
Xue Jie (*Daemonoropsis resina*)
Xue Yu Tan (*Crinis carbonisatus*)

Yan Hu Suo (*Corydalidis rhizoma*)
Yang Qi Shi (*Actinolitum*)
Ye Jiao Teng (*Polygoni multiflori caulis*)
Ye Ju Hua (*Chrysanthemi indici flos*)
Ye Shan Shen (wild mountain *Ginseng radix*)
Yi Mu Cao (*Leonuri herba*)
Yi Tang (*Maltose*)
Yi Yi Ren (*Coicis semen*)
Yi Zhi Ren (*Alpiniae oxyphyllae fructus*)
Yin Chai Hu (*Stellariae radix*)
Yin Chen Hao (*Artemisiae scopariae herba*)
Yin Er (*Tremellae*)
Yin Yang Huo (*Epimedii herba*)
Ying Su Ke (*Papaveris somniferi pericarpium*)
Yu Jin (*Curcumae radix*)
Yu Li Ren (*Pruni semen*)

Yu Mi Xu (*Maydis stigma*)
Yu Xing Cao (*Houttuyniae herba cum radice*)
Yu Zhu (*Polygonati odorati rhizoma*)
Yuan Hua (*Genkwa flos*)*
Yuan Zhi (*Polygalae radix*)
Yue Ji Hua (*Rosae chinensis flos*)

Zao Jiao (*Gleditsiae fructus*)
Zao Xin Tu (*Terra flava usta*)
Ze Lan (*Lycopi herba*)
Ze Xie (*Alismatis rhizoma*)
Zhe Bei Mu (*Fritillariae thunbergii bulbus*)
Zhe Chong (*Eupolyphaga seu opisthoplatia*)*
Zhen Zhu (*Margarita usta*)
Zhen Zhu Mu (*Concha margaritifera usta*)
Zhi Gan Cao (*Glycyrrhizae radix preparata*)
Zhi Ke (*Aurantii fructus*)
Zhi Ma Huang (honey-toasted *Ephedrae herba*)
Zhi Mu (*Anemarrhenae rhizoma*)
Zhi Nan Xing (processed *Arisaematis rhizoma*)
Zhi Shi (*Aurantii fructus immaturus*)
Zhi Zi (*Gardeniae fructus*)
Zhu Li (*Bambusae succus*)
Zhu Ling (*Polyporus*)
Zhu Ma Gen (*Boehmeriae radix*)
Zhu Ru (*Bambusae caulis in taeniam*)
Zhu Sha (*Cinnabaris*)*
Zhu Ye (*Bambusae folium*)
Zhu Ye Juan Xin (*Bambusae viride folium*)
Zi Bei Chi (*Erosaria caputserpentis*)
Zi Cao (*Arnebiae/Lithospermi radix*)
Zi He Che (*Placenta hominis*)
Zi Shi Ying (*Fluoritum*)
Zi Su Geng (*Perillae caulis et flos*)
Zi Su Ye (*Perillae folium*)
Zi Wan (*Asteris radix*)
Zi Zhu Cao (*Callicarpae folium*)
Zong Lü (*Stipulae trachycarpi fibra*)
Zhu Dan Zhi (*Pulvis bovis*)

Banned toxic herbs are marked with an asterisk (*).
Banned and protected substances are marked with two asterisks (**).

Bibliography

Modern texts

Bensky D, Barolet R 1990 Chinese herbal medicine, formulas and strategies. Eastland Press, Seattle WA

Bensky D, Gamble A 1986 Chinese herbal medicine, materia medica. Eastland Press, Seattle WA

Cheng Bao Tao 1991 Clinical application of the Dr Zhang Zhong Jing's formulas (Zhong Jing Fang Yu Lin Chuang). China Medical Technology Publishing House, Beijing

Ding Guang Di 1982 Combination and application of Chinese herbal medicine (Zhong Yao de Pei Wu Yu Ying Yong). People's Medical Publishing House, Beijing

Guang An Men hospital attached to China Academy of Traditional Chinese Medicine 1980 Wei Wen Gui's experience on ophthalmopathy (Wei Wen Gui Yan Ke Lin Chuang Jing Yan Xuan). China Medical Technology Publishing House, Beijing

Jiangsu College of New Medicine 1977 Encyclopedia of Traditional Chinese Materia Medica (Zhong Yao Da Ci Dian). Shanghai People's Press, Shanghai

Li Bao Shuen et al 1990 Distinguished doctors and distinguished formulas (Min Yi Min Fang Lu). Hua Yi Publishing House, Beijing

Luo Yuan Kai 1990 Discussion on medicine (Luo Yuan Kai Lun Yi Ji). People's Medical Publishing House, Beijing

Maciocia G 1989 The foundations of Chinese medicine. Churchill Livingstone, London

Maciocia G 1994 The practice of Chinese medicine. Churchill Livingstone, London

Xu Ji Qun, Wang Mian Zhi et al 1985 Chinese herbal formulas (Fang Ji Xue). Science and Technology Publishing House, Shanghai

Yan Zheng Hua, Weng Wei Jian, Gao Xue Min et al 1979 Chinese herbal medicine (Zhong Yao Xue). Beijing College of Traditional Chinese Medicine, Beijing

Yin Jian, Guo Li Gong et al 1993 Modern pharmacological research on Chinese herbal medicine and applications (Zhong Yao Xian Dai Yan Jiu Yu Lin Chuang Ying Yong). Xue Yuan Publishing House, Beijing

Zhu Shen Yu et al 1982 The clinical experience of Dr Shi Jin Mo (Shi Jin Mo Lin Chuang Jing Yan Ji). People's Medical Publishing House, Beijing

Ancient classics

Gao Shi Shi 1983, first published in 1699 Lectures on medicine (Yi Xue Zhen Zhuan). People's Medical Publishing House, Beijing

Han Tian Jue 1989, first published in 1522 Han's understanding of medicine (Han Shi Yi Tong). People's Medical Publishing House, Beijing

Li Shi Zhen 1982, first published in 1596 Grand materia medicia (Ben Cao Gang Mu). People's Medical Publishing House, Beijing

Origin of medicine (Yi Xue Qi Yuan) 1978, first published c. 1200. People's Medical Publishing House, Beijing

Sun Si Miao 1994, first published c. AD 670 The thousand ducat formula (Qian Jin Yao Fang). Ji Lin People's Publishing House, Shen Yang

Wang Qing Ren 1991, first published in 1830 Corrections of errors among physicians (Yi Lin Gai Cuo). People's Medical Publishing House, Beijing

The Yellow Emperor's Classic of Internal Medicine—simple questions (Huang Di Nei Jing Su Wen) 1990, first published c. 100 BC. People's Medical Publishing House, Beijing

You Yi (You Zai Jing) 1991, first published c. 1730 Study note on medicine (Yi Xue Du Shu Ji). People's Medical Publishing House, Beijing

Zhang Ji (Zhang Zhong Jing) 1963, first published c. AD 200 (Essentials from the Golden Cabinet (Jin Gui Yao Lue Fang Lun). People's Medical Publishing House, Beijing

Zhang Ji (Zhang Zhong Jing) 1963, first published c. AD 200 Discussion on cold induced diseases (Shang Han Lun). People's Medical Publishing House, Beijing

Zhang Jie Bin (Zhang Jing Yue) 1982, first published in 1624 Classic of categories (Lei Jing). People's Medical Publishing House, Beijing

Zhang Jie Bin (Zhang Jing Yue) 1982, first published in 1624 Complete book of Jing Yue (Jing Yue Quan Shu). People's Medical Publishing House, Beijing

Zhang Zhi Cong 1983, first published in 1670 Discussion on syndromes at Lu Shan Tang School (Lü Shan Tang Lei Bian). People's Medical Publishing House, Beijing

Other sources of knowledge of Chinese herbal medicine

Chen Yan 1843, first published in 1174 Discussion on illnesses, syndromes and formulas related to the unification of the three etiologies (San Yi Ji Yi Bing Zheng Fang Lun). Lian Hua Guan Press, Shanghai

Cheng Zhong Ling 1990, first published in 1732 Medical revelations (Yi Xue Xin Wu). China Press of Traditional Chinese Medicine, Beijing

Li Gao 1976, first published in 1247 Discussion on the Spleen and Stomach (Pi Wei Lun). People's Health Publishing House, Beijing

The People's Welfare Pharmacies 1925, first published c. 1080 Formulary of the Tai Ping Hui Min Bureau (Tai Ping Hui Min He Ji Ju Fang). Shanghai Xiao Jing Shan Fang Publishing House, Shanghai

Qian Yi 1935–37, first published in 1119 Craft of medicinal treatment for the disorders of children (Xiao Er Yao Zheng Zhi Jue). Shanghai Commerce Press, Shanghai

Wang Ang 1990, first published in 1682 Analytic collection of medical formulas (Yi Fang Ji Jie). China Press of Traditional Chinese Medicine, Beijing

Wang Ken Tang 1990, first published in 1602 Standards of syndromes and treatment (Zheng Zhi Zhun Sheng). China Press of Traditional Chinese Medicine, Beijing

Wang Meng Ying 1990, first published in 1852 Warp and woof of warm-induced diseases (Wen Re Jing Wei). China Press of Traditional Chinese Medicine, Beijing

Wang Tao 1898, first published in 752 Arcane essential from the Imperial Library (Wai Tai Mi Yao). Shanghai Book Publishing House, Shanghai

Wu Ju Tong 1998, first published in 1798 Systematic differentiation of warm-induced diseases (Wen Bing Tiao Bian). People's Medical Publishing House, Beijing

Wu Kun 1990, first published in 1584 Investigations of medical formulas (Yi Fang Kao). China Press of Traditional Chinese Medicine, Beijing

Yan Yong He 1982, first published in 1253 Formulas to aid the living (Ji Sheng Fang). Guang Ling Classics Publishing House, Yang Zhou

Yifan Yang Lectures and study note on Chinese herbal medicine (not published)

Yifan Yang Lectures and study note on Chinese herbal formula (not published)

Zhang Xi Chun 1956, first published during 1909–24 Records of experiences in medicine with reference to the Western medicine (Yi Xue Zhong Zhong Can Xi Lu). China Academy of New Medicine, Beijing

Zheng Mei Jian 1917, first published in 1838 Jade key to many towers (Chong Lou Yu Yao). Zhang Fu Ji Publishing House, Shanghai

Zhu Dan Xi 1959, first published in 1481 Dan Xi's understanding of medicine (Dan Xi Xin Fa). Shanghai Science and Technology Press, Shanghai

Index

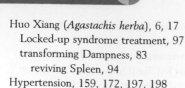

Printed and bound by CPI Group (UK) Ltd, Croydon, CR0 4YY

Printed and bound by CPI Group (UK) Ltd, Croydon, CR0 4YY

03/10/2024

01040365-0002